Schizophrenia
Concepts and clinical management

Kraepelin, who in 1896 first defined the disorder now known as schizophrenia, appreciated that there were many difficulties with the concept, and believed that, since the cause of the disorder was essentially unknown, there could be no rational treatment. In spite of advances in the intervening century, particularly in understanding the biological basis of schizophrenia, scientific knowledge has not been matched by advances in patient management, and some healthcare issues, particularly those relating to risk assessment and treatment costs, present ever increasing problems.

This authoritative text provides a wide-ranging survey of the disorder, including an up-to-date account of what is known about the underlying biology. The main part of the book covers clinical aspects, including, differential and dual diagnosis, and treatment and management problems, particularly in relation to care in the community. Topics covered include brain imaging, genetics, pharmacology and neuropsychology, as well as a chapter on health economics. Much clinical and media attention has focused on violence and other antisocial behaviour associated with schizophrenia, and a final chapter discusses forensic issues.

The authors have extensive clinical experience with schizophrenia patients, and this book, which is unusual in its breadth and its concern for social and community issues, will be a valuable reference for all psychiatrists, and other health professionals involved in the management of schizophrenia.

EVE C. JOHNSTONE is Professor of Psychiatry and Head of Department at the University of Edinburgh, and an internationally-renowned authority on schizophrenia.

MARTIN S. HUMPHREYS, FIONA H. LANG, STEPHEN M. LAWRIE and ROBERT SANDLER were all at the University of Edinburgh and involved in clinical and research work with Eve Johnstone as this book was prepared.

Publishers' Note

The Publishers acknowledge their debt to the late George Winokur, MD, who, in the last years of his life, worked with them to develop this book, and three further volumes, as the first titles in a new series under his editorship, to be called *Concepts in Clinical Psychiatry*. Dr Winokur was not, unfortunately, able to read any of these works in their final form.

Dr Winokur's contribution to contemporary psychiatry, and in particular his dedication to a medical model for psychiatric disorders, was distinctive, and his editorial style was inimitable. These four volumes are a tribute to his vision for psychiatry as a clinical discipline founded on the principles of scientific evidence and clinical judgement.

The Anxiety Disorders
by Russell Noyes, Jr, and Rudolf Hoehn-Saric

Delusional Disorder
Paranoia and related illnesses
by Alistair Munro

Schizophrenia
Concepts and clinical management
by Eve C. Johnstone, Martin S. Humphreys, Fiona H. Lang, Stephen M. Lawrie and Robert Sandler

Somatoform and Dissociative Disorders
by William R. Yates, Carol S. North and Richard D. Wetzel

Schizophrenia
Concepts and clinical management

Eve C. Johnstone, Martin S. Humphreys,
Fiona H. Lang, Stephen M. Lawrie
and Robert Sandler

Department of Psychiatry, University of Edinburgh, UK

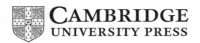
CAMBRIDGE
UNIVERSITY PRESS

PUBLISHED BY THE PRESS SYNDICATE OF THE UNIVERSITY OF CAMBRIDGE
The Pitt Building, Trumpington Street, Cambridge, United Kingdom

CAMBRIDGE UNIVERSITY PRESS
The Edinburgh Building, Cambridge CB2 2RU, UK http://www.cup.cam.ac.uk
40 West 20th Street, New York, NY 10011-4211, USA http://www.cup.org
10 Stamford Road, Oakleigh, Melbourne 3166, Australia

First published 1999

Printed in the United Kingdom at the University Press, Cambridge

Typeset in Times 10/13 pt [VN]

A catalogue record for this book is available from the British Library

Library of Congress Cataloguing in Publication data

Schizophrenia : concepts and clinical management / Eve C. Johnstone . . . [et al.].
    p.   cm.
  Includes index.
  ISBN 0 521 58084 6
  1. Schizophrenia.   I. Johnstone, Eve C.
  [DNLM: 1. Schizophrenia.   WM 203 S337749 1999]
RC514.S3347   1999
616.89'82–dc21   98—24801   CIP
DNLM/DLC
for Library of Congress

ISBN 0 521 58084 6 hardback

Every effort has been made in preparing this book to provide accurate and up-to-date information which is in accord with accepted standards and practice at the time of publication. Nevertheless, the authors, editors and publisher can make no warranties that the information contained herein is totally free from error, not least because clinical standards are constantly changing through research and regulation. The authors, editors and publisher therefore disclaim all liability for direct or consequential damages resulting from the use of material contained in this book. Readers are strongly advised to pay careful attention to information provided by the manufacturer of any drugs or equipment that they plan to use.

Contents

Preface

The disorder which came to be known as schizophrenia was defined more than 100 years ago by Emil Kraepelin (1896). Although his was a substantial advance, Kraepelin himself appreciated that there were many difficulties with the concept. He believed it to be a disease entity with a tangible underlying morbid process, but could neither define nor demonstrate that process. For that reason the condition was defined on purely clinical grounds, and in the successive editions of his textbook he revised the boundaries of the disorder in an attempt to clarify the concept. He considered (Kraepelin, 1919) that since the cause of the disorder was essentially unknown, there could be no rational treatment. The many attempts to advance from this position may be described as modestly successful. Today, some of the problematic issues are much as they were in Kraepelin's time; some areas show great improvement and some new difficulties have been added. There are certainly some unsolved controversies.

In recent years there has been a great deal of interest in schizophrenia and much has been written about it. This further volume seems worthwhile, because in spite of the amount that has been written, many issues are unresolved and some matters, particularly those relating to risk and to cost present ever-increasing problems. Practical and at least partially effective steps have been taken to clarify the diagnostic uncertainties and ambiguities that our predecessors faced (Chapters 2 and 3) but the central difficulty of the lack of an effective validating criterion in the absence of clarification of the 'tangible morbid underlying process' is with us still. Since early this century a great deal of research effort has been directed towards clarification of the 'tangible underlying morbid process' and towards devising effective management strategies, even although without understanding of the underlying process they could not be rationally based.

For the first 50 years relatively little progress was made, although a large number of areas were pursued. In general, studies of the problem of schizophrenia were not based upon clear theoretical constructs but involved the application of new methods of investigation as they developed (Johnstone, 1994). Since the 1950s, however, there have been some major advances. As far as the management of the disorder is concerned, the first of these was the introduction of antipsychotic agents into psychiatric practice by Delay & Deniker in 1952. The introduction of a form of treatment which could clearly be shown to relieve the most florid features of the condition radically altered psychiatric practice and provided a route which allowed the study of neural mechanisms relevant to schizophrenia to begin. Like so many treatment advances in psychiatry, the introduction of chlorpromazine was entirely serendipitous. Indeed, as various chapters of this volume show, the development of the scientific investigations of schizophrenia over the last 50 years provides relatively few examples of well thought out, cohesive, persistently pursued plans of hypothesis driven research ending in major new findings.

Nonetheless, over the last 20 years there have been substantial advances in understanding the biological basis of schizophrenia, and this is an area where there seems to be considerable potential for further success. Although it is evident that the findings that have been made have not always been pursued or clarified as much as they might have been, scientific advances have not really been matched by advances in patient management. Patients have not benefitted as much from the introduction of traditional or 'typical' antipsychotics as was hoped at the time, and indeed the hyperbole that has attended the introduction of some of the newer antipsychotic drugs is difficult to reconcile with recent deeply distressing descriptions of the state of services for psychotic patients in London (King's Fund, 1997). Concern about some well publicized cases (see Chapter 9) has provoked major public debate, and it may well be that policy changes will result.

The introduction of antipsychotic agents has provided a basis for investigating neural mechanisms in schizophrenia, as well as being the cornerstone of the management of the disorder. As is described in Chapter 4, the mode of action of antipsychotic agents seemed for a time to be a rock of established fact amidst a sea of uncertainty, but further advances, particularly the introduction of newer antipsychotic agents, have shown that the picture is much more complex than was at one time believed. It is now clear that a primary abnormality of dopaminergic transmission does not provide the neurochemical basis for the symptoms of all patients with schizophrenia, and that we do not understand the complex interplay between neurotransmitters and receptors in health or in disease. Much research work continues to be carried out in this area, the understanding of which underpins the huge financial investment of the pharmaceutical industry in developing more effective antipsychotic agents.

This is one of the new areas of controversy. New antipsychotic agents are probably more effective than traditional drugs and certainly they have less troublesome side-effects. They are, however, much more expensive than conventional antipsychotics. In the past the treatment of schizophrenia was relatively uncontroversial because there was very little real choice. There were many antipsychotic preparations, but there was not a great deal to choose between them, and if patients did not do well they usually spent a lot of time as inpatients. In many countries, including the UK and the USA, this policy has been changed. The hospital closure programme has been extensive and alternatives to inpatient care such as day hospitals, hostels, etc. have been provided. With the provision of these alternatives and the option of new generation antipsychotics, health economic issues (described in Chapter 12) have been raised. It is possible to compare different modes of care in health economics terms, and it is only recently that the full costs of schizophrenia have been faced.

The work on neuropathology, brain structure and imaging described in Chapter 5 has advanced considerably over the last 20 years, but it is clear that using the techniques and resources available, it could have advanced further. This has perhaps been the most rewarding area for researchers in schizophrenia over the last two decades and the challenge described by Weinberger (1995) of finding evidence that would implicate the brain in schizophrenia has been overcome. The challenge is now to understand the mechanisms which allow development of the lesions which have been demonstrated in the brain, and here progress has been much more limited. All of the microscopic work has been encouraging rather than definitive, and the field is bedevilled by inadequate sample sizes and conflicting methods. Policies of hospital closure have meant that collection of post-mortem samples, which was never easy, has become more difficult and it is unlikely that any research group working alone could make adequate progress. The need for collaboration is obvious but it will not be easy. In 25 years of experience in this area, I have been involved in every type of biological and clinical investigation in schizophrenic patients, and there have certainly been some anxiety-provoking and awkward moments – none more difficult, however, than seeking post-modern permission (for research purposes) from newly bereaved, often elderly relatives of deceased schizophrenic patients, some of whom may have ended their own lives. Research nurses are sometimes employed in this task, but the yield is better if a doctor who knew the patient goes to the relatives' home. It is easier to make that effort to advance the situation of your own group than to help a professional rival, even although the aims of both may be the same. Adequate sample sizes and shared protocols in imaging studies are less problematic, but in that field too there are gaps which adequate planning and foresight could surely have overcome. To clarify the issues, larger samples, especially including more women, are required and studies which go beyond saying that schizophrenic patients differ significantly from normal subjects and which address issues of specificity could be done with the case material and techniques now available. If sample sizes were to be adequate they would be expensive, and as they would be clarifying established matters rather than raising new issues, they might not be held to be at the 'cutting edge' of science and therefore might not have high priority for funding.

Similar criticisms apply to some of the work on epidemiological issues. In particular, studies of the season of birth, epidemics of influenza, ethnicity and perinatal events have all been interpreted as offering support for the idea that insults of various kinds very early in life may result in the later development of schizophrenia. The mechanism by which this might occur is, however, a matter of speculation. We have no real idea at all about the type of obstetric difficulty which is most relevant to the later development of schizophrenia, and yet maternity records (of varying detail and quality but some very detailed) have been kept in this country and in others for a very long time.

Genetic studies are well known to be bedevilled by small sample sizes. Large numbers of related affected and unaffected individuals are required. This applies to genetic studies in all areas, but problems of case definition are much greater in schizophrenia than in disorders such as cystic fibrosis or diabetes where there are biochemical markers for the disease. We do not know what the boundaries of the phenotype of schizophrenia are. Ideally we should have samples of broad and narrow phenotypic definition. Even with very good collection systems, adequate samples of narrow definition will be hard to find. Again, persuading families distressed by discussing the hereditary taint of mental illness that appears to affect them, to encourage all relatives to cooperate fully is not easy, and is most readily done by someone who knows the unhappy details. This is another area where the tendency to be possessive about samples that you know others might well not have been able to obtain has to be overcome. This field could move forward with the techniques available now if sufficient samples were available.

Management issues seem to have greater problems. The details of research work are of course not really in the public domain, but management issues are, and as was pointed out in Chapter 8, the public is 'alarm minded and action orientated' and health service delivery is a matter which has changed in a circular fashion as each approach has fallen into disrepute. Many changes which have taken place have not been based on any clear rationale and there seems to have been a tendency to assume that changes made will be for the better. Any account of current service delivery (e.g. King's Fund, 1997) will show the error of this assumption, and it is clear that for a large number of patients comprehensive services are not being provided. In this area of health care management the greatest fault seems not so much to be a lack of knowledge, but rather a failure to apply what is known.

Chapter 9 deals with the worrying matter of the association between disturbed behaviour, mental illness in general, and schizophrenia in particular. Some work has been done which gives an indication of the predictors of violent behaviour but the evidence currently available concerns very small numbers of patients. As it does appear that the risk of disturbed behaviour (and this includes self-harm as well as harm to others) is symptom related and therefore may be changed by treatment, this is an issue of great importance, and yet adequate studies have not been done. The need for large-scale population based longitudinal studies is clear and again these would have to involve many collaborators in order to succeed.

Issues relating to family interventions lack the dramatic urgency of those concerning assaults and violent deaths, but the same theme of studies too small to be adequately interpreted occurs. There seems to be good evidence that family interventions and social skills offer definite benefits to patients with schizophrenia and their families, but the mechanism of achieving these benefits is unclear (see Chapter 11). We do not know what the essential elements of an effective family intervention actually are. The development of various psychosocial management approaches has not been based upon objective evidence of effectiveness. The situation is that comprehensive programmes of treatment in this area are not widely available, and that there has been wastage of professional resources and indeed of patients' time.

In reading about all of this work the magnitude and intractability of the problems associated with schizophrenia leave an overwhelming impression. Of course there have been advances and for someone like me, with a long involvement in this field of work, it has been enormously exciting and rewarding, and yet of course, at times heartbreakingly sad, because the advances are not really doing anything for the patients, who were good enough to give the samples, have the scans and participate in the trials. We have been able to implicate the brain in schizophrenia and it does seem reasonably likely that we will come to understand the mechanisms underlying the disorder. New techniques may develop, new insights may appear, and yet in the meantime progress could be achieved with the tools to hand if our studies were more efficiently conducted. When considered as a whole, the programme of research conducted into schizophrenia over the last 20 years has a very unplanned quality. And of course, taken as a whole, it was unplanned. Research, in the UK and elsewhere, is funded in terms of discrete, fairly short-term projects, carried out by specified groups of individuals. In general, there is no clear obligation to fit in with the work of others. This system has its merits, but although 'bottom up' research is tried and tested and collaborative schemes imposed from above have obvious difficulties, perhaps the time for a rethinking of funding schemes and some 'top down' investigation has come.

EVE C. JOHNSTONE

References

Delay, J. & Deniker, P. (1952). Le traitement des psychoses par une méthode neurolyptique derivée de l'hibernothérapie. In *Congrés de Médecins Aliénistes et Neurologistes de France*, ed. P. Cossa, pp. 497–502. Paris and Luxembourg: Masson Editeus Libraires de L'Academie de Médecine.

Johnstone, E. C. (1994). *Searching for the Causes of Schizophrenia*. Oxford: Oxford University Press.

King's Fund (1997). *London's Mental Health*. London: King's Fund.

Kraepelin, E. (1896). *Psychiatrie, ein Lehrbuch für Studierende und Artze*, 5th edn. Leipzig: Barth.

Kraepelin, E. (1919). *Dementia Praecox* (translated by R. M. Barclay. Edited by G. M. Robertson. Facsimile edition published by Krieger: New York, 1971).

Weinberger, D. R. (1995). From neuropathology to neurodevelopment. *Lancet*, **346**, 552–7.

1
Introduction

Any attempt at a historical narrative of schizophrenia must acknowledge a rather uncertain beginning (Turner, 1995) as there is an unresolved debate as to whether schizophrenia existed before the eighteenth century (Hare, 1988; Jeste et al., 1985). While psychiatric concepts were well developed in ancient Greece (Adams, 1856), the core categories of Greek psychiatry were phrenitis, mania, melancholia and paranoia (Roccatagliata, 1973) and descriptions to which a diagnosis of schizophrenia could reasonably be applied did not occur until very much later. Although Willis (1683) and Kinnear (1727) left reports of symptomatology which could have been due to schizophrenic illness, the first unambiguous accounts were written by two separate authors, Haslam and Pinel in 1809. Throughout the nine-teenth century, many attempts were made to classify insanity. In 1860 Morel introduced the term *démence précoce* to describe an adolescent patient, once bright and active, who had slowly lapsed into a state of withdrawal.

He gradually lost his cheerfulness, became gloomy, taciturn and showed a tendency towards solitude – the young patient progressively forgot everything he had lear-ned, his so brilliant intellectual faculties underwent, in time, a very distressing arrest. A kind of torpor akin to hebetude replaced the earlier activity and when I saw him I concluded that the fatal translation to the state of *démence précoce* was about to take place... A sudden paralysis of the faculties, a *démence précoce*, indicated that this patient had reached the end of the part of his intellectual life that he could control.

Emil Kraepelin (1856–1927) is generally considered to have defined (as dementia praecox) the disease concept which came to be known as schizo-phrenia. He was Professor of Psychiatry in Heidelberg and later in Munich and wrote nine editions of his *Lehrbuch der Psychiatrie* (*Textbook of Psychiatry*), published between 1893 and 1927. In the first three editions of

1

his book he was concerned to move away from the earlier nineteenth century nosological concepts which he criticized as unreliable from a clinical and especially prognostic point of view (Hoff, 1995). The term dementia praecox was not used in these editions and it was in the fourth to eighth editions of *Lehrbuch der Psychiatrie* (1893–1915) that Kraepelin created a nosological system and finalized his concept of natural disease entities.

In the fifth (1896) and sixth (1899) editions he developed the concept of dementia praecox and the separation of dementia praecox with a poor prognosis and manic depressive illness with a good or at least a better prognosis. Kraepelin described hebephrenic, catatonic and paranoid forms of the illness. In defining dementia praecox he had drawn together hebephrenia as described by Hecker (1871), catatonia as described by Kahlbaum (1874) and his own dementia paranoides, regarding them as manifestations of the same disorder, which typically had its onset in early adult life and had a poor outcome. Although the patient's individual personality could promote the development of the psychotic illness, it was not a central factor. He considered delusions, hallucinations and catatonic features to be important characteristics of the disorder.

In defining the disease entity of dementia praecox he was following the pattern of definition of concepts of disease which had arisen since the work of Sydenham in the seventeenth century (Sydenham, 1696). In the ancient world, symptoms and signs, e.g. fever, asthma, rashes, joint pains, were themselves regarded as diseases to be studied separately, and it was really only with Sydenham's work in the seventeenth century that the idea of disease as a syndrome, i.e. a constellation of symptoms having a characteristic prognosis, became established. It is still the case that an adequate definition for all disorders that may be regarded as diseases is hard to find (Kendall, 1975). Although from the time of Sydenham diseases were defined on a syndromal basis, with the increasing popularity of post-mortem examination in the nineteenth century, disease became defined by pathological findings rather than by the clinical picture, and later technological development has allowed diseases to be defined in a variety of different terms, e.g. bacteriological, biochemical and molecular biological. As these new methods of definition of disease have developed, the older ones have persisted to some extent, so that any medical textbook will list diseases defined in terms of varied concepts which may have little or no relationship to one another. The development of morbid anatomy and histology in the nineteenth century, and later that of physiology and biochemistry, showed that many diseases defined as syndromes were in fact associated with identifiable lesions. This led to the view that the demonstration of such an identifiable lesion was the defining characteristic of disease.

There are many problems with this clear-cut and initially appealing view, especially perhaps as far as psychiatry is concerned. The principal model of disease in psychiatry remains the 'syndrome model', i.e. a cluster of symptoms and signs which are associated with a characteristic course over time; however, in psychiatry no physical basis has been defined for most major syndromes. Many psychiatrists have, however, taken the view that disorders defined on a syndromal basis would in time be found to be based upon an identifiable lesion. For example, Kurt Schneider (1950) saw no difficulty in accepting the idea that the word illness should only be used in situations in which 'some actual morbid change' or 'defective structure' was present in the body. In this context he stated that he did not regard either neurotic states or personality disorders as illness, but simply as 'abnormal varieties of sane mental life'. He still, however, considered schizophrenia and manic depressive psychosis as illness, along with organic and toxic psychoses, on the basis of the assumption that in time they would prove to have an 'underlying morbid physical condition'.

This was certainly Kraepelin's view of dementia praecox and although he defined the condition on the basis of the characteristic course and outcome of a cluster of symptoms and signs, he stated that this was a disorder of which if 'every detail' were known, a specific anatomical pathology with a specific aetiology would be found. In grouping together the mental diseases of early adult life which were associated with a poor outcome, Kraepelin considered that he was defining a clinical syndrome which represented a disease of the brain, the nature of which would eventually be revealed by appropriate investigations.

In 1911 Eugen Bleuler published his *Dementia praecox or the Group of Schizophrenias* and it is his term of schizophrenia which has received general acceptance (Bleuler, 1950). Although Bleuler considered that he was developing Kraepelin's concept, in fact he changed it substantially. Bleuler was influenced by psychoanalytic schools of thought and saw schizophrenia in psychological terms as much as in the neuropathological ones envisaged by Kraepelin. His term schizophrenia, meaning split mind, was intended to describe what he called a loosening of the associations between the different functions of the mind, so that thoughts became disconnected and the coordination between emotional, cognitive and volitional processes became poor. He considered thought disorder, affective disturbance, autism and ambivalence to be the fundamental symptoms of schizophrenia and that the more clear-cut phenomena of hallucinations, delusions and catatonic features emphasized by Kraepelin were secondary features. This view led him to conclude that schizophrenia could be diagnosed when there was no evidence that hallucinations or delusions had ever occurred, and he thus added simple schizophrenia to the hebephrenic, catatonic and paranoid forms recognized by Kraepelin. Bleuler's ideas became influential in some centres, particularly in the United States, but Kraepelin's concept of dementia praecox, including the idea of an as yet unknown underlying morbid physical condition, never lost its domination in many European countries.

The lack of common ground between these two concepts was illustrated by the findings of the US–UK diagnostic project (Cooper et al., 1972). In this comparative study, 250 consecutive admissions between the ages of 20 and 59 were studied in New York and London. Information was obtained from patients and their relatives by structured interviews and a diagnosis using nomenclature from the *International Classification of Diseases* (ICD) (WHO, 1967) was assigned to each patient. The project diagnoses obtained in this way were compared with the diagnoses given independently to the same patients by the hospital staff. In the New York series 61.5% of the patients were given a hospital diagnosis of schizophrenia, whereas in the London series the proportion was 33.9%. However, in terms of the project diagnoses, the percentages were 29.2 and 35.1, i.e. clearly similar. By contrast, 31.5% of the London sample received a hospital diagnosis of manic depressive disorder, but only 5.2% of the New York sample were given such a diagnosis. Clearly, therefore, the concept of schizophrenia in New York at that time was wider than that employed in London.

Findings such as these encouraged the formulation of operational rules for defining psychiatric disorders, including schizophrenia, for example the St. Louis criteria (Feighner et al., 1972); DSM III, DSM IIIR, DSM IV, (APA 1980, 1987, 1994). The introduction of operational definitions for schizophrenia has clarified the syndrome and reaffirmed the importance of delusions and hallucinations as well as thought disorder, but cannot address the matter of 'the underlying morbid physical condition'.

When he defined dementia praecox, Kraepelin seemed to have the idea that the underlying deficit in the condition led to the destruction of cortical neurones, possibly by a process of 'auto-intoxication' (Hoff, 1995). In his book *Dementia Praecox* (1919) he did, however, express the view that 'the causes of dementia praecox are, at the present time still mapped in impenetrable darkness'. Nonetheless, he devoted a chapter of this book to morbid anatomy in which he quoted the work of Alzheimer and Nissl. Although he believed that the causes of dementia praecox were unknown, Kraepelin considered that hereditary factors and 'injury to the germ' could be relevant. He postulated that 'such activities as are peculiar to the higher psychic stages of development' might be ascribed to the small-celled layers of the cortex noted by Alzheimer and stated 'We see therefore in all the domains of psychic life the ancestral activities offering a greater power of the resistance to the morbid process than the psychic faculties belonging to the highest degrees of development'.

The idea of a neurodevelopmental basis for schizophrenia has recently had considerable support (Weinberger, 1986; Murray & Lewis, 1987; Weinberger, 1995a) but Kraepelin was not the only psychiatrist working one hundred or more years ago who thought along these lines. Sir Thomas Clouston saw his concept of adolescent insanity as being part of Kraepelin's disease entity of dementia praecox. Clouston included adolescent insanity within his general concept of developmental insanity and in his Morison Lecture of 1890 (Clouston, 1891) he described investigations of palatal structures in over 2000 individuals including normal controls and sufferers from adolescent insanity, as well as criminals, epileptics, idiots and imbeciles and those with 'acquired insanity'. He interpreted these findings as indicating that adolescent insanity represented a form of developmental defect of ectodermal tissue.

The search for the 'underlying morbid physical conditions' of schizophrenia has continued ever since the time of Clouston and Kraepelin. Many early investigations of the biological basis of schizophrenia concentrated on neuropathology, and indeed the notion that the neuropathological changes were determined by maldevelopment of the brain was widespread (Mackenzie, 1912; Turner, 1912; Rosanoff, 1914; Southard, 1915). The early histological work of Alzheimer (1897, 1913); Wernicke (1900), and Klippel & Lhermitte (1909) described changes such as 'lacunae', pyknotic neuronal atrophy, focal demyelination and 'metachromatic bodies'. This work was, however, all carried out when histological techniques were in their infancy and when the need for controlling the effects of fixation and staining, and indeed for controlled experiments, was not appreciated. In 1924 Dunlap carried out a careful comparison of the brains of eight schizophrenic patients aged under 45 at death with the brains of five normal individuals selected for having a cause of death unlikely to have influenced the structure of the brain. Cell counts in the areas where abnormalities had been described in earlier studies were carried out by three independent observers, all of whom were in good agreement and found no differences between patients and controls. Neuropathological studies of schizophrenia did continue (Vogt & Vogt, 1948) but Dunlap's study cast a shadow of scepticism over this area of work which persisted for many years (David, 1957).

Much of the early search for the biological basis of schizophrenia concerned the structure of the brain, but a number of other areas of investigation were pursued. On the whole these were not based upon clear theoretical constructs but involved the application to the problem of schizophrenia of new methods of biological investigation as they became available. Areas of early study included nitrogen metabolism (Gjessing, 1938), the circulatory system (Lewis, 1923; Shattock, 1950) and gonadal dysfunction (Mott, 1919; Hemphill et al., 1944; Blair et al., 1952). In general the results of the various studies did not show consistent findings. In the 1960s work relating to the 'pink spot' in the urine of patients with schizophrenia was described (Friedhoff & van Winkel, 1962; Bourdillon et al., 1965). This 'pink spot' was due to the presence of 3,4 dimethyl-oxyphenylethylamine (DMPE) in the urine of schizophrenics. This led to the development of the transmethylation hypothesis which proposed that abnormal methylation of cactetholamines might be of aetiological importance in schizophrenia. However the work of Keuhl et al. (1966) and Hollister & Friedhoff (1966) showed no support for this possibility. The many sources of possible artefact in studying schizophrenic patients, who at the period in question were almost all cared for in large mental hospitals, had not been appreciated during the conduct of much of this early work, but they were well described by Kety in 1959.

Parallel to the neuropathological search for structural brain abnormalities in schizophrenia described above was a series of investigations examining brain structure by neuroradiological means. Pneumoencephalography had been introduced by Dandy in 1919 and in 1927 Jacobi & Winkler reported a study in which 18 of 19 schizophrenic patients showed 'unquestionable' internal hydrocephalus. A number of other studies showing similar conclusions were reported (for review see Johnstone, 1994). Some of the pneumoencephalographic studies were small and uncontrolled but others were large and evidently well conducted. In general, in spite of a negative investigation by Storey (1966), the finding of ventricular enlargement in schizophrenia, and within groups of schizophrenic patients of an association between such enlargement and features of deterioration and defect was confirmed.

By the 1960s the pneumoencephalographic studies provided the strongest available evidence that there was a biological basis for schizophrenia, and yet at that time this evidence was largely ignored. It is difficult now to understand why this should have been so, but following the Second World War there was an upsurge of interest in psychodynamic and social psychiatry. The prevailing view at that time was that schizophrenia was caused by a fault in the mother–child relationship. Indeed in the late/middle part of this century this had gained the status of orthodoxy (Hirsch & Weinberger, 1995). Other work at this time (Myerson, 1939; Martin, 1955; Wing & Brown, 1961) indicated that the psychological and social impairments of patients with schizophrenia were partly the result of the circumstances in the institutions in which the patients then lived. The efficacy of antipsychotic drugs in treating acute episodes of schizophrenia had been clearly demonstrated in the 1960s (NIMH, 1964). Initially there was great optimism about their use and it seemed possible that most patients could be discharged from mental hospitals (Jones, 1987) and that no particular provision in the community would be required (Tooth & Brooke, 1961; Taylor, 1962).

It is easy to see that against this background there would seem to be little purpose in looking for a biological basis for schizophrenia, and that the possibility of a structural, genetic or developmental cause would have seemed unlikely. By the 1970s it was clear that these optimistic views were misplaced, but scientific advances made at that time and since greatly enhanced the possibilities of investigating the biological basis or 'underlying morbid physical condition' of schizophrenia. There have been major technical advances, in pharmacology, in both structural and functional imaging and in genetics. The current state of knowledge in each of these areas will be described in more detail in subsequent chapters, but their development over recent years will be briefly summarized here.

In 1952, chlorpromazine was introduced into psychiatric practice on an empirical basis by Delay & Deniker. By the late 1950s it was clear that this drug was actively anti-schizophrenic and not simply a more effective sedative than had previously been available. This discovery of a class of drugs which relieved the fundamental symptoms of schizophrenia was an enormous advance. At the time of their introduction the mechanism by which these drugs produced their antipsychotic effect was not understood at all, but in 1963 Carlsson & Lindquist suggested that they might act by blocking dopamine (DA) receptors in the brain. The subsequent development of in vitro assay systems for dopamine receptors has allowed extensive study of the dopamine antagonist effect of antipsychotic drugs (Kebabian et al., 1972; Miller et al., 1974; Seeman et al., 1976). Dopamine receptors were shown to exist in at least two major subtypes, D_1 and D_2, by Kebabian & Calne in 1979. Subsequent work showed that the very high correlation between dopamine receptor affinity and clinical antipsychotic potency (Seeman et al., 1976) concerned D_2 and not D_1 receptors (Seeman, 1980; Richelson & Nelson, 1984). D_2 receptor blockade came to be considered as having an essential or even exclusive role in mediating the antipsychotic activity of neuroleptic drugs. This naturally led to consideration of the possibility that dopaminergic (essentially D_2) mechanisms were disturbed in schizophrenia, and was one of the two main lines of evidence on which the so-called 'dopamine' hypothesis of schizophrenia (i.e. that schizophrenia resulted from excessive dopaminergic activity at certain sites in the brain) was based.

The other main line of evidence was the fact that amphetamine and other dopamine releasing drugs, if used by non-psychotic individuals, could induce a schizophrenia-like paranoid state (Connell, 1958; Griffiths et al., 1972; Angrist et al., 1974). Studies of dopaminergic function in schizophrenic patients, however, have generally not yielded evidence of excessive activity (Bowers, 1974; Post et al., 1975: Bird et al., 1977; Owen et al., 1978; Crow et al., 1979). Post-mortem studies of the brains of schizophrenics showed an increased density of dopamine D_2 receptors (Lee et al., 1978; Owen et al., 1981). It was difficult to know whether this effect was directly related to the schizophrenic illness or was an artefact induced by antipsychotic medication. Although a few patients who were not thought to have had antipsychotic medication were included in these studies, the numbers were necessarily small and the complete absence of administration of antipsychotic medication in this situation can never be established with certainty. Later, receptor densities were measured by means of positron emission tomography (PET), and again it was suggested that schizophrenic patients who were drug naive had increased dopamine D_2 density in their brains (Wong et al., 1986).

Conflicting results have been found and the balance of the evidence at present is that there is no difference in D_2 receptor density between drug-naive schizophrenics and controls (Nordstrom et al., 1993; Carlsson, 1995). A very large amount of research effort has been expended upon studying dopaminergic mechanisms in relation to schizophrenia and antipsychotic medication. This work has established beyond reasonable doubt that the principal relevant mode of action of typical antipsychotic drugs is blockade of D_2 receptors, but the hope that this line of investigation would shed light upon the underlying mechanism or biological basis of schizophrenia has not been realized.

For many years the development of new antipsychotic drugs was influenced by the dopamine hypothesis of schizophrenia and by the fact that all effective antipsychotic drugs exhibited some degree of dopamine receptor (D_2) antagonism. The demonstration (Kane et al., 1988) that clozapine (classed as an 'atypical' antipsychotic agent on the basis that it has a low propensity to induce extrapyramidal side-effects), has enhanced antipsychotic activity in patients resistant to the effects of 'typical' drugs such as haloperidol or chlorpromazine made the position with regard to the relationship between D_2 blockade and schizophrenia much less clear-cut. Clozapine has a modest affinity for D_1 and D_2 receptors and a broad range of effects on other neurotransmitter receptors, including other dopamine receptor subtypes, serotonin and alpha-adrenergic receptors (Kane & McGlashan, 1995). At the present time the pharmacological basis which enables antipsychotic drugs to exhibit 'atypicality' (i.e. a low propensity to induce extrapyramidal side-effects) with or without greater efficacy to alleviate the symptoms of schizophrenia than their counterparts (Waddington, 1995) is unknown, although a number of 'atypical' drugs other than clozapine have been introduced, e.g. risperidone, zotepine, sertindole, amperozide, olanzapine.

As far as the shedding of pharmacological light upon the biological basis of schizophrenia is concerned, a critical issue that remains to be resolved is the extent to which the putative basis(es) of such atypicality can be accommodated within, or else prove supplementary or even contradictory to, the dopamine receptor hypothesis (Meltzer, 1992). A position that seemed reasonably clear for 15 years has become clouded by doubts and contradictions. While the mechanisms of action of antipsychotics remain likely to reveal something of the nature of the condition they are used to treat, the wide-ranging effects of the newer drugs provide a wealth of possibilities but no direct route to the biological basis of schizophrenia.

As noted earlier, structural imaging using pneumoencephalography was first used to demonstrate structural brain changes in schizophrenia in 1927, and differences between patients and control subjects were established in a number of studies. Investigations by this method were limited by the fact that the American Roentgen Ray Society in 1929 declared that it was unethical to use normal controls in pneumoencaphlographic studies. However, the introduction of computer-assisted tomography (CT) in 1973 by Hounsfield provided a non-invasive technique which allowed controlled studies to be conducted. Schizophrenic patients were shown in 1976 to have ventricular enlargement as compared with age-matched normal subjects (Johnstone et al., 1976). Subsequent studies have largely confirmed this finding, although there have been some discordant results. The later introduction of magnetic resonance imaging (MRI) provided improved resolution, and the ability to distinguish grey and white matter. Raz & Raz (1990) performed a meta-analysis of CT and MRI studies in schizophrenia. They defined 'effect size' as the ratio of the difference between mean ventricular volume in patients and controls divided by the pooled standard deviation for each study. They found that the 'effect size' for the various studies was normally distributed with a mean value of approximately 0.6 standard deviations. Thus, there is convincing evidence for larger ventricular volume in patients as compared with normal individuals, but the magnitude of the effect is relatively small, so that the failure of some individual studies to find a significant difference is not unexpected. Enlargement of the ventricles, of course, implies a reduction in the volume of cerebral tissue and the MRI studies have indicated a reduction in volume, largely in grey matter and most consistently in the temporal lobes (Suddath et al., 1990; Shenton et al., 1992; Zipursky et al., 1992; Lawrie & Abukmeil, 1998). Structural imaging does not provide information at a cellular level and these studies have provoked a renewed interest in the neuropathology of schizophrenia.

Morphometric studies (Bogerts et al., 1985; Pakkenberg, 1987; Bruton et al., 1990) have shown reductions in brain tissue and cytoarchitectural studies have shown anomalies of laminar organization in most patients (Jakob & Beckman, 1986; Arnold et al., 1991; Benes et al., 1991). These findings have been interpreted in neurodevelopmental terms and together with evidence concerning perinatal events (Gunter-Genta et al., 1994), minor physical anomalies (Green et al., 1994) and childhood development in individuals destined to develop schizophrenia in adult life (Done et al., 1994), have been put forward as the basis for the neurodevelopmental hypothesis of schizophrenia (Weinberger, 1995b). Weinberger (1995b) is probably justified in his claim that there no longer can be any doubt that there is underlying brain pathology in a large proportion of cases of schizophrenia, but certainly many of the findings described above require further clarification and replication. If the neurodevelopmental hypothesis of schizophrenia is correct, the mechanisms which permit relatively early compensation for the lesion and initiate clinical decompensation may be expected to be revealed in time.

Functional imaging techniques, including positron emission tomography (PET), single photon emission tomography (SPET) and functional MRI (FMRI) may be used to establish the relationship between disordered neural activity and the clinical features of schizophrenia. Regional cerebral blood flow (rCBF) may be measured with any of these techniques. Simple motor tasks or sensor experiences are associated with increases in rCBF in the relevant primary motor or sensory areas, indicating that rCBF is an index of local neuronal activity. The earliest studies of rCBF in schizophrenia (Ingvar & Franzen, 1974) revealed relative frontal cortical underactivity as compared with post central cortical lesions. Later studies showed somewhat conflicting results, but the balance of the evidence by the late 1980s was that schizophrenic patients exhibit abnormal rCBF in the resting state and that different schizophrenic patients exhibit different patterns of abnormality. In a PET study of medicated schizophrenic patients with stable symptoms, Liddle et al. (1992) demonstrated that the syndrome patterns of (a) psychomotor poverty (b) reality distortion and (c) disorganization was each associated with a specific pattern of rCBF in association cortex of frontal parietal and temporal lobes and in related subcortical nuclei. These patterns indicate imbalances between neuronal activity at diverse interconnected brain sites rather than abnormal function at a single location. During the performance of executive tasks (e.g. Wisconsin Card Sort Test) schizophrenic patients exhibit impaired frontal activation (Weinberger et al., 1986), while during memory tests there is some evidence of impaired temporal activation (Ganguli et al., 1995). These findings and others, such as those of Frith et al. (1995), who found that in a word generation test the activation of the left prefrontal cortex seen in schizophrenics was not accompanied by the reduction in rCBF in the left superior temporal gyrus seen in controls, would be consistent with the view that the characteristic feature of schizophrenia is disturbed connectivity between cerebral areas. The physical basis for this disturbed connectivity remains a matter for speculation.

The genetic aspects of schizophrenia and other psychoses have been the focus of considerable attention in the past few years. The idea that mental disorders run in families is a very old one and Kraepelin (1907) considered heredity to be a prominent factor in relation to liability to dementia praecox. The familiality of schizophrenia has continued to receive investigation since that time (Falconer, 1965; Shields, 1977) and in an elegant series of studies (Rosenthal et al., 1971; Kety et al., 1975) it was demonstrated that this familial tendency to develop the disorder was due not to shared environment but to shared genetic material.

Genetic studies of schizophrenia have received a major impetus from the recent advances that have been made in molecular genetics. Until the advent of modern molecular genetics, investigations were limited by the few informative markers in any given family. Only 'classical' markers such as human leucocyte antigen system (HLA) colour blindness or blood group polymorphisms were used. The use of restriction endonucleases has uncovered a considerable amount of previously inaccessible genetic variation. This variation detected by restriction fragment length polymorphisms (RFLPs) has dramatically increased the number of potentially informative markers in any given pedigree. The success of RFLP linkage methods in locating the loci for several important Mendelian disorders, most notably Huntington's disease, Duchenne's muscular dystrophy and cystic fibrosis, has given great encouragement to molecular geneticists (Kendler, 1987). In schizophrenia, however, the pattern of transmission is complex and although some multigeneration pedigrees with a Mendelian-like appearance are found, they are very much the exception to the rule (Asherson et al., 1995). It seems likely that at a molecular level schizophrenia will turn out to be heterogeneous. We do not know whether we are searching for one gene of major effect, several genes of moderate effect or many genes each of only a small effect. Nonetheless, it has been estimated that as much as 80% of the variance in liability to schizophrenia is of genetic origin (McGuffin et al., 1984; Farmer et al., 1987), and although studies of the genetics of schizophrenia have not been as fruitful as seemed likely at one time, it is a field of investigation that will continue.

Over the last 20 years, therefore, there have been substantial advances in understanding the biological basis of schizophrenia and this is an area of study where there is much activity and great potential for further success.

The scientific advances have not really been matched by improvements in patient management. The introduction of newer 'atypical' antipsychotics has provided drugs with less severe side-effects, but their efficacy remains limited and the adverse effects are still a problem.

The evidence for enhanced therapeutic efficacy, except in restricted patient groups, is not strong (Owens, 1996). In spite of recent improvements for most patients, the treatments available rarely produce full recovery, and many patients continue to struggle with considerable psychosocial and vocational disability. Further advances are sorely needed to alleviate the enormous personal suffering, family burden and societal costs associated with the disease. It is often the case that welcome advances in treatment arouse unrealistic expectations in those providing care. While the introduction of typical neuroleptics in the 1950s was a great advance, patients did not in the long run benefit as much as was hoped, and ideas that they would be able to be discharged into the community with few further problems have proved sadly mistaken. Concerns about some well publicized cases of very disturbed behaviour in schizophrenic patients in the community have provoked major public debate about the appropriateness or otherwise of our current methods of management. Our understanding of the biological basis of schizophrenia is improving, available treatments are advancing, and it seems probable that our enhanced biological understanding will in time provide rational and more effective treatments. Current concern about plans of management is likely to bring improvement in delivery of care.

The timescale of worthwhile gains in these areas can only be estimated at present. Improvements in understanding, treatment and management will be very valuable, and at least when in an optimistic frame of mind, it is possible to think that these can be foreseen, albeit dimly. Prevention of this dreadful disease would, of course, be the ultimate goal. Sadly at present it is difficult to say anything about how and when this will be achieved.

References

Adams, F. (1856). *Aretaeus, the Cappadocian. The Extant Works.* Edited and translated by F. Adams. Boston: Mulford House.

Alzheimer, A. (1897). Beitrage zur pathologischen anatomie der hirnrinde und zur anatomischen grundlage der psychosen. *Monatsschrift für Psychiatrie und Neurologie*, **2**, 82–120.

Alzheimer, A. (1913). Beitrage zur pathologischen anatomie der Dementia Praecox. *Allgemeine Zeitschrift für Psychiatrie*, **70**, 810–12.

Angrist, B., Sathanathan, C., Wilk, S. & Gershon, S. (1974). Amphetamine psychosis, behavioural and biochemical aspects. *Journal of Psychiatric Research*, **11**, 13–23.

Arnold, S. E., Hyman, B. T., Van Hösen, G. W. & Damasio, A. R. (1991). Some cytoarchitectural abnormalities of the entorhinal cortex in schizophrenia. *Archives of General Psychiatry*, **48**, 625–32.

Asherson, P., Mant, R. & McGuffin, P. (1995). Genetics & schizophrenia. In *Schizophrenia*, ed. S. R. Hirsch & D. R. Weinberger, pp. 253–92. Oxford: Blackwell Science Ltd.

Benes, F. M., McSporran, J., Bird, E. D., San Giovanni, J. P. & Vincent, S. L. (1991). Deficits in small interneurons in prefrontal and cingulate cortices of schizophrenic and schizoaffective patients. *Archives of General Psychiatry*, **48**, 996–1001.

Bird, E. C., Spokes, E. G., Barnes, J., Mackay, A. V. P., Iversen, L. L. & Shepherd, M. (1977). Increased brain dopamine and reduced glutamic acid decarboxylase and choline acetyl transferase in schizophrenia and related psychoses. *Lancet*, **ii**, 1157–9.

Blair, J. H., Smiffen, R. C., Cranswick, E. H., Jaffe, W. & Kline, N. S. (1952). The question of histopathological changes in the testes of schizophrenia. *Journal of Mental Science*, **98**, 464–5.

Bleuler, E. (1950). *Dementia Praecox or the Group of Schizophrenias.* Translated by J. Zinkin. New York: International Universities Press.

Bogerts, B., Meerts, E. & Schonfeldt-Bausch, R. (1985). Basal ganglia and limbic system pathology in schizophrenia: a morphometric study of brain volume and shrinkage. *Archives of General Psychiatry*, **42**, 784–91.

Bourdillon, R. E., Clarke, C. A., Ridges, A. P., Sheppard, P. M., Harper, P. &

Leslie, S. A. (1965). 'Pink spot' in the urine of schizophrenics. *Nature* (London), **208**, 453.

Bowers, M. B. (1974). Central dopamine turnover in schizophrenic syndromes. *Archives of General Psychiatry*, **31**, 50–4.

Bruton, C. J., Crow, T. J., Frith, C. D., Johnstone, E. C., Owens, D. G. C. & Roberts, G. W. (1990). Schizophrenia and the brain: a prospective clinico-neuropathological study. *Psychological Medicine*, **20**, 285–304.

Carlsson, A. (1995). The dopamine theory revisited. In *Schizophrenia*, ed. S. R. Hirsch & D. R. Weinberger, pp. 379–400. Oxford: Blackwell Science Ltd.

Carlsson, A. & Lindqvist, M. (1963). Effect of chlopromazine and haloperidol on formation of 3-methoxy-tyramine and normetanephrine in mouse brain. *Acta Pharmacologica et Toxicologica*, **20**, 140–4.

Clouston, T. S. (1891). *The Neuroses of Development, Being the Morison Lectures of 1890*. Edinburgh: Oliver & Boyd.

Connell, P. H. (1958). *Amphetamine psychosis*. Maudsley Monography No. 5. London: Chapman & Hall.

Cooper, L. E., Kendell, R. E., Gurland, B. J., Sharpe, L., Copeland, J. R. M. & Simon, R. (1972). *Psychiatric diagnosis in New York and London*. Maudsley Monograph No. 20. London: Oxford University Press.

Crow, T. J., Cross, A. J. & Owen, F. (1979). Monoamine mechanisms in chronic schizophrenia: post mortem neurochemical findings. *British Journal of Psychiatry*, **134**, 249–56.

Dandy, W. E. (1919). Roentgenography of the brain after injection of air into the cerebral ventricles. *American Journal of Roentgenography*, **6**, 26.

David, G. B. (1957). The pathological anatomy of the schizophrenias. In *Schizophrenia, Somatic Aspects*, ed. D. Richter, pp. 93–130. New York: Pergamon.

Delay, J. & Deniker, P. (1952). Le traitment des psychoses par une méthode neurolytique derivée de l'hibernothérapie. In *Congrés de Médecines Aliénistes et neurologistes de France*, Paris and Luxembourg: Masson Editeurs Libraires de L'Academie de Médecine.

Done, D. J., Crow, T. J., Johnstone, E. C. & Sacker, A. (1994). Childhood antecedents of schizophrenia and affective illness: social adjustment at ages 7 and 11. *British Medical Journal*, **309**, 699–703.

Dunlap, C. B. (1924). Dementia praecox: some preliminary observations on brains from carefully selected cases and a consideration of certain sources of error. *American Journal of Psychiatry*, **80**, 403–21.

Falconer, D. S. (1965). The inheritance of liability to certain diseases estimated from the incidence among relatives. *Archives of Human Genetics*, **29**, 51–76.

Farmer, A. E., McGuffin, P. & Gottesman, I. I. (1987). Twin Concordance for DSM-III schizophrenia: scrutinising the validity of the definition. *Archives of General Psychiatry*, **44**, 634–41.

Feighner, J. P., Robins, E., Guze, S., Woodruff, R. A., Winokur, G. & Munoz, R. (1972). Diagnostic criteria for use in psychiatric research. *Archives of General Psychiatry*, **26**, 57–62.

Friedhoff, A. J. & Van Winkle, E. (1962). Isolation and characterisation of the compound from the urine of schizophrenics. *Nature*, **194**, 897.

Frith, C. D., Friston, K. J., Herold, S. et al. (1995). Regional brain activity in chronic schizophrenic patients during the performance of a verbal fluency task. *British Journal of Psychiatry*, **167**, 343–9.

Ganguli, R., Mintuin, M. & Carter, C. (1995). The functional neuroanatomy of memory in schizophrenia: an O^{15} H_2O PET study during supraspan memory performance. *Schizophrenia Research*, **15**, 82–3.

Gjessing, R. (1938). Disturbances of somatic functions in catatonia with a periodic course and their compensation. *Journal of Mental Science*, **84**, 608–21.

Green, M. F., Satz, P. & Christensen, C. (1994). Minor physical anomalis in schizophrenic patients, bipolar patients and their siblings. *Schizophrenia Bulletin*, **20**, 433–40.

Griffiths, L. D., Cavanagh, J., Held, J. & Oates, J. A. (1972). Dextramphetamine: evaluation of psychotomimetic properties in man. *Archives of General Psychiatry*, **26**, 97–100.

Gunther-Genta, F., Bovet, P. & Honfeld, P. (1994). Obstetric complications and schizophrenia: a case-control study. *British Journal of Psychiatry*, **164**, 165–70.

Hare, E. H. (1988). Schizophrenia as a recent disease. *British Journal of Psychiatry*, **153**, 521–31.

Haslam, J. (1809). *Observations on Madness and Melancholy*. London: Rivington.

Hecker, E. (1871). Hebephrenie ein Beitrag zur klinischen psychiatrie. *Archiv für pathologische Anatomie und Physiologie und für klinische Medizin*, **52**, 394–429.

Hemphill, R. E., Reiss, M. & Taylor, A. L. (1944). A study of the histology of the testis in schizophrenia and other mental disorders. *Journal of Mental Science*, **90**, 681–95.

Hirsch, S. R. & Weinberger, D. R. (1995). *Preface. In Schizophrenia*, pp. xiii–xiv. Oxford: Blackwell Science Ltd.

Hoff, P. (1995). Kraepelin. In *A History of Clinical Psychiatry – the Origin and History of Psychiatric Disorders*, ed. G. Berrios & R. Porter, pp. 263–79. London: the Athlone Press.

Hollister, L. E. & Friedhoff, A. J. (1966). Effects of 3:4 dimethoxyphenylethylamine in man. *Nature (London)*, **210**, 1377.

Hounsfield, G. N. (1973). Computerised transverse axial scanning (tomography) Part I: Description of the system. *British Journal of Radiology*, **46**, 1016–22.

Ingvar, D. H. & Franzen, G. (1974). Abnormalities of cerebral blood flow distribution in patients with chronic schizophrenia. *Acta Psychiatrica Scandinavica*, **50**, 425–62.

Jacobi, W. & Winkler, H. (1927). Encephalographische studien an chronisch schizophrenen. *Archiv. für Psychiatrie und Nervenkrankheiten*, **81**, 299–332.

Jakob, H. & Beckman, H. (1986). Prenatal developmental disturbances in the limbic allocortex in schizophrenics. *Journal of Neural Transmission*, **65**, 303–26.

Jeste, D. R., Carman, R., Lodr, J. B. & Wyatt, R. J. (1985). Did schizophrenia exist before the eighteenth century? *Comprehensive Psychiatry*, **26**, 493–503.

Johnstone, E. C. (1994). *Searching for the Causes of Schizophrenia*. Oxford: Oxford University Press.

Johnstone, E. C., Crow, T. J., Frith, C. D., Husband, J. & Kreel, L. (1976). Cerebral ventricular size and cognitive impairment in chronic schizophrenia. *Lancet*, **ii**, 924–6.

Jones, K. (1987). Why a crisis situation? What has heppened? In *Schizophrenia*, ed. K. Herbst, pp. 47–52. London: Mental Health Foundation.

Kahlbaum, K. L. (1874). *Die Katatonie order das Spannungirresein. Eine Klinische Form Psychischer Krankheit*. Berlin: Hirschwald.

Kane, J. M. & McGlashan, T. H. (1995). Treatment of schizophrenia. *Lancet*, **346**,

820–5.

Kane, J. M., Honigfeld, G. Singer. J. & Meltzer, H. (1988). Clozapine for the treatment resistant schizophrenic: a double blind comparison versus chlorpromazine/benzotropine. *Archives of General Psychiatry*, **45**, 789–96.

Kebabian, J. W. & Calne, D. B. (1979). Multiple receptors for dopamine. *Nature*, **277**, 93–6.

Kebabian, J. W., Petzold, G. L. & Greengard, P. (1972). Dopamine sensitive adenylate cyclase in caudate nucleus of rat brain and its similarity to the 'dopamine receptor'. *Proceedings of the National Academy of Sciences (USA)*, **69**, 2145–9.

Kendell, R. E. (1975). *The Role of Diagnosis in Psychiatry*. Oxford: Blackwell Scientific Publications.

Kendler, K. S. (1987). The feasibility of linkage studies in schizophrenia. In *Biological Perspectives of Schizophrenia*, ed. H. Helmchen & F. A. Henn, pp. 19–32. Chichester: Wiley.

Kety, S. (1959). Biochemical theories of schizophrenia I and II. *Science*, **129**, 1528–90.

Kety, S. G., Rosenthal, D. D., Wender, P. I. L., Schilsinger, F. & Jacobsen, B. (1975). Mental illness in the biological and adoptive families of adopted individuals who become schizophrenic. In *Genetic Research in Psychiatry*, ed. R. R. Fieve., D. Rosenthal & H. Bill, pp. 147–65. Baltimore: John Hopkins University Press.

Keuhl, F. A., Osmond, R. E. & Vendenheuvel, W. J. A. (1966). Occurrence of 3,4 dimethoxyphenyl-acetic acid in urines of normal and schizophrenic individuals. *Nature (London)*, **211**, 606.

Kinnear, W. (1727). Cited by R. Hunter & I. MacAlpine. *Three Hundred Years of Psychiatry*, 1535–1860. Oxford: Oxford University Press.

Klippel, M. & Lhermitte, J. (1909). Un cas de démence précoce a type catatonique avec autopsie. *Revue Neurologique*, **17**, 157–8.

Kraepelin, E. (1893–1915). *Lehrbuch der Psychiatrie* Editions 1–8. (1883), Leipzig: Abel; (1887) Leipzig: Abel (1889) Leipzig: Abel; Leipzig: Abel (1893); (1896) Leipzig: Barth; (1899), Leipzig: Barth; (1903/1904) Leipzig: Barth; (1909/1910/1913/1915) (4 vols) Leipzig: Barth.

Kraepelin, E. (1907). *Lehrbuch der Psychiatrie* (Translated by A. R. Diefendorf). Macmillan: New York.

Kraepelin, E. (1919). *Dementia Praecox*. Translated by R. M. Barclay. Edited by G. M. Robertson. Facsimile edition published by Kriefer: New York, 1971.

Lawrie, S. M. & Abukmeil, S. S. (1998). Brain abnormality in schizophrenia *British Journal of Psychiatry*, **172**, 110–20.

Lee, T., Seeman, P., Tourtellotte, W. W., Farley, I. J. & Hornykiewicz, O. (1978). Binding of ^3H neuroleptics and ^3H apomorphine in schizophrenic brains. *Nature (London)*, **274**, 897–900.

Lewis, N. D. C. (1923). The constitutional factors in dementia praecox with particular attention to the circulatory system and to some of the endocrine glands. *Nervous and Mental Diseases Monographs* No. 35. New York: Nervous and Mental Disease Publishing Co.

Liddle, P. F., Friston, K. J., Frith, C. D. & Frackowiack, R. (1992). Cerebral blood flow and mental processes in schizophrenia. *Journal of Royal Society of Medicine*, **85**, 224–7.

McGuffin, P., Farmer, A. E., Gottesman, I., Murray, R. M. & Reveley, A. M. (1984). Twin concordance for operationally defined schizophrenia.

Confirmation of familiality and heritability. *Archives of General Psychiatry*, **41**, 541–5.

Mackenzie, I. (1912). The physical basis of mental disease. *Journal of Mental Science*, **58**, 465–77.

Martin, D. (1955). Institutionalisation. *Lancet*, **ii**, 1188–90.

Meltzer, H. Y. (1992). *Novel Antipsychotic Drugs.* New York: Raven Press.

Miller, R. J., Horn, A. S. & Iversen, L. L. (1974). The action of neuroleptic drugs on dopamine stimulated adenosine cyclase 3'5' monophosphate production in rat neostriatum and limbic forebrain. *Molecular Pharmacology*, **10**, 759–66.

Morel, B. A. (1860). *Traite des maladies mentales.* Paris: Masson.

Mott, F. W. (1919). Normal and morbid conditions of the testes from birth to old age in 100 asylum and hospital cases. *British Medical Journal*, **ii**, 655–8.

Murray, R. M. & Lewis, S. W. (1987). Is schizophrenia a neurodevelopmental disorder? *British Medical Journal*, **295**, 681–2.

Myerson, A. (1939). Theory and principles of the 'total push' method in the treatment of chronic schizophrenia. *American Journal of Psychiatry*, **95**, 1197–204.

NIMH (National Institute of Mental Health) Psychopharmacology Service Center Collaborative Study Group (1964). Phenothiazine treatment of acute schizophrenia. *Archives of General Psychiatry*, **10**, 246–61.

Nordstrom, A. L., Farde, L. & Halldin, C. (1993). High $5HT_2$ receptor occupancy in clozapine treated patients. *Psychopharmacology*, **110**, 365–7.

Owen, F., Cross, A. J., Crow, T. J., Langdon, A., Poulter, M. & Riley, G. J. (1978). Increased dopamine receptor sensitivity in schizophrenia. *Lancet*, **ii**, 223–6.

Owen, F., Cross, A. J., Crow, T. J., Lofthouse, R. & Poulter, M. (1981). Neurotransmitter receptor in the brain in schizophrenia. *Acta Psychiatrica Scandinavica*, **62**, (Suppl 291). 20–6.

Owens, D. G. C. (1996). Adverse effects of antipsychotic agents. Do newer agents offer advantages? *Drugs*, **6**, 895–930.

Pakkenberg, B. (1987). Post-mortem study of chronic schizophrenic brains. *British Journal of Psychiatry*, **151**, 744–52.

Pinel, P. (1809). *Traité medico-philosophique sur l'aliénation mental* 2nd edn. Paris: Brosson.

Post, R. M., Fink, E. Carpenter, W. T. & Goodwin, F. K. (1975). Cerebrospinal fluid amine metabolism in acute schizophrenia. *Archives of General Psychiatry*, **32**, 1013–69.

Raz, S. & Raz, N. (1990). Structural brain abnormalities in the major psychoses: a quantitative review of the evidence from computerized imaging. *Psychological Bulletin*, **108**, 93–108.

Richelson, E. & Nelson, A. (1984). Antagonism by neuroleptics of neurotransmitter receptors of normal human brain in vitro. *European Journal of Pharmacology*, **103**, 197–204.

Roccatagliata, G. (1973). *Storia della Psichiatria Antica.* Milan: Ulrica Hoepli. English translation by B. Simon. (1978). *Mind and Madness in Ancient Greece.* London: Cornell University Press.

Rosanoff, A. J. (1914). Dissimilar heredity in mental disease. *American Journal of Insanity*, **LXX**, I.

Rosenthal, D., Wender, P. H., Kety, S. S., Welner, J. & Schulsinger, F. (1971). The adopted away offspring of schizophrenia. *American Journal of Psychiatry*, **128**, 397–411.

Schneider, K. (1950). *Die Psychopathischen Persön lichkeiten.* Translation of the 9th edition by Hamilton, M. W. (1958). Castle: London.

Seeman, P. (1980). Brain dopamine receptors. *Pharmacological Reviews,* **32,** 229–313.

Seeman, P., Lee, T., Chau-Wong, M. & Wong, K. (1976). Antipsychotic drug doses and neuroleptic dopamine receptors. *Nature* (London), **261,** 717–19.

Shattock, F. M. (1950). The somatic manifestations of schizophrenia: a clinical study of their significance. *Journal of Mental Science,* **96,** 32–142.

Shenton, M. E., Kikinis, R., Jolenz, F. A. et al. (1992). Abnormalities of the left temporal lobe and thought disorder in schizophrenia: a quantitative magnetic resonance imaging study. *New England Journal of Medicine,* **327,** 604–12.

Shields, J. (1977). High risk for schizophrenia: genetic considerations. *Psychological Medecine,* **7,** 7–10.

Southard E. E. (1915). On the topographical distribution of cortex lesions and anomalies in dementia praecox with some account of their functional significance. II. *American Journal of Insanity,* **71,** 603–71.

Storey, P. B. (1966). Lumbar air encephalography in chronic schizophrenia: a controlled experiment. *British Journal of Psychiatry,* **112,** 135–44.

Suddath, R. L., Christie, G. W., Torrey, E. F., Casanova, M. F. & Weinberger, D. R. (1990). Anatomical abnormalities in the brains of monozygotic twins discordant for schizophrenia. *New England Journal of Medicine,* **322,** 789–94.

Sydenham, T. (1696). *The Whole Works of that Excellent Physician Dr. Thomas Sydenham.* Translated by J. Pechy. London: Richard Wellington & Edward Castle.

Taylor, the Lord. (1962). The public, parliament and mental health. In *Aspects of Psychiatric Research,* ed. D. Richter, J. M. Tanner, Lord Taylor & P. L. Zangmill. London: Oxford University Press.

Tooth, G. C. & Brooke, E. M. (1961). Trends in the mental hospital population and their effect on future planning. *Lancet,* **i,** 710–13.

Turner, J. (1912). The classification of insanity. *Journal of Mental Science,* **58,** 1–25.

Turner, T. (1995). Schizophrenia – social section. In *A History of Clinical Psychiatry – The Origin and History of Psychiatric Disorders,* ed. G. Berrios & R. Porter, pp. 349–59. London: The Athlone Press.

Vogt, C. & Vogt, O. (1948). Über anatomische Substrate Bernerkungen zu pathoanatomischen Befunden bei Schizophrenie. *Ärzliche Forschungen,* **3,** 1–7.

Waddington, J. L. (1995). The clinical pharmacology of antipsychotic drugs in schizophrenia. In *Schizophrenia,* ed. S. R. Hirsch & D. R. Weinberger, pp. 341–57. Oxford: Blackwell Science Ltd.

Weinberger, D. R. (1986). The pathogenesis of schizophrenia: a neurodevelopmental disorder. In *The Neurology of Schizophrenia,* ed. H. A. Nasrallah & D. R. Weinberger, pp. 397–406. Amsterdam: Elsevier.

Weinberger, D. R. (1995a). From neuropathology to neurodevelopment. *Lancet,* **346,** 552–7.

Weinberger, D. R. (1995b). Schizophrenia as a neurodevelopmental disorder. In *Schizophrenia,* ed. S. R. Hirsch & D. R. Weinberger, pp. 293–323. Oxford: Blackwell Science Ltd.

Weinberger, D. R., Berman, K. F. & Zec, R. F. (1986). Physiologic dysfunction of dorsolateral prefrontal cortex in schizophrenia. *Archives of General*

Psychiatry, **43**, 114–24.

Wernicke, C. (1900). *Grundriss der Psychiatrie*. Leipzig: Johannes Barth.

Willis, T. (1683). *Two Discourses Concerning the Soul of Brutes*. London: Dring.

Wing, J. K. & Brown, G. W. (1961). Social treatment of chronic schizophrenia: a comparative study of three mental hospitals. *Journal of Mental Science*, **107**, 847–61.

Wong, D. F., Wagner, H. N. & Tune, L. E. (1986). Positron emission tomography reveals elevated D_2 dopamine receptors in drug-naive schizophrenics. *Science*, **234**, 1558–62.

World Health Organization. (1967). *Manual of the International Statistical Classification of Diseases, Injuries and Causes of Death (ICD.8)*. Geneva: WHO.

Zipursky, R. B., Lim, K. O., Sullivan, E. V., Brown B. W. & Pfefferbaum, A. (1992). Widespread cerebral grey matter volume deficits in schizophrenia. *Archives of General Psychiatry*, **49**, 195–205.

2
Diagnostic issues: concepts of the disorder

Introduction

As has been stated in Chapter 1, in defining the concept of dementia praecox, which we have come to know as schizophrenia, Kraepelin (1896) was describing the characteristic course and outcome of a cluster of symptoms and signs. He believed that this cluster of symptoms and signs had a specific anatomical pathology with a specific aetiology, even although essentially nothing was known of either the pathology or aetiology during his lifetime. In the last 20 years an increasing body of knowledge supportive of the hypothesis that schizophrenia is a disorder associated with pathological changes in the central nervous system has developed, and this is described in detail in Chapter 3 of this book. A specific lesion diagnostic of the condition, i.e. found in all those suffering from the disorder and not in other people, is yet to be determined and the cause of those changes which are found is still a matter for speculation.

In terms of a diagnostic test for the condition therefore, we are no further forward than Kraepelin and his contemporaries and like them, in diagnosing schizophrenia we have to rely on our ability to define the boundaries of that cluster of symptoms and signs suggestive of the disorder which will in fact have the characteristic course and outcome which are considered to be a validating criterion for schizophrenia.

In the 100 plus years since Kraepelin wrote the fifth edition of *Lehrbuch der Psychiatrie* there have been a number of shifts of opinion about what constitutes the cluster of symptoms and signs which makes the diagnosis of schizophrenia appropriate, i.e. likely to be validated by outcome.

Kraepelin himself, like Kahlbaum (1874) regarded general paralysis of the insane as a model for a disease based on unity of cause, course and outcome. He considered that a tangible morbid process in the brain would be found in dementia praecox (schizophrenia) and he was clear that in defining it he was describing a form of insanity. Essentially his concept embraced Kahlbaum's catatonia (1874), Hecker's hebephrenia (1871) and his own dementia paranoides. The symptoms that he emphasized included auditory and tactile hallucinations, delusions, formal thought disorder, incoherence, blunted affect, negativism, stereotypes and lack of insight. He was very much aware of the diversity of the clinical presentation and the twists and turns of the course.

The presentation of clinical details in the large domain of dementia praecox meets with considerable difficulties because a delineation of the different clinical pictures can only be accomplished artificially. There is certainly a whole series of phases which frequently return, but between them are such numerous transitions that in spite of all efforts it appears impossible at present to delimit them sharply and to assign each case without objection to a different form.
(Kraepelin. *Dementia Praecox*, 1919).

While Kraepelin's views were still being defined and to a degree struggling to reach acceptance, Bleuler (1950) published his text *Dementia Praecox or the Group of Schizophrenias*, and described a very different concept of the disorder. Bleuler's concept was not influenced by the idea of some tangible morbid (if unknown) underlying process in the way that Kraepelin's was and his view of the central cluster of signs and symptoms which defined the condition had very little common ground with that of Kraepelin. As noted above, for Kraepelin delusions, hallucinations, catatonia and disturbances of behaviour were central features of the disorder. For Bleuler disorders of affectivity, ambivalence, autism, attention and will were fundamental features which could be observed in every case, and hallucinations, delusions, catatonia and behavioural disturbances were secondary phenomena which might or might not be present. For him the diagnosis of schizophrenia could be made even if delusions or hallucinations had never been known to be present at any time, and on the basis of this idea he added simple and latent forms to the catatonic, paranoid and hebephrenic subtypes already described by Kraepelin.

These near-nineteenth century differences of opinion have relevance for the arguments about diagnostic practice that have taken place in more recent decades, and indeed for some of the diagnostic and conceptual difficulties that face us still. Although he included blunted affect and negativism in his descriptions of the clinical features of schizophrenia, Kraepelin laid emphasis upon hallucinations, delusions, incoherence of speech and catatonic phenomena, all of which would nowadays be included among the 'positive' features of schizophrenia. Bleuler's fundamental features would be classed as 'negative' symptoms, although neither he nor Kraepelin employed these terms. The positive/negative symptom terminology originated with Hughlings Jackson (1869), who classified as negative symptoms those losses of function that he hypothesized were directly due to some anatomical lesion. In contrast, positive symptoms were excessive behaviours generated by a still intact neurophysiological system disinhibited by the original lesions. Hughlings Jackson applied the model to both neurological and psychiatric disorders. The modern psychiatric use of the term (Fish, 1962; Wing, 1978; Crow, 1980) disregards Jackson's theoretical framework but retains his descriptive emphasis on behavioural excesses and deficits, so that positive features are those which are pathological by their presence (e.g. delusions, hallucinations), while negative features represent the loss of some normal function.

In general, positive features are relatively easy to assess. With a few exceptions such as hypnagogic hallucinations and unusual subcultural beliefs, phenomena like delusions and hallucinations do not occur in well people. They can usually be described in such a way that there is no great difficulty in making a decision about their presence or absence, or indeed grading their severity. Thus when it comes to delineating the boundaries of the cluster of symptoms and signs which in Kraepelin's view would define an illness as dementia praecox/schizophrenia, the problems are not in specifying the presence/absence, or indeed severity of the features, but in the fact that the validation in terms of a deteriorating course and poor outcome did not always occur (indeed 13% of Kraepelin's own cases were said to show recovery) and the tangible morbid process thought to underlie these features could not be established in spite of intensive research effort extending over very many years.

The problems with Bleuler's concept were different. Although it is easy enough to make the case that the defect state characterized by negative features and cognitive impairments which so cripples some individuals who have suffered psychotic episodes is the hallmark of schizophrenia, this state can be hard to define. If severe, it is readily recognized but difficult to describe. The negative features most often used in modern assessments include lack of animation, flattening of affect, slowness, paucity of speech. Clearly in mild degree these features shade into normality and in more severe degrees they occur in a variety of other disorders, including depression (McGlashan & Carpenter, 1976) and the extrapyramidal syndromes produced by antipsychotic drugs (Rifkin et al., 1975). The conceptual and methodological problems associated with negative symptoms as they are currently described have been discussed with particular clarity by Sommers (1985). She emphasized the conceptual ambiguity of negative symptoms and described evidence that the various elements included within our general concept of negative symptoms may occur not only in depression and in states induced by antipsychotic drugs, but in association with schizoid and schizotypal personality, and as a result of a non-responsive milieu. Sommers was, of course, referring to negative features as now considered, and it is obvious that these considerations would apply still more strongly to Bleuler's fundamental symptoms of disordered affectivity, ambivalence, autism, attention and will, for these features are indeed difficult to define. They are intangible qualities which are hard to separate from the range of normality, particularly the range of normality in uncertain, socially unsophisticated young people of the age of maximum risk of schizophrenia (24.3 years in males; 27.5 years in females – Hafner et al., 1991).

Subsequent development of Kraepelin ideas and the general concept of positive features

Kraepelin's views of the clinical features of dementia praecox/schizophrenia gained wide acceptance in Europe and never really lost their dominance there. As noted, however, the principal problem for Kraepelin's concept was that although he had set out to define from within the broad class of psychotic illness, associated with no demonstrable underlying lesion, a cluster of symptoms and signs which predicted the characteristically poor outcome of dementia praecox/schizophrenia (which would in due course be found to have a tangible morbid underlying process), not all cases with the cluster did have a poor prognosis and we are still struggling to define the tangible morbid process. A widespread reaction to this situation was to try to redefine the boundaries of the central cluster of signs and symptoms diagnostic of schizophrenia. The classifications of Kleist (1947) and Leonhard (1957) are examples of this and describe more and more tightly defined subgroupings of schizophrenia (e.g. Kleist, 1947; seven typical and one atypical forms of schizophrenia; Leonhard, 1957; four subgroups of schizophrenia). These definitions of subgroups and later studies of symptomatology and course of illness (e.g. Strauss et al., 1974; Bilder et al., 1985; Carpenter et al., 1988) were motivated by a wish to identify subcategories of schizophrenic patients whose prognosis could be shown to be predictable in various respects.

The Norwegian psychiatrist Langfeldt (1939) sought to distinguish between patients who had true dementia praecox/schizophrenia and those who had what he called schizophreniform psychosis. The underlying idea was that the study of schizophrenia was distorted because samples of patients included both genuine cases of the disorder and those who were superficially similar but did not really have the condition, so that their outcome was better and investigations would never reveal the underlying morbid condition in them. This idea has obvious attractions and was enthusiastically received. Langfeldt (1939) presented evidence which had some methodological weaknesses but was said to show that true 'process' schizophrenia and schizophreniform psychoses had different outcomes and different responses to the physical treatments available at the time, i.e. ECT and insulin coma therapy. In the United States a number of scales (e.g. Phillips Scale, Kantor Scale) separated 'true' process schizophrenia from non-process schizophrenia (schizophreniform states). Clear demarcation between the two was not demonstrated, but the view that there are 'lesser' psychoses superficially resembling schizophrenia but without the poor prognosis, without any underlying physical abnormality to be demon-strated, and for which the appropriate treatment is essentially psycho-therapeutic, has persisted, e.g. Stromgren (1989). Empirical evidence for these views is lacking (for review see Johnstone et al., 1996).

Kurt Schneider (1959) was also involved in work related to defining the cardinal features of schizophrenia. He described a number of 'features of the first rank' whose presence he considered to be pathognomonic of schizophrenia in the absence of coarse brain disease such as temporal lobe epilepsy (Table 2.1).

It is evident that many of these experiences can be interpreted as a result of the failure to distinguish between ideas and impulses arising from within the subject's own mind and perceptions arising from stimuli in the external world – the so-called 'loss of ego boundaries' (Kendell, 1988), but for Schneider they had no particular theoretical significance of this kind – he merely regarded them as a practical guide to diagnosis on the basis of the idea that if any one was clearly present in the absence of organic brain disease, then the diagnosis could be considered to be that of schizophrenia. He accepted that some patients with schizophrenia never exhibited these symptoms and that all of them could at times occur in organic psychoses but considered that it was useful to distinguish them from what he called symptoms of the second rank, e.g. perplexity, emotional blunting and hallucinations and delusions of other kinds. Schneider's concepts have remained popular in Europe and in the United Kingdom and the PSE/Catego system (Wing et al., 1974) used in WHO and other studies has been influenced by them – the so-called 'nuclear' schizophrenic symptoms in the PSE/Catego system having a great deal of common ground with Schneider's first rank symptoms. Schneider did not particularly relate his

Table 2.1. *Kurt Schneider's first rank symptoms of schizophrenia*

1. Auditory hallucinations taking the form of a voice or voices repeating the subject's thoughts out loud (gedankenlautwerden or écho de la penseé).
2. Auditory hallucinations discussing the subject or arguing about him/her and referring to him/her in the third person.
3. Auditory hallucinations discussing the patient's thoughts as or before they occur.
4. Auditory hallucinations taking the form of a commentary upon the subject's thoughts or behaviour.
5. The experience of intrusion of alien ideas or thoughts into the subject's mind as a result of the action of some external agency (Thought insertion).
6. The experience that the subject's thinking is no longer confined within his/her own mind but is shared by or is accessible to other people (Thought broadcasting).
7. The experience of being bereft of thought as a result of the removal of the subject's thoughts from the mind by some person or influence (Thought withdrawal).
8. The experience that actions, sensations, bodily movements, emotions or thought processes are generated by an outside agency that usurps the will of the subject (Passivity experiences).
9. Primary delusions (also known as delusional perceptions): beliefs arising suddenly 'out of a clear blue sky' from a normal perception which would seem commonplace and unrelated to others but which nevertheless generates an unshakeable delusional conviction.

work to treatment response and although Langfeldt (1939) did consider that 'true' schizophrenia failed to respond to physical treatments whereas schizophreniform states did, this work of course predated the introduction of effective antipsychotic agents in the 1950s. Although initially Delay & Deniker's view (1952) that these drugs had a specific action against schizophrenic symptoms and were not merely super sedatives was not widely accepted, by the 1960s it was evident that drugs such as phenothiazines like chlorpromazine, and butyrophenones like haloperidol had a specific antipsychotic effect. They were initially introduced on an empirical basis but by the 1960s evidence relating them to dopaminergic transmission unfolded.

Soon after antipsychotics were introduced into psychiatric practice, it was suggested that their antipsychotic effect was related to their ability to induce extrapyramidal effects (Flugel, 1953; Deniker, 1960). After the discovery (Ehringer & Horneykiewicz, 1960) that dopamine is depleted in the brains of patients dying of Parkinson's disease, selective effects of antipsychotic drugs on central dopamine turnover were described (Carlsson & Lindqvist, 1963) and attributed to dopamine receptor blockade. In vitro methods of studying dopamine receptors became available in the 1970s

(Kebabian et al., 1972; Burt et al., 1977) and it was possible to relate the antipsychotic potency of drugs like phenothiazines and butyrophenones to their ability to block dopamine receptors (Seeman et al., 1976).

The relevance of dopaminergic blockade for antipsychotic effect and the fact that dopamine agonists like amphetamines can produce a schizo-phrenia-like psychosis reversible by antipsychotic drugs (Angrist et al., 1974) generated the so-called dopamine hypothesis, which postulated that dopaminergic mechanisms were intimately involved in schizophrenia and that indeed dopamine release was increased in schizophrenic patients (Matthysse, 1973; Snyder, 1973). Subsequent work did not support their view that there was increased dopamine turnover in schizophrenia (Crow et al., 1979), although the evidence for the importance of D_2 receptor blockade in the antipsychotic action of traditional 'neuroleptic' drugs remained strong (Iversen, 1985). A study of the antipsychotic effects of the two isomers of flupenthixol – one of which blocks dopamine receptors while the other does not – (Johnstone et al., 1978) showed that the anti-psychotic effect of the dopamine blocking isomer was considerable in respect of positive symptoms but minimal as far as negative symptoms were concerned (Figure 2.1).

It is, of course, evident from Figure 2.1 that being less severe at the outset, negative symptoms had much less room to improve than had positive symptoms, but other work has shown that negative symptoms are affected very little by traditional antipsychotic agents, or indeed by phar-macological methods generally (Pogue-Geile & Zubin, 1988). In the later 1970s the idea that D_2 receptor blockade was the essential feature of antipsychotic agents was widely held, and indeed the view that the symp-toms which were most central to the diagnosis of schizophrenia were most strikingly reversed by such drugs was suggested (Johnstone, 1979). This line of thinking could be interpreted as considering that symptom reversal by D_2 blockade could be a guide to the core cluster of symptoms sought by Kraepelin as predictive of the characteristic outcome of dementia praecox/ schizophrenia. Evidence against such notions was, however, rapidly forth-coming. Not only are first rank features relatively poor predictors of outcome in schizophrenia (Kendell et al., 1979), but the psychotropic effects of antipsychotic agents are by no means confined to schizophrenia. Antipsychotics with a broad spectrum of pharmacological actions are effective in mania (Prien et al., 1972) but so is the selective D_2 dopamine blocker pimozide (Cookson et al., 1982). Antipsychotics have also been shown to be beneficial in severe depression, delirious states and Gilles de la Tourette syndrome (for review see Johnstone, 1987).

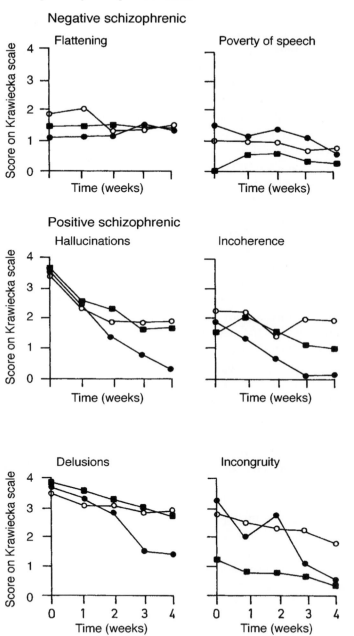

Figure 2.1. Clinical effects of the isomers of flupenthixol. ■ placebo, ● α (cis) flupenthixol, ○ β (trans) flupenthixol. (From Johnstone et al., 1978.)

In the late 1970s and early 1980s selective D_2 dopamine receptor blockade was the desired goal of the pharmaceutical industry as far as new antipsychotics were concerned, but as time progressed it became evident that D_2 receptor blockade was not necessarily associated with improvement in clinical features and that more selective D_2 blockers were not necessarily clinically any more useful (Johnstone, 1994). The demonstration by Kane et al. in 1988 that clozapine, which has wide ranging pharmacological effects, was more effective in treating 'treatment resistant' schizophrenia than traditional antipsychotics turned emphasis away from the classical dopamine hypothesis (Owens, 1996). When the greater efficacy of D_2 blockers in relieving positive symptoms as opposed to negative symptoms was first demonstrated (Figure 2.1) the idea that the basis of these two groups of symptoms might differ developed. This idea contributed to the view that there were two syndromes in schizophrenia which represented more than one disease process (Crow, 1980). By that time it had become apparent that in schizophrenia there was evidence of structural changes in the brain (as indicated by neuroradiological and post mortem studies) and neurochemical changes (as suggested by the responsiveness of episodes of illness to neuroleptic medication). Crow developed the hypothesis that positive symptoms such as hallucinations and delusions were associated with a neurochemical disturbance which was at least potentially reversible and responsive to neuroleptic drugs, whereas negative symptoms such as affective flattening and poverty of speech were more closely related to structural, perhaps irreversible changes in the brain (Crow et al., 1982). The hypothesis was not that there were two separate types of schizophrenia illness, but that there were two syndromes with different dimensions of pathology within the disease process. The suggested correlates of the Type I syndrome (associated with positive symptoms) and the Type II syndrome associated with negative symptoms are shown in Table 2.2.

It is interesting that although the work on which this hypothesis was based involved clinical assessments which included ratings of incoherence of speech and incongruity of affect (Johnstone et al., 1978; Owens & Johnstone, 1980) the place of these clinical features within the Type I/Type II dichotomy was not specified. Relative to the other symptoms and signs assessed in these studies, incoherence and incongruity were not common but they did occur. The work of Crow (1980) was further developed by Liddle (1987), who suggested that in addition to the symptoms characteristic of the Type I and Type II syndromes, there was a third entity relating to disorganization of behaviour and including incoherent speech and incongruity of affect. These three dimensions of schizophrenic symptomatology

Table 2.2. *Crow's two syndromes in schizophrenia*

	TYPE I	TYPE II
Characteristic symptoms	Delusions; hallucinations	Flattening of affect; poverty of speech; loss of drive
Type of illness in which most commonly seen	Acute episodes of schizophrenia	Chronic schizophrenia (defect state)
Response to typical antipsychotics	Good	Poor
Intellectual impairment	Absent	Sometimes present
Irreversible involuntary movements	Absent	Sometimes present
Postulated pathological process	?increased numbers of D_2 dopamine receptors	Cell loss in some brain areas including medial temporal lobe

have been replicated in the work of Arndt et al. (1991, Van der Does et al. (1993) and Johnstone & Frith (1996). Liddle's work was further developed by studying patterns of cerebral blood flow using positron emission tomography in relation to the three syndromes of schizophrenic symptomatology he had earlier described. The patterns of cerebral blood flow differed between the three syndromes (Liddle et al., 1992). The psychomotor poverty syndrome (poverty of speech, flattening of affect, psychomotor retardation) was associated with underactivity of prefrontal cortex and parietal cortex on the left, the disorganization syndrome, with underactivity of the right prefrontal cortex, and delusions and hallucinations were associated with overactivity in the left medial temporal lobe and left lateral frontal lobe. In each case the cerebral sites involved included those activated in well individuals during performance of the type of mental processing that is implicated in the corresponding syndrome – e.g. psychomotor poverty is associated with impaired ability to generate words – maximum cerebral activation observed in healthy individuals during word generation is seen in the left prefrontal cortex.

This type of work allows us to delineate patterns of cerebral activity associated with specific neurophysiological tests or mental acts in the well and in those affected by mental disorders. It allows us to see the neurophysiological basis of the symptoms which are components of the cluster of clinical features which Kraepelin thought predicted the cause and outcome typical of dementia praecox/schizophrenia. We are beginning to approach the 'tangible morbid process' (which represents a dynamic imbalance between activity in different cerebral areas rather than isolated local deficits or increases in activity) but the information is essentially about neuro-physiological correlates of symptoms and the validation of the symptom clusters in terms of outcome or indeed demonstrable pathological change in the CNS remains elusive.

Subsequent development of Bleulerian ideas

Although Kraepelin's views retained their popularity in Europe until the 1960s and 1970s, Bleuler's ideas held sway in the United States. His concept of schizophrenia as an essentially psychological disorder, possibly with a psychogenic basis, rather than a pathological condition of the nervous system, was compatible with the psychoanalytic orientation prevailing in the USA at that time. It was shown in the study of Cooper et al. in 1972 that the diagnosis of schizophrenia was very much more frequently employed in the USA than in the UK and this was due to the fact that the New York psychiatrists in the American arm of the project had a concept of schizophrenia so broad that it included patients who in the UK would have been regarded as having depressive or manic psychoses, or even neurotic ill-nesses or personality disorders. Indeed, in the 1950s the idea that illness which did not at first glance appear psychotic at all actually represented a form of schizophrenia was put forward in the work of Hoch & Polatin (1949), who described what they called 'pseudoneurotic schizophrenia'. It became clear from the *International Pilot Study of Schizophrenia* (IPSS) (WHO, 1973) that psychiatrists both in the USA (Washington) and the USSR (Moscow) had a wider concept of schizophrenia than their col-leagues in the other countries involved (Columbia, Czechoslovakia, Den-mark, India, Nigeria, Taiwan and the United Kingdom). The breadth of this concept was due, at least in part, to the use of Bleuler's least differenti-ated subtypes of schizophrenia (simple and latent) (Wing, 1978, 1995). After the publication of the IPSS study (WHO, 1973) the need for operational definitions of schizophrenia was increasingly recognized. Numbers of them were developed, e.g. St. Louis (Feighner et al., 1972) and the Research Diagnostic Criteria (RDC) (Spitzer et al., 1975). Later versions of both WHO and American Psychiatric Association criteria (ICD 10, WHO 1992; DSM IV, APA 1994) also took this form. All require clear evidence of psychosis either current or past, and all but the St. Louis criteria specify particular kinds of hallucinatory experience or delusional ideation. While not entirely embracing Kraepelin's views, all of these definitions differ from Bleulerian ideas in terms of the fact that their central features are not those regarded as fundamental by Bleuler but rather those which he saw as secondary phenomena. Until recently, Bleulerian concepts were much in the shadows, having been shown to be difficult to define, unreliable, and possibly the basis for the major differences in diagnostic practice across the world which were seen as having perhaps held back advances in understanding of schizophrenia. Certain aspects of areas of current research interest have, however, somewhat unexpectedly at least for some, brought them closer to centre stage once more.

The development of non-invasive cerebral imaging techniques in the early 1970s and the demonstration in schizophrenic patients of enlarged cerebral ventricles which correlated with cognitive deficits (Johnstone et al., 1976) was initially interpreted as being in keeping with Kraepelin's concepts and as indicating a neurodegenerative process. The idea was that the brain was relatively normal until the illness struck in early adulthood, from which point any pathological changes inflicted upon the brain by the illness would become more pronounced with the progression of the disorder over time. Such progression has not, however, been shown by follow up studies (Degreef et al., 1991; Illowsky et al., 1988) and the possibility that the structural changes in the brain represent a neurodevelopmental rather than a neurodegenerative process has received increasing interest (Weinberger, 1986; Murray & Lewis, 1987; Frangou & Murray, 1996). Central to this view is the idea that abnormalities such as minor physical anomalies (Green et al., 1994) and subtle neurological abnormalities (Walker & Lewine, 1990) occur premorbidly in those destined to develop schizophrenia. The methodological difficulties of blindly assessing the premorbid state of those who have developed schizophrenia are obvious, but the work of Done et al. (1991 and 1994) and Jones et al. (1994) examining records of the large British birth cohorts (1958 cohort in the case of Done et al. and 1964 cohort in the case of Jones et al.) allowed the childhood performance of individuals who went on to develop schizophrenia to be compared with that of those who did not. Premorbid cognitive and social deficits in pre-schizophrenia were found. Although it is certainly true that the psychosis when it develops is very different from these subtle abnormalities which do not constitute an easily recognizable pattern (Rutter, 1990) the notion that, in those with schizophrenia, disorders of communication and of the development of social relations precede the presence of florid psychotic symptoms shares common ground with Bleuler's view that the fundamental features of schizophrenia are disturbances of affectivity, ambivalence, autism, attention and will, and that hallucinations, delusions, etc. are secondary phenomena.

Another area of investigation which has heightened interest in

Bleulerian concepts is that of psychiatric genetics. As discussed in Chapter 7 the familial aspects of schizophrenia have long been known. It has been estimated that most of the variance in liability to the disorder (perhaps 80% or more) is accounted for by genetic factors, but it is evident from studies of twins discordant for schizophrenia (Gottesman & Bertelsen, 1989) that genotypes which give rise to schizophrenia may not be expressed as the disease. The significance of some published genetic studies of schizophrenia (e.g. Blackwood et al., 1989) depends upon the inclusion of persons affected by e.g. manic depressive illness. Similarly, Kendler et al. (1985a) reported a lifetime risk of 3.7% among first degree relatives of schizophrenic patients using DSM III criteria but found that this increased to 8.6% when other non-affective psychoses and schizoaffective psychoses were included. It thus became evident that as far as genetic studies of schizophrenia are concerned, the boundaries of the phenotype are far from clear. Siever & Gundersen (1983) and Kendler et al. (1985a) drew attention to the work of Bleuler and his colleagues which pointed out that the relatives of schizophrenic patients could display asociality and mild psychotic like symptomatology which resembled in character if not severity the features manifested by their affected family members. The adoptive studies of Kety, Rosenthal and colleagues (Kety et al., 1975) showed these minor features to be apparent in relatives of schizophrenic probands and studies of the clinical profiles of these individuals were used to develop the criteria for schizotypal personality disorder of DSM III (APA, 1980). The relatives of schizophrenic patients who have schizotypal personality disorder are primarily characterized by negative or deficit like symptoms (Lenzenweger & Dworkin, 1984; Lyons et al., 1992). They could probably be embraced by Bleulerian concepts of schizophrenia, and they certainly would be included as affected in some current linkage studies of schizophrenia. It is widely accepted that for theoretical reasons relating to the uncertainty of the boundaries of the phenotype of schizophrenia, as well as for practical reasons concerning the difficulties of finding sufficient affected related individuals, that it is wise to draw a wide net in identifying probands. Bleuler's concepts are thus kept alive, although they are not employed in any of the operational definitions used to identify individuals as suffering from schizophrenia for research, or indeed general diagnostic purposes.

Having discussed the difficulties of defining the core of symptoms and signs central to the diagnosis of schizophrenia, it is important to consider those prodromal or atypical forms that lie on the edge of the core.

Prodromal symptoms

As has been described, the large British birth cohort studies have been used to provide evidence that those destined to develop schizophrenia show group differences in various aspects of childhood performance as compared with those who will remain well (Done et al., 1994; Jones et al., 1994). These differences do not concern symptoms but relate to simple measures of behaviour as assessed by school teachers, made about 20 years before the individuals concerned could be expected to become ill. Such work does not, therefore, offer any assessment of the kind of symptoms which may present as prodromal of a schizophrenic psychosis. Similarly, the work of Foerster et al. (1991), which on the basis of maternal interviews showed schizophrenic men to have manifested more premorbid impairments than either schizophrenic women or men with affective illness, concerned long standing premorbid traits rather than prodromal symptomatology. In work available to date such symptoms can really only be assessed on the basis of the patients' accounts once they have become ill. The Northwick Park First Episodes study (Johnstone et al., 1986) concerns a wide range of aspects of 253 first episodes of schizophrenic illness. The clinical work on which this study is based was principally done by Macmillan (1984) and it is evident that some patients were able to describe symptoms such as anxiety, obsessional features, suspiciousness and ideas of reference in the months leading up to their admission, but in many cases it was not easy in retrospect to separate features at the beginning of the illness from prodromal ones.

Although in this study a very acute illness onset (where the interval between complete well being and florid illness was stated to be five days or less) did occur in 31 patients, subacute (interval 7–30 days) and insidious onsets (interval > 30 days) were more common, and in 89 patients the features were at times so lacking in clarity that grading of the onset in these terms was not possible. The interval between onset of the florid illness and admission to hospital was in many cases surprisingly long (Johnstone et al., 1986) and in 66 cases more than one year elapsed between onset and admission. In retrospect the patients could not often give a clear account of this period, and certainly it was not usually possible to obtain from them a chronological account of their symptoms over this time. Details of the patients' behaviour during this period were obtained from their relatives and potentially dangerous behaviour, inappropriate sexual behaviour, inexplicable damage to property and behaviour that was bizarre in other ways, were all frequent. Subsequent further examination of the available data concerning this period (Humphreys et al., 1994) revealed that approximately 20% of the sample (52 patients out of 253) behaved in a way that was threatening to the lives of others during the pre-admission period. Later accounts made it clear that this behaviour was associated with delusions or hallucinations in some cases but not others. Sometimes patients later spoke of carrying out these antisocial acts in the light of delusional beliefs or misperceptions which they had denied at the time. Social withdrawal, loss of interest in school or work, deterioration in hygiene and grooming, unusual behaviour or outbursts of anger are listed as possible prodromal features of schizophrenia by DSM IV (APA, 1994) and clinical experience would support the view that such features do occur in some individuals in the year or so preceding the development of florid schizophrenic features. They do, of course, occur in other young adults as well and at present there is little information about the relative frequency of such phenomena in pre-schizophrenics and in others.

A study currently being conducted in the Department of Psychiatry, University of Edinburgh, is likely in due course to provide such information. It is a prospective study of the development of schizophrenia in 200 individuals aged 16 to 22 years at high risk of developing the disorder because they have two affected close relatives. There is a control group of individuals with matching age, sex and social background who have no family history of serious mental disorder. Use of the Structured Interview for Schizotypy (SIS) (Kendler et al., 1989) has revealed symptomatic and mental state differences between the high risk subjects and controls which are significant in the first 100 subjects tested (Hodges et al., 1999). These concern abnormalities of speech and affective response and reported sensitivity, rather than perceptual abnormalities and over valued ideas, but of course only a relatively small proportion of the high risk subjects will ever actually develop psychosis and we cannot know from these results what the pro-dromal features in those who become schizophrenic are actually going to be. It is anticipated that this matter will be clarified when the full results of the study are available in two years' time, as psychosis is developing in individuals who have been prior assessed on one or more occasions.

Forms of established rather than prodromal psychotic illness which lie on the margins of the diagnosis of schizophrenia may be divided into: (a) those in which the affective elements seem to be too great for a diagnosis of schizophrenia to be made, i.e. the schizo-affective disorders; (b) those in which the symptomatology seems to be too restricted (generally to a circumscribed set of delusions) for the diagnosis to be appropriate, i.e. delusional or paranoid states; and (c) those in which the symptomatology is not sufficiently sustained or sufficiently clearly present to justify the diagnosis (transient and partial psychoses).

Schizo-affective psychosis

Schizo-affective psychosis was originally described by Kasanin in 1933. The term is widely used and it can be very helpful in clinical practice when introducing the issue of the diagnosis of a psychosis in a young adult to the distressed family, but it is rarely clearly defined and the level of agreement across various definitions of this and related terms is low (Brockington & Leff, 1979). A number of studies have, however, been conducted using outcome or treatment response (currently the best if imperfect validating criteria for the diagnosis of either affective psychosis or schizophrenia) to try to decide whether schizo-affective illness should be included with schizophrenic or with affective illness. Conclusive results were generally not to be found and the issue was examined again by Johnstone et al. (1992) in a study involving 326 consecutively admitted patients with non organic psychosis to whom no diagnostic classification was applied and who were followed up after two and a half years. Detailed assessments of outcome were made. Thereafter details of the index admission were used for diagnostic classifications according to DSM and Catego (Wing et al., 1974) criteria. Significant differences were established between those fulfilling criteria for schizophrenic and affective psychosis, but the general conclusion of the study was that the diagnostic classifications used were of limited value in predicting outcome in functional psychosis. Significant differences between those fulfilling specified criteria for schizo-affective illness and other diagnostic groups were not established, and general scrutiny of the results in this study indicated that the findings in the schizo-affective cases lay between those of schizophrenic and affectively ill patients.

Psychoses of restricted symptomatology

What I have termed psychoses of restricted symptomatology would include those disorders which would fulfil DSM IV (APA, 1994) criteria for delusional disorder; that is, disorders characterized by persistent non bizarre delusions with or without hallucinations, it being specified that the criteria for schizophrenia have never been met. This classification would include specific delusional states such as erotomania (de Clerambault syndrome), delusions of jealousy and monosymptomatic hypochondriacal psychoses. These circumscribed conditions are generally considered separate from schizophrenia but the position is less clear cut as far as paranoia and paraphrenia are concerned.

The independence of paranoia and paraphrenia from schizophrenia and affective psychoses has been the subject of debate since Kraepelin's day. Paranoia was used by him to describe psychoses characterized by chronic systematized delusions but with no other disturbance of cognition or affect, while paraphrenia (a concept introduced by Kraepelin in the later editions of his textbook) was a chronic delusional state accompanied by prominent auditory hallucinations but which was not accompanied by the development of a defect state, despite a protracted course. Family studies conducted by Kendler et al. (1985a,b) have suggested that paranoia is separate from schizophrenia. Nonetheless, it is evident that the borderlines between paranoia and paraphrenia and schizophrenia are not well defined. In particular, whether paraphrenia is a separate entity or whether it is schizophrenia with the characteristics of the late onset form of that disorder, is far from clear. Issues of gender and age are important here. Paraphrenia of late onset is much commoner in women (Kay & Roth, 1961; Post, 1966). The mean age of onset of schizophrenia is lower in men than in women. In men onsets peak sharply between 20 and 24, thereafter remaining more or less constant at a lower level, while women have a less prominent peak in their twenties, followed by a statistically significant second peak in the years 45 to 49 (Häfner, 1993). Schizophrenic illnesses with onset at ages 35 to 59 have different phenomenology from those of younger patients, with systematized delusions of persecution, being significantly commoner in those with later onsets. It is postulated by Häfner (1993) that oestrogen levels in women delay the onset of the condition by raising the vulnerability threshold. The protective effect wanes at the menopause, thus accounting for the second peak of onset at a time when the characteristics of the illness would be different. These issues have been discussed in relation to the question of the relative frequency of schizophrenia in males and females. Some studies have reported a higher lifetime risk in men (Böok, 1978; Hagnell, 1989) but if cohorts are followed up until old age, numbers of women affected match, or even exceed, those of men, provided cases of late onset paraphrenia are included (Helgason & Magnusson, 1989; Jablensky, 1995). It may therefore be that paraphrenia is the form that schizophrenia takes in cases where the onset is late and that the late onsets which are known to occur in women do so for constitutional, possibly hormonal reasons. If this is so, then the cluster of symptoms and signs central to the diagnosis (and presumed to result from a tangible morbid process) must be able to be modified by age and gender related factors.

Transient and partial psychoses

There is extensive reference, particularly in the European literature, to concepts of psychosis that are too brief or where the psychotic phenomena are not expressed with sufficient conviction to allow the diagnosis of schizophrenia. The diagnostic classifications reactive psychosis (Wimmer, 1916), *bouffee delirante* (Legrain, 1886), and cycloid psychosis (Leonhard, 1959) are all attempts to separate 'lesser' psychoses from schizophrenia. The same is true of DSM IV's brief reactive psychosis (APA, 1994) and ICD 10's psychogenic paranoid psychosis. The assumption underlying the diagnosis of these disorders is that they represent syndromes which have a favourable outcome in comparison with schizophrenia. Such assumptions have been tested by follow up studies of first psychotic episodes (e.g. Kane et al., 1982; Nyman & Jonsson, 1983; Macmillan et al., 1986) and by genetic studies in which fairly brief psychoses have been compared with similar data from unequivocal schizophrenics (e.g. Astrup et al., 1962; Tsuang et al., 1976; Kendler et al., 1985b). Results have on the whole been conflicting. In a recent study (Johnstone et al., 1996) an unselected sample of patients assessed for a study of psychotic illness were followed up for two and a half years and those who could not readily be assigned to a major psychiatric category were compared with those who did fulfil diagnostic criteria for schizophrenia or affective disorder. Patients were classed as 'transient' where it was the fleeting nature of the symptoms that was the bar to diagnosis and 'partial' where it was the lack of firm conviction. Differences between the 'partials' and the more typical cases of schizophrenia were few but the 'transient' cases fared significantly better at follow up. These illnesses appeared to some extent to remit fully and to be associated with relatively little social decline. Their phenomenology was not typical of schizophrenic or indeed of affective illness, and cases where there was a possibility of an organic basis to the condition had been excluded from the sample.

Conclusion

Little more than description can be offered regarding the atypical or prodromal forms of symptomatology which lie at the periphery of the core features of schizophrenia. This is to be expected, because the present state of knowledge of the relationship of that core to the validating criteria of poor outcome and response to treatment, and indeed to the tangible morbid process (or processes) believed to underlie the disorder remains unclear. As far as defining the clinical boundaries of schizophrenia/dementia praecox is concerned, we have not moved very far in the last 100 years. We still have the same difficulty that Kraepelin had; we believe we are defining an entity which will be shown to have a tangible underlying morbid process, but we cannot demonstrate the process. Things are better for us than they were for Kraepelin, who in 1919 wrote 'the causes of dementia praecox are at the present time still mapped in impenetrable darkness'. As is clearly described in Chapters 4, 5, 6 and 7, the darkness does not seem so impenetrable any more, but the dawn will have to break more fully before we can be clear about the central cluster of clinical features which mean that someone should be diagnosed as having schizophrenia.

References

American Psychiatric Association. (1994). DSM IV: *Diagnostic & Statistical Manual of Mental Disorders.* 4th edn. Washington DC: APA.

American Psychiatric Association. Committee on Nomenclature & Statistics. (1980). *Diagnostic and Statistical Manual of Mental Disorders.* (Third edition). Washington, DC: APA.

Angrist, B., Sathanathan, G., Wilk, S. & Gershon, S. (1974). Amphetamine psychosis, behavioural and biochemical aspects. *Journal of Psychiatric Research,* **11**, 13–23.

Arndt, S., Alliger, R. J. & Andreasen, N. C. (1991). The destruction of positive and negative symptoms; the failure of a two dimensional model. *British Journal of Psychiatry,* **58**, 317–22.

Astrup, C., Fossum, A. & Holmboe, R. (1962). *Prognosis in Functional Psychoses.* Springfield, Illinois: Thomas.

Bilder, R. M., Mukherjee, S., Reider, R. O. & Pandurangi, A. K. (1985). Symptomatic and neuropsychological components of defect states. *Schizophrenia Bulletin,* **11**, 409–19.

Blackwood, D. H. R., Muir, W. J., St. Clair, D. M. & Evans, H. J. (1989). Schizophrenia and chromosomes. *Lancet,* **ii**, 1459.

Bleuler, E. (1950). *Dementia Praecox or the Group of Schizophrenias.* Translated by J. Zinkin. New York: International Universities Press.

Böök, J. A., Wettenberg, L. & Modrewska, K. (1978). Schizophrenia in a North Swedish geographical isolate, 1900–1977: epidemiology, genetics and biochemistry. *Clinical Genetics,* **14**, 373–94.

Brockington, I. F. & Leff, J. P. (1979). Schizoaffective psychosis: definitions and incidence. *Psychological Medicine,* **9**, 91–9.

Burt, D. R., Creese, I. & Snyder, S. H. (1977). Antischizophrenic drugs: chronic treatment elevates dopamine receptor binding in the brain. *Science,* **196**, 326–8.

Carlsson, A. & Lindqvist, M. (1963). Effect of chlorpromazine and haloperidol on formation of 3-methoxy-tyramine and normetanephrine in mouse brain. *Acta Pharmacologica et Toxicoligica,* **20**, 140–4.

Carpenter, W. T., Heinrichs, D. W. & Wagman, A. M. I. (1988). Deficit and non deficit forms of schizophrenia: the concept. *American Journal of Psychiatry*, **145**, 578–83.

Cookson, I. C., Silverstone, T. & Rees, L. (1982). Plasma prolactin and growth hormone levels in manic patients treated with pimozide. *British Journal of Psychiatry*, **140**, 274–9.

Cooper, J. E., Kendell, R. E., Gurland, B. J., Sharpe, L., Copeland, J. R. M. & Simon, R. (1972). *Psychiatric diagnosis in New York and London. Maudsley Monography 20*. Oxford: Oxford University Press.

Crow, T. J. (1980). Molecular pathology of schizophrenia: more than one disease process. *British Medical Journal*, **280**, 66–8.

Crow, T. J., Cross, A. J. & Owen, F. (1979). Monoamine mechanisms in chronic schizophrenia: post mortem neurochemical findings. *British Journal of Psychiatry*, **134**, 249–56.

Crow, T. J., Cross, A. J., Johnstone, E. C. & Owen, F. (1982). Two syndromes of schizophrenia and their pathogenesis. In *Schizophrenia as a Brain Disease*, ed. F. A. Henn & H. A. Nasrallah, pp. 196–234. New York: Oxford University Press.

Degreef, G., Ashtari, M., Wu, H. W., Borenstein, M., Geisler, L. & Lieberman, J. (1991). Follow up study in first episode schizophrenia. *Schizophrenia Research*, **5**, 204–6.

Delay, J. & Deniker, P. (1952). Le traitment des psychoses par une méthode neurolytique derivée de l'hibernothérapie. In *Neurologistes de France*, ed. P. Cossa, pp. 497–502. Paris & Luxembourg: Masson et Cie, Libraires de L'Academie de medicine.

Done, D. J., Johnstone, E. C., Frith, C. D., Golding, J., Shepherd, P. M. & Crow, T. J. (1991). Complications of pregnancy and delivery in relation to psychosis in adult life. Data from the British perinatal mortality survey sample. *British Medical Journal*, **302**, 1576–80.

Done, D. J., Crow, T. J., Johnstone, E. C. & Sacker, A. (1994). Childhood antecedents of schizophrenia and affective illness: social adjustment at ages 7 and 11. *British Medical Journal*, **309**, 699–703.

Ehringer, H. & Horneykiewicz, O. (1960). Verteilung von Noradrenalin and Dopamin (3 hydroxytrypamin) in Gehirn des Menschen und ihr verhalten bein erkrankungen des extrapyramidalen systems. *Klin Wochenschr*, **38**, 1236–9.

Feighner, J. P., Robins, E., Guze, S., Woodruff, R. A., Winokur, G. & Munoz, R. (1972). Diagnostic criteria for use in psychiatric research. *Archives of General Psychiatry*, **26**, 57–62.

Fish, F. (1962). *Sschizophrenia*. Bristol: Wright.

Flugel, F. (1953). Therapeutique par medication neuroleptique obtenue en realisant systematique des états Parkinsoniformes. *L'Encephale*, **45**, 1090–2.

Foerster, A., Lewis, S., Owen, M. & Murray, R. (1991). Premorbid adjustment and personality in psychosis: effects of sex and diagnosis. *British Journal of Psychiatry*, **158**, 171–6.

Frangou, S. & Murray, R. M. (1996). Imaging as a tool in exploring the neurodevelopment and genetics of schizophrenia. In *Biological Psychiatry*, ed. E. C. Johnstone. *British Medical Bulletin 52(3)*.

Gottesman, I. I. & Bertelsen, A. (1989). Confirming unexpressed genotypes for schizophrenia – risks in the offspring of Fischer's Danish identical and fraternal discordant twins. *Archives of General Psychiatry*, **46**, 867–72.

Green, M. F., Satz, P. & Christensen, C. (1994). Minor physical anomalies in schizophrenic patients, bipolar patients and their siblings. *Schizophrenia Bulletin*, **20**, 433–40.

Häfner, H. (1993). What is schizophrenia? *Neurology, Psychiatry and Brain Research*, **2**, 36–52.

Häfner, H., Behrens, S., De Vry, K. & Gattaz, W. F. (1991). Oestradiol enhances the vulnerability threshold for schizophrenia in women by an early effect on dopaminergic neurotransmission. *European Archives of Psychiatry and Clinical Neuroscience*, **241**, 65–8.

Hagnell, O. (1989). Repeated incidence and prevalence studies of mental disorders in a total population followed during 25 years. The Lundby Study, Sweden. *Acta Psychiatrica Scandinavica*, **79** (suppl. 348), 61–78.

Hecker, E. (1871). Hebephrenie ein Beitrag zur klinischen psychiatrie. *Archiv für pathologische Anatomie und Physiologie und für klinische Medizin*, **52**, 394–429.

Helgason, T. & Magnusson, H. (1989). The first 80 years of life. A psychiatric epidemiological study. *Acta Psychiatrica Scandinavica*, **79** (Suppl. 348), 85–94.

Hoch, P. & Polatin, P. (1949). Pseudoneurotic forms of schizophrenia. *Psychiatric Quarterly*, **23**, 248–56.

Hodges, A., Byrne, M., Grant, E. & Johnstone, E. (1999). Subject at risk of schizophrenia. *British Journal of Psychiatry*, **173**, (in press).

Hughlings Jackson, J. (1869). Certain points in the study and classification of diseases of the nervous system. Reprinted in Taylor, J. (1932). *Selected writings of John Hughlings Jackson*, Vol. 2. London: Hodder & Stoughton.

Humphreys, M., Johnstone, E. & Macmillan, F. (1994). Offending among first episode schizophrenics. *Journal of Forensic Psychiatry*, **5**, 51–61.

Illowsky, B. P., Juliano, D. M., Bigelow, L. B. & Weinberger, D. R. (1988). The stability of CT scan findings in schizophrenia: results of an eight year follow up study. *Journal of Neurology, Neurosurgery and Psychiatry*, **51**, 209–13.

Iversen, L. L. (1985). Mechanism of action of antipsychotic drugs: retrospect and prospect. In *Psychopharmacology. Recent Advances and Future Prospects*, ed. S. D. Iversen. Oxford: Oxford University Press.

Jablensky, A. (1995). Schizophrenia: the epidemiological horizon. In *Schizophrenia*, eds. S. R. Hirsch & D. R. Weinberg, pp. 206–52. Oxford: Blackwell.

Johnstone, E. C. (1979). The clinical implications of dopamine receptor blockade in acute schizophrenia. In *Proceedings of International Symposium on Neuroleptics and Schizophrenia*, ed. J. Simister. Letchworth: Lundbeck.

Johnstone, E. C. (1987). Physical treatments. In *Recurrent and Chronic Psychoses*, ed. T. J. Crow. *British Medical Bulletin*, **43(3)**, Churchill Livingston.

Johnstone, E. C. (1994). *Searching for the Causes of Schizophrenia*. Questions and answers derived from the large clinical studies, pp. 46–58. Oxford: Oxford University Press.

Johnstone, E. C. & Frith, C. D. (1996). Validation of three dimensions of schizophrenic symptoms in a large unselected sample of patients. *Psychological Medicine*, **26**, 669–79.

Johnstone, E. C., Crow, T. J., Frith, C. D., Husband, J. & Kreel, L. (1976). Cerebral ventricular size and cognitive impairment in chronic schizophrenia. *Lancet*, **ii**, 924–6.

Johnstone, E. C., Crow, T. J., Frith, C. D., Carney, M. W. P. & Price, J. S. (1978). Mechanism of the antipsychotic effect in the treatment of acute schizophrenia. *Lancet*, **i**, 848–51.

Johnstone, E. C., Crow, T. J., Johnson, A. L. & Macmillan, J. F. (1986). The Northwick Park Study of First Episodes of Schizophrenia. 1. Presentation of the illness and problems relating to admission. *British Journal of Psychiatry*, **148**, 115–20.

Johnstone, E. C., Frith, C. D., Crow, T. J., Owens, D. G. C., Done, D. J., Baldwin, E. J. & Charlette, A. (1992). The Northwick Park 'Functional' Psychosis Study: diagnosis and outcome. *Psychological Medicine*, **22**, 331–46.

Johnstone, E. C., Connelly, J., Frith, C. D., Lambert, M. T. & Owens, D. G. C. (1996). The nature of 'transient' and 'partial' psychoses: findings from the Northwick Park 'Functional' Psychosis Study. *Psychological Medicine*, **26**, 361–9.

Jones, P., Rodgers, B., Murray, R. & Marmot, M. (1994). Child development risk factors for adult schizophrenia in the British 1964 birth cohort. *Lancet*, **344**, 1389–402.

Kahlbaum, K. L. (1874). *Die Katatonie order das Spannungurresein. Eine Klinisch Form Psychischer Krankeit*. Berlin: Hirschwald.

Kane, J. H., Rifkin, A., Quitkin, F., Nayak, D. & Ramos Lorenzi, J. (1982). Fluphenazine vs. placebo in patients with remitted acute first episode schizophrenia. *Archives of General Psychiatry*, **39**, 70–3.

Kane, J., Honigfeld, G., Singer, J. and Meltzer, H. (1988). Clozapine for the treatment resistant schizophrenic: a double blind comparison versus chlorpromazine/benztropine. *Archives of General Psychiatry*, **45**, 789–96.

Kasanin, J. (1933). The acute schizoaffective psychoses. *American Journal of Psychiatry*, **90**, 97–126.

Kay, D. W. K. & Roth, M. (1961). Environmental and hereditary factors in the schizophrenias of old age ('late paraphrenia') and their bearing on the general problem of causation in schizophrenia. *Journal of Mental Science*, **107**, 649–86.

Kebabian, J. W., Petzold, G. L. & Greengard, P. (1972). Dopamine sensitive adenylate cyclase in caudate nucleus of rat brain and its similarity to the 'dopamine receptor'. *Proceedings of the National Academy of Sciences (USA)*, **69**, 2145–9.

Kendell, R. E. (1988). Schizophrenia. In *Companion to Psychiatric Studies*, ed. R. E. Kendell & A. K. Zealley, pp. 310–34. Churchill Livingstone: Edinburgh.

Kendell, R. E., Brockington, I. F. & Leff, J. P. (1979). Prognostic implications of six alternative definitions of Schizophrenia. *Archives of General Psychiatry*, **25**, 25–31.

Kendler, K. S., Masterton, C. C. & Davis, K. L. (1985a). Psychiatric illness in first degree relatives of patients with paranoid psychosis, schizophrenia and medical illness. *British Journal of Psychiatry*, **147**, 524–31.

Kendler, K. S., Gruenberg, A. M. & Tsuang, M. T. (1985b). Psychiatric illness in first degree relatives of schizophrenics and surgical control patients. *Archives of General Psychiatry*, **42**, 770–9.

Kendler, K. S., Lieberman, J. A. & Walsh, D. A. (1989). The structured interview for schizotypy (SIS). A preliminary report. *Schizophrenia Bulletin*, **15**, 559–71.

Kety, S. S., Rosenthal, D., Wender, P. I. L., Schulsinger, F. & Jacobsen, B. (1975). Mental illness in the biologic and adoptive families of adopted individuals who become schizophrenic. In *Genetic Research in Schizophrenia*, ed. R. R. Fieve, D. Rosenthal & H. Brill, pp. 147–65. Baltimore: Johns Hopkins University Press.

Kleist, K. (1947). *Fortschrik der Psychiatrie.* Frankfurt: A. M. Kramer.

Kraepelin, E. (1896). *Lehrbuch der Psychiatrie* 5th edn. Leipzig: Barth.

Kraepelin, E. (1919). *Dementia Praecox.* Translated by R. M. Barclay. Edited by G. M. Robertson, Facsimile Edition. Published by Krieger: New York, 1971.

Langfeldt, T. G. (1939). *The Schizophreniform States.* Copenhagen: Munksgaard.

Legrain, M. (1886). *Du délire chez les dégéneres.* Paris: Libraire A. Deshaye et E. Lecrosnier.

Lenzenweger, M. A. & Dworkin, R. H. (1984). Symptoms and genetics of schizophrenia: implications for diagnosis. *American Journal of Psychiatry,* **141,** 1541–6.

Leonhard, K. (1957). *Aufteilung der endogenen Psychosen.* (*Classification of Endogenous Psychoses*), 1st edn. Berlin: Akademie Verlag.

Liddle, P. F. (1987). The symptoms of chronic schizophrenia: a re–examination of the positive–negative dichotomy. *British Journal of Psychiatry,* **151,** 145–51.

Liddle, P. F., Friston, K. J., Frith, C. D. & Frackowiak, R. (1992). Central blood flow and mental processes in schizophrenia. *Journal of Royal Society of Medicine,* **85,** 224–7.

Lyons, M., Tsuang, M., Faraone, S. & Kremen, W. S. (1992). Characteristics of schizotypal subjects related to schizophrenic versus affective probands: symptomatology, co-morbidity and familial psychopathology. *Society of Biological Psychiatry 47th Annual Meeting,* **31,** 68A. Washington, DC.

McGlashan, T. H. & Carpenter, W. T. (1976). Post psychotic depression in schizophrenia. *Archives of General Psychiatry,* **33,** 231–9.

Macmillan, J. F. (1984). The First Schizophrenic Illness – presentation and short term outcome incorporating a trial of prophylactic neuroleptic maintenance therapy versus placebo. M.D. Thesis: University of Edinburgh.

Macmillan, J. F., Crow, T. J., Johnson, A. L. & Johnstone, E. C. (1986). The Northwick Park Study of First Episodes of Schizophrenia. III Short term outcome in trial entrants and trial eligible patients. *British Journal of Psychiatry,* **148,** 128–33.

Matthysse, S. (1973). Antipsychotic drug actions, a clue to the neuropathology of schizophrenia? *Federation Proceedings,* **32,** 200–5.

Murray, R. M. & Lewis, S. W. (1987). Is schizophrenia a neurodevelopmental disorder? *British Medical Journal,* **295,** 681–2.

Nyman, A. K. & Jonsson, H. (1983). Differential evaluation of outcome in schizophrenia. *Acta Psychiatrica Scandinavica,* **68,** 458–75.

Owens, D. G. C. (1996). Adverse effects of antipsychotic agents – do fewer agents offer advantages? *Drugs,* **59,** 895–930.

Owens, D. G. C. & Johnstone, E. C. (1980). The disabilities of chronic schizophrenia – their nature and factors contributing to their development. *British Journal of Psychiatry,* **136,** 384–95.

Pogue-Geile, M. F. & Zubin, J. (1988). Negative symptomatology and schizophrenia: a conceptual and empirical review. *International Journal of Mental Health,* **16,** 3–45.

Post, F. (1966). *Persistent Persecutory States in The Elderly.* Oxford: Pergamon.

Prien, R. F., Caffey, E. M. & Klett, C. J. (1972). Comparison of lithium carbonate and chlorpromazine in mania. *Archives of General Psychiatry,* **26,** 146–53.

Rifkin, A., Quitkin, F. & Klein, D. F. (1975). Akinesia. *Archives of General Psychiatry,* **32,** 672–4.

Rutter, M. (1990). Changing patterns of psychiatric disorders during adolescence. In *Adolescence and Psychiatry,* ed. J. Bancroft & J. Machover Ranish, pp. 124–45. The Kinsey Institute Series. Oxford: Oxford University Press.

Schneider, K. (1959). *Clinical Psychopathology*. New York: Grune and Stratton.

Siever, L. J. & Gunderson, J. G. (1983). The search for a schizotypal personality: historical origins and current status. *Comprehensive Psychiatry*, **24**, 99–212.

Snyder, S. H. (1973). Amphetamine psychosis: a model of schizophrenia mediated by catecholamines. *American Journal of Psychiatry*, **120**, 61–7.

Sommers, A. A. (1985). 'Negative symptoms', conceptual and methodological problems. *Schizophrenia Bulletin*, **11**, 364–78.

Spitzer, R. L., Endicott, J. & Robins, E. (1975). *Research Diagnostic Criteria for a Selected Group of Functional Psychoses*, 2nd edn. New York: Biometrics Research Division.

Strauss, J. S., Carpenter, W. J. & Bartko, J. P. (1974). The diagnosis and understanding of schizophrenia. III Speculation on the process that underlies schizophrenic symptoms and signs. *Schizophrenia Bulletin*, **1**, 61–76.

Stromgren, E. (1989). The development of the concept of reactive psychosis. *British Journal of Psychiatry*, **154** Suppl. 4, 47–50.

Tsuang, M. T., Dempsey, G. M. & Rauscher, F. (1976). A study of 'atypical schizophrenia'. Comparison with schizophrenia and affective disorder by sex, age of admission, precipitant outcome and family history. *Archives of General Psychiatry*, **33**, 1157–60.

Van der Does, A. J. W., Dingemans, P., Maj Linszen, D. H., Neigter, M. A. & Scholte, W. T. (1993). Symptoms dimensions and cognitive and social functioning in recent onset schizophrenia. *Psychological Medicine*, **23**, 745–53.

Walker, E. & Lewine, R. J. (1990). Prediction of adult-onset schizophrenia from childhood home movies of the patients. *American Journal of Psychiatry*, **147**, 1052–6.

Weinberger, D. R. (1986). The pathogenesis of schizophrenia: a neurodevelopmental disorder. In *The Neurology of Schizophrenia*, ed. H. A. Nasrallah & D. R. Weinberger, pp. 397–406. Amsterdam: Elsevier.

Wimmer, A. (1916). Psykogene Sindssygdomsformer. In *St. Hans Hospital 1816–1915*, ed. A. Wimmer, pp. 85–216. Kovenhaven: Gad.

Wing, J. K. (1978). *Reasoning about Madness*. Oxford: Oxford University Press.

Wing, J. K. (1995). Concepts of schizophrenia. In *Schizophrenia*, ed. S. R. Hirsh & D. R. Weinberger, pp. 3–14. Oxford: Blackwell.

Wing, J. K., Cooper, J. E. & Sartorius, N. (1974). *The Description and Classification of Psychiatric Symptoms. An Instruction Manual for The PSE and Catego Systems*. Cambridge: Cambridge University Press.

World Health Organization (1973). *WHO Report of the International Pilot Study of Schizophrenia*. Vol. I. Geneva: WHO.

World Health Organization (1992). *The ICD-10 Classification of Mental and Behavioural Disorders: Clinical Descriptions and Diagnostic Guidelines*. Geneva: WHO.

3

Diagnostic issues: aspects of differential diagnosis

Introduction

As will be clear from Chapter 2, there is no diagnostic test for schizophrenia. The diagnosis is made using operational criteria which depend upon the patient's description of his/her mental content, observation of the features of his mental state, and information with regard to his/her general functioning and behaviour. There has been much debate about the particular features which are important and relevant. At present, generally accepted international criteria such as ICD-10 (WHO, 1992) and DSM IV (APA, 1994) are widely used and reasonably high rates of inter-rater reliability can be obtained using these and other operational criteria. Clinical judgement still needs to be employed with regard to whether or not specific features are present, but on the whole, reasonable agreement can be achieved among trained staff that a patient does or does not conform to operational criteria for the diagnosis of schizophrenia.

The question of the extent to which such diagnoses will ever be able to be validated by objective biological correlates remains open. A question that can be addressed at the present time is the extent to which less than typical cases can be misclassified according to standard operational criteria. Such presentations may generally be divided into those where the initial clinical picture is schizophrenic but where this diagnosis is not supported by subsequent events – 'false positives' – and those where the initial picture is suggestive of some other diagnosis, either functional or organic, but where in due course operational criteria for schizophrenia are fulfilled – 'false negatives'. In addition there are certain circumstances where diagnosis is made difficult because of particular features of the affected individual. Examples of this would be language or cultural difficulties, the presence of concomitant substance misuse, communication difficulties relating to muteness or deafness, and the situation of the learning disabled patient.

Presentation where the initial clinical picture is schizophrenic but where this is not supported by later events: ('false positives')

Schizophrenia is a common disorder and it is bound at times to occur by chance in people who have organic disease of the central nervous system or of some other part of the body, and indeed there are many reports of apparently typical schizophrenic illnesses arising in association with organic brain disease (Davison & Bagley, 1969). As indicated above, such an association could be fortuitous but alternative explanations (a) that the organic CNS disorder 'causes' the psychosis and (b) that the organic CNS psychosis 'precipitates' true schizophrenia, are also possible. It is unlikely that fortuitous association accounts for all of the cases, because schizophrenia is associated with an increased risk of death (Baldwin, 1979; Herrman et al., 1983). While some of this increased mortality is clearly secondary to the psychosis (i.e. that resulting from the enhanced risk of trauma and poisoning associated with this disorder (Anderson et al., 1991)), or the enhanced risk of infections formerly found in patients with schizophrenia (Baldwin, 1979), not all of the organic disease described by Davison & Bagley (1969) or in later accounts (Johnstone et al., 1987; 1988; Feinstein & Ron, 1990) could plausibly be considered to result from any of the social or environmental disadvantages suffered by those with mental disorders. It must therefore be that some sort of causative association between the organic disease and the psychosis exists, i.e. that one or other, or both of the alternative explanations above are sometimes correct. Studies in this area have recently been reviewed by Lewis (1995), who concluded that about 3% of newly presenting cases of schizophrenia are secondary to organic physical disease. Johnstone et al. (1987) reported 6% of their 268 cases of first episode schizophrenia as being secondary to organic disease, but included in that figure five cases where the disorder was related to substance use (alcohol, illicit or prescribed drugs). The nature of the 10 remaining cases is shown in Table 3.1. These cases are therefore not frequent but are by no means gross rarities, and will arise in the day to day practice of most psychiatrists.

In the study of Johnstone et al. (1987) patients had been referred on to the research team as probable cases of schizophrenia by collaborating psychiatrists to whom the organic diagnosis was not apparent. They had, however, been asked to make referrals at an early stage and detailed investigations had not been carried out. Nonetheless, the question is obviously raised that if organic disease was initially overlooked but later discovered in 10 cases, in how many others was it never discovered? This is

Table 3.1. *Organic diseases associated with psychoses initially diagnosed as schizophrenia*

Organic disorder	Number of cases
Syphilis	3
Sarcoidosis	2
Carcinoma of the lung	1
Autoimmune multisystem disease	1
Epilepsy resulting from cerebral cysticercosis	1
Chronic thyroid disease with acute thyrotoxicosis	1
Head injury with hemiparesis	1

Note: From Johnstone et al. (1987).

unanswerable, but the entire first episode sample was followed up for two years and no further organic disease was demonstrated during that time, and those who were admitted to Northwick Park Hospital (about 20% of the total) were followed up again after eight years (Geddes et al., 1994), and again nothing was found. It might be expected that most diseases which could underlie schizophrenia-like psychosis would, if present, have become apparent during time periods of this nature, but of course we cannot exclude the possibility that some disorder that we are just not considering, or the nature of which is not yet known, is present in some of these patients and relevant to their psychosis.

The important issue is that diseases that are known, and especially those that might be treatable, are not overlooked. Reviews (e.g. Lewis, 1995) point out that in most series of cases of schizophrenia with underlying organic illness, patients are rather older at onset and are less likely to have a family history of schizophrenia than the generality of affected individuals, but these characteristics are not helpful in the individual case. Phenomenoligically there is a very large overlap between the organically based patients and the generality of cases (Cutting, 1987; Johnstone et al., 1988; Feinstein & Ron, 1990).

I met all of the patients described in Johnstone et al. (1987). In the notes I made at the time, I commented upon the strikingly poor response to antipsychotic medication of some of these patients. Treatment resistance to antipsychotic agents has become a more fashionable theme since that time, in the wake of the introduction of 'atypical' antipsychotics (Kane et al., 1988; Mercer et al., 1997). Many schizophrenic patients respond poorly, but the patients with sarcoidosis and a woman who was eventually found to have carcinoma of the lung seemed (Johnstone et al., 1987) to be entirely unaffected by antipsychotics, apart from perhaps being mildly sedated, and a woman with multi-system autoimmune disease deteriorated steadily from the point of view of her mental state. Series of cases like those mentioned here, where schizophrenia appears to develop in the setting of organic diseases, arouse much interest. In part this is because the issue of appropriate treatment of the primary condition is obviously important, but at least some of the interest relates to the possibility that the causation of the generality of schizophrenia might be illuminated by the study of such cases. On the whole this has not happened, and indeed the diverse nature of the underlying causes in the series described makes it difficult to envisage any final common pathway by which they might give rise to an often very similar pattern of symptomatology. At a practical level, the gratifying response to appropriate treatment of cases such as patients with thyroid disease and cerebral cystcercosis in the report by Johnstone et al. (1987) underlines the importance of adequate investigation in patients where there is any possibility of organic disease. My own experience of this area has certainly been that even when the primary diagnosis is not one where a very satisfactory response to specific treatment may be anticipated, the relatives, and the patients (where they are able to comprehend the situation) are pleased that the nature of the illness is understood, and express relief that the underlying condition has not been overlooked.

Davison & Bagley (1969) carefully reviewed the links between schizophrenia-like psychoses and the various organic diagnoses which they considered could underlie them, and concluded that in the case of a number of disorders, including cerebral syphilis and cerebral tumours, the co-occurrence of the two exceeded chance expectations. The evidence for similar conclusions regarding the disorders relevant for the patients they described was reviewed by Johnstone et al. (1987). A number of diagnoses which are suggested as leading to secondary schizophrenia are described in case reports, and such evidence is difficult to evaluate, because as schizophrenia is a common diagnosis, it must occur in association with other disorders by chance alone.

No evidence of a stronger nature is available when the links between HIV/AIDS and schizophrenia and new variant Creutzfeldt–Jakob disease and schizophrenia are considered. The possible importance of both of these disorders as underlying causes of psychotic illness was not appreciated at the time that most of the work on secondary schizophrenia described above was carried out, and the issues can only be examined in relation to anecdotal reports. Infection with Human Immunodeficiency Virus (HIV) may be associated with a wide range of psychiatric problems (Catalan,

1990) and this includes psychotic illness which may resemble schizophrenia. Such disorders could be manifestations of the organic brain disease associated with HIV/AIDS, and while features of an organic brain syndrome may be present, they do not always occur. The nature of the relationship between the schizophrenia-like psychosis and HIV/AIDS remains unclear and the possibility of a chance association remains.

In 1996, the new variant Creutzfeldt–Jakob disease (CJD) was described. This condition affects much younger people than those described as having CJD in the past. As it may possibly be associated with the past ingestion of beef infected with bovine spongiform encaphlopathy, the issue has been associated with much public concern, particularly in relation to the possibility that the small number of cases so far reported (Will et al., 1996; Zeidler et al., 1997) may represent the tip of an iceberg, and that increasing numbers of our young people may be about to succumb to a devastating and evidently inevitably fatal disease. A number of the young people affected by new varient CJD were initially seen by psychiatrists, and while in most cases the manifestations were anxiety and depression which were fairly rapidly succeeded by generally deteriorating function and the development of neurological signs, in one of the early cases the initial features were of a paranoid illness which would certainly have fulfilled at least some operational criteria for schizophrenia (Zeidler et al., 1997). At present the frequency of new varient CJD is yet to be established, and we can have no idea of whether a presentation which could initially appear to be that of schizophrenia will be an extreme rarity amounting to a curiosity, or an issue which will merit practical clinical consideration. Clearly we must hope for the former possibility.

As far as schizophrenia is concerned, 'false positive' diagnoses generally refer to situations such as those described above, where the picture has appeared to be that of schizophrenia but where some other diagnosis of an organic nature (usually with the availability of diagnostic support in terms of laboratory tests) was subsequently shown to be appropriate. It will be clear, for reasons described in Chapter 2, that the superseding of a schizophrenic diagnosis by that of another 'functional' psychiatric disorder cannot occur in quite the same way. The main possible alternative diagnosis is that of affective psychosis, and in the absence of a diagnostic test for either schizophrenia or affective illness, disputes as to whether an individual psychotic episode should 'really' be diagnosed as one or other condition cannot be satisfactorily resolved. The phenomenology of subsequent episodes and the general course taken by the illness are often used to clarify situations where there has initially been diagnostic doubt.

In 1954 Lewis & Pietrowski noted that while half of their series of 122 patients with schizophrenia had been diagnosed as having manic depressive illness in a previous episode, it was uncommon for patients initially diagnosed as schizophrenic to be reclassified as affective in a subsequent episode. Nonetheless, it does occur, and Sheldrick et al. (1977) reported a change to a diagnosis of affective illness from a previous diagnosis of schizophrenia in 12 cases. These authors went on to examine the follow up of the International Pilot Study of schizophrenia (WHO, 1973) and found a switch to a diagnosis of affective disorder in 3% of cases. It is, of course, possible that affective illnesses occur in the course of some schizophrenic illnesses. Indeed it is known that they do. The phenomenon of post psychotic depression was described in the 1920s (Mayer-Gross, 1920) and the occurrence of depressive symptoms in schizophrenic patients when they are not actively psychotic is increasingly reported (McGlashan & Carpenter, 1976; Hirsch et al., 1989; Siris, 1991). Nonetheless, in the material of Sheldrick et al. (1977) there was no instance of a patient reverting to schizophrenic symptomatology and a diagnosis of schizophrenia after having suffered a psychotic relapse with affective symptoms. The data are therefore less consistent with the possibility of one disease entity being replaced by another or superimposed upon another, than with the situation of an illness, which subsequent events would clarify as affective, initially having features which supported a diagnosis of schizophrenia.

Presentations where the initial clinical picture is suggestive of some other diagnosis but where in due course operational criteria for schizophrenia are fulfilled ('false negatives')

Such situations are not uncommon. As has been described in Chapter 2, nonspecific symptoms of various kinds occur in those at risk of developing schizophrenia who are not yet ill (Hodges et al., 1999), the prodromal states of schizophrenia include features which may suggest a variety of other diagnoses (Chapter 2) and the situation whereby a typically schizophrenic psychosis presents in an individual who has previously had a diagnosis of affective psychosis must be familiar to most practising psychiatrists. In part, this diagnostic uncertainty is likely to relate to the reluctance of clinicians, particularly perhaps those of an older generation, to diagnose schizophrenia in a first episode unless the situation is absolutely unequivocal. Although the possibility that delay in introducing antipsychotic agents may have detrimental effects upon the long term prognosis of schizophrenia (Crow et al., 1986) is currently receiving a good deal of interest

(Wyatt et al., 1997) there is no real reason to believe that delay in diagnosis as schizophrenia, rather than some other type of psychosis, is harmful to patients.

The situation whereby schizophrenia presents as a behavioural disturbance which is not necessarily recognized as illness at all, is different. A substantial proportion of schizophrenic patients have had involvement with the police (Mackay & Wright, 1984) and this applies even to their first episode (Macmillan & Johnson, 1987). Humphreys et al. (1994) examined the offending behaviour of the individuals who participated in the Northwick Park First Episodes Study (Johnstone et al., 1986) in the five years before their admission (and first diagnosis of schizophrenia, or indeed psychotic illness of any kind). Thirty one patients had convictions recorded during that time, and while in some cases there was no reason to believe that the offences were related to psychiatric illness, in 13 cases the offending behaviour appeared to be the result of delusions which were not revealed at the time. Clearly situations such as that described in one woman with unrevealed delusions of poisoning, where conviction resulted from her repeated theft of food which she considered to be uncontaminated, are not just and can never be other than detrimental to those involved.

Circumstances which can give rise to diagnostic difficulty

Substance misuse and schizophrenia

The role of some substances of abuse in precipitating psychotic symptomatology is undoubted. Intoxication with hallucinogenic substances such as lysergic acid diethylamide (LSD) is associated with sensory distortions, hallucinations and sometimes intense emotions of a frightening nature. These generally resolve over a matter of days, but characteristically acute and transient flashbacks may occur months after drug use has ceased (Horowitz, 1969). The fact that amphetamines can produce a state (albeit a temporary one) resembling paranoid schizophrenia (Connell, 1958; Griffiths et al., 1972; Angrist & Gershon, 1970) in mentally well individuals was one of the lines of evidence on which the dopamine hypothesis of schizophrenia was based. Paranoid symptoms of a similar nature may accompany the use of cocaine and methylenedioxymethylamphetamine (MDMA or Ecstasy). In all of these instances the symptoms usually resolve over days to weeks, at the most.

The nature of the association between cannabis use and schizophrenia-like psychosis has caused more controversy. Acute psychotic reactions to cannabis may occur (Tennant & Groesbeck, 1972). The use of cannabis has been stated to be an independent risk factor in the development of schizophrenia. Evidence for this comes from a prospective study of Swedish conscripts who were followed up over a 15 year period (Andreasson et al., 1987). The relative risk for developing schizophrenia was 2.4 for cannabis users and 6 for heavy users when compared with non users at conscription. Whether there is a 'cannabis psychosis', an entity separate from schizophrenia and indeed from affective psychosis, is doubtful. Certainly this view has been put forward (Imade & Ebie, 1991), and indeed the diagnosis has been quite widely made. The thinking behind the making of this diagnosis has, at least in some cases, been coloured by the view that a cannabis psychosis might be less serious and the outlook less pessimistic than is the case in schizophrenic illness. The recent literature is against such ideas. The use of cannabis among schizophrenic patients is associated with greater severity of psychotic symptoms and earlier and more frequent relapses (Linszen et al., 1994; Martinez-Arevalo et al., 1994). Comorbidity of substance misuse and schizophrenia, so-called 'dual diagnosis' (Regier et al., 1990) has received increasing attention in recent years. The problems relate to alcohol (Drake et al., 1993) as well as to the drugs mentioned above. The effects of alcohol withdrawal in producing transient psychotic states are, of course, very well known (Victor, 1966), but the effects of alcohol in producing persistent psychotic states, although long described (Victor & Hope, 1958) are more controversial (Glass, 1989). The intensification of the difficulties of schizophrenic patients where there is concomitant alcohol use has been established in the United Kingdom (Menezes et al., 1996) as well as in the United States (Drake & Wallach, 1989; Regier et al., 1990), where much of the earlier work was done. It is evident that both drug misuse and alcohol misuse in schizophrenic patients are associated with a detrimental effect on the course and prognosis of the psychotic illness (Cantwell & Harrison, 1996). Whether or not these substances cause independent psychotic states or precipitate psychosis in vulnerable individuals is less certain, but from the point of view of management issues schizophrenic young men with co-morbid substance use and chaotic lifestyles represent a very major problem (Johnson et al., 1997). Current thinking would tend to be that differentiating schizophrenia *per se* from a similar psychosis implicated by drug and/or alcohol use is less important than acknowledging the problems of substance use in schizophrenia patients and in providing a service that will accommodate complex difficulties of affected individuals. The poor compliance, disturbed behaviour and social instability of these patients may mean that some traditional psychiatric services are reluctant to accept them and find them very difficult to manage (Cantwell & Harrison, 1996).

Language and cultural difficulties

Relatively high rates of the diagnosis of schizophrenia in immigrant population have been known to occur for a long time (Odegaard, 1932; Cochrane, 1977). The possibilities of diagnostic bias and misclassification have received extensive consideration (Lipsedge & Littlewood, 1979). The importance of the whole issue was, however, very much highlighted by exceptionally high (up to tenfold in comparison with the local White population) first admission and first contact rates for schizophrenia in African Caribbeans born in the UK (Harrison et al., 1988; Wessely et al., 1991). The potential importance of this finding as a possible clue to the aetiology of schizophrenia has meant that later studies (e.g. Bhugra et al., 1997) have been most careful to exclude the possibility of misdiagnosis. The very high rates have not been substantiated by later work and may well have related to difficulties in establishing the size and age structure of the African Carib-bean population, but the rate still appears to be twice that in the White population and a degree of validation in terms of a poor prognosis is present, in that the relapse rates in both the work of Birchwood et al. (1992) and Bhugra et al. (1997) are significantly higher than they are in the White (European) subjects studied. Thus, although it seems, from a commonsense point of view, possible that a patient who is not fluent in the language(s) of those who care for him, and may entertain cultural or religious beliefs that they do not share and that carers indeed have no knowledge of may wrongly be diagnosed as psychotic, the extensive work that has been conducted in the UK indicates that this is not the explanation for the high rates of psychosis in immigrants. How frequently it does actually occur is unknown, but from a practical point of view it is important to remember that for the most skilled of psychiatrists diagnosis in a patient whose language and culture are unfamiliar can never be easy, and the help of someone from the patient's own community who will understand what is said and will appreciate the limits of normality of non-Western subcultural or religious beliefs, is likely to be of considerable assistance.

Deafness

A high prevalence of deafness among patients with late onset schizophrenia was noted in the 1960s (Post, 1966), and this has been confirmed in the subsequent studies which have addressed this issue (Cooper et al., 1974; Grahame, 1982; Hassett et al., 1992). Cooper's (1974) study compared rates and types of deafness in patients with late onset paranoid illness with those with manic depressive illness of similarly late onset, and related these to rates of deafness in the general population. The rates in the affectively ill patients were only marginally above those of the general population but rates of deafness in the paranoid patients were much higher. It appeared that in the paranoid patients the deafness was inclined to antedate the psychosis, although this was not true of the affectively ill. While the association between deafness and late onset schizophrenia has been well replicated, the reason for this association has received little formal exploration. The idea that is usually advanced is that in a predisposed personality, deafness enhances a tendency to social isolation, so that partially heard conversations are easily misinterpreted and may form the basis of ideas of reference, and that this situation leads on to the development of paranoid psychosis. While this is plausible, other explanations are, of course, possible.

Although the communication difficulties associated with the deafness of some patients with late paraphrenia may increase their social isolation and promote the development of paranoid beliefs, these difficulties do not interfere with the diagnostic process. Generally such patients do not have problems in conveying their ideas to others. The situation is very different in people with profound prelingual deafness (Denmark, 1985). Children with profound deafness from birth or an early age cannot develop speech and language normally through learning, and will always have limited speech and verbal language skills. Such people are likely to rely upon manual methods of communication, i.e. sign language and finger spelling (Denmark, 1973). In the United Kingdom psychiatric services for the deaf began in the 1960s and the main centre is in Lancashire (Denmark & Warren, 1972). Mental illness certainly does occur in the prelingually deaf and specific diagnoses can appropriately be made. Indeed, standardized diagnoses can be assisted by use of a British Sign Language translation of the Present State Examination (Thacker, 1994). The great difficulties of assessing and treating mental illness in the profoundly deaf, even when using staff who are skilled in manual methods of communication, have been clearly described (Denmark & Eldridge, 1969). They are illustrated by the fact that in a sample of 250 referrals to a tertiary psychiatric service for the deaf (Denmark, 1985) the reason for referral in almost 80% of cases was to clarify whether or not the individual was suffering from a mental illness, although many referrals came from consultant psychiatrists. 40% of the patients did have mental illnesses, more than half of which were diagnosed as schizophrenia, and some of them had got into great difficulties, including being involved in criminal charges. The problems presented by schizophrenia in the profoundly deaf are grave and cannot be appropriately dealt with by those who do not have relevant communication skills. As in other situations where understanding between the psychiatrist and patient cannot be established, the essential elements of management are to remember that inexplicable behaviour may be due to psychosis, and that the situation will be greatly helped by the assistance of someone who can communicate effectively with the patient.

Learning disability

The association between learning disability and schizophrenia has been studied for a long time (Greene, 1930; O'Gorman, 1954) and the historical aspects are the subject of an elegant review by Turner (1989). Relatively recent studies (Reid, 1972; Corbett, 1979) suggest a prevalence figure of about 3% for both current and past illness (i.e. approximately three times the rate in the general population). These figures are based upon studies of people whose learning disability is not severe, and it has been suggested (Forrest & Ogunremi, 1984) that they may be an underestimate because the communication problems of those with more severe learning disability present considerable difficulties for the assessment of psychopathology. It has been established (Meadows et al., 1991) that standardized interviews and criteria for schizophrenia can be successfully applied to those with IQs of 50–70 and that the clinical phenomena in individuals in this intelligence range are similar to those in the generality of cases of schizophrenia. Nonetheless, it is reported (Meadows et al., 1991) that in the learning disabled the emergence of bizarre speech and behaviour can wrongly be attributed to the learning disability itself, leading to delayed or inappropriate treatment. In the study of Doody et al., (1998) described below, such delays between emergence of symptomatology and diagnosis of psychotic illness appeared to occur. It has been suggested that in individuals whose disability is such that they do not have verbal skills, changes in behaviour with an emphasis on posture, movement and social interaction may be considered as a means of assessing mental state including features of psychosis (Fraser et al., 1986). Whether or not an illness which could be appropriately classed as schizophrenia can develop in such individuals is probably not a useful question at the present time, but if the 'tangible morbid underlying process' of the disorder (Chapter 2) is found, it would be sensible to consider it again.

A study comparing individuals with co-morbid learning disability and schizophrenia, with matched cases of (a) schizophrenia and (b) learning disability is currently being conducted in the Edinburgh University Department of Psychiatry (Doody et al., 1995; Doody et al., 1998). Interesting results concerning the occurrence among the co-morbid of a highly familial form of schizophrenia, associated in a significant percentage of cases, with demonstrable chromosomal abnormality (Doody et al., 1998) have been found. Further exploration of these findigs may provide clues to the genetic basis of the disorder. Of relevance to the present issue of communication difficulties leading to diagnostic problems in schizophrenia are not only the delay in diagnosis demonstrated in this study, but also the recurrent difficulties in placement, inconsistent treatment management, and offending behaviour of the co-morbid patients.

Conclusion

In the absence of a diagnostic test for schizophrenia, not all issues relating to differential diagnosis will be able to be resolved, although they may well continue to form the basis of many teaching case conferences and presentations. From a practical clinical point of view, serious consequences of diagnostic difficulties are not commonplace, although they certainly occur. While treatable organic disorders only infrequently underlie schizophrenia-like psychosis, the importance of accurate diagnosis is obvious. Complicating substance misuse is much more frequent. It is not difficult to detect but is at times unwisely ignored in the drawing up of care programmes, where success will be undermined by omissions of this kind. It is not easy to estimate the frequency with which communication difficulties of the various kinds described prevent or delay accurate diagnosis of schizophrenia. The importance of remembering this possibility, so that psychotic individuals who cannot communicate their disturbing experiences to those around them are not left without appropriate management, afraid, unable to care for themselves and perhaps in conflict with the Law, is very clear.

References

American Psychiatric Association 1994. *Diagnostic and Statistical Manual of Mental Disorders (4th edition), DSM 4*. Washington DC: APA.
Anderson, C., Connelly, J., Johnstone, E. C. & Owens, D. G. C. (1991). Cause of death V. In *Disabilities and Circumstances of Schizophrenic Patients – A*

Follow up Study. British Journal of Psychiatry, **159** (Suppl 13), 30–3.

Andreasson, S., Allebeck, P., Engstrom, A. & Rydberg, U. (1987). Cannabis and schizophrenia: a longitudinal study of Swedish conscripts. *Lancet,* **ii,** 1483–5.

Angrist, B. & Gershon, S. (1970). The phenomenology of experimentally induced amphetamine psychosis – preliminary observations. *Biological Psychiatry,* **2,** 95–107.

Baldwin, J. A. (1979). Schizophrenia presenting as physical disease. *Psychological Medicine,* **9,** 611–18.

Bhugra, D., Leff, J., Mallett, R., Der, G., Corridan, B. & Rudge, S. (1997). Incidence and outcome of schizophrenia in Whites, African-Caribbeans and Asians in London. *Psychological Medicine,* **27,** 791–8.

Birchwood, M., Cochrane, R., Macmillan, F., Copestake, S., Kucharska, J. & Cariss, M. (1992). The influence of ethnicity and family structure on relapse in first episode schizophrenia. A comparison of Asian, Afro Caribbean and White patients. *British Journal of Psychiatry,* **161,** 783–90.

Cantwell, R. & Harrison, G. (1996). Substance misuse in the severely mentally ill. *Advances in Psychiatric Treatment,* **2,** 117–24.

Catalan, J. (1990). HIV and AIDS related psychiatric disorder: what can the psychiatrist do? In *Difficulties and Dilemmas in the Management of Psychiatric Patients,* ed. K. Hawton & P. Cowen, pp. 205–17. Oxford: Oxford University Press.

Cochrane, R. (1977). Mental illness in immigrants to England and Wales: an analysis of mental hospital admissions. *Social Psychiatry,* **12,** 23–35.

Connell, P. H. (1958). Amphetamine psychosis. *Maudsley Monograph No. 5.* London: Chapman and Hall.

Cooper, A. F., Garside, R. F. & Kay, D. W. K. (1974). A comparison of deaf and non deaf patients with paranoid and affective psychoses. *British Journal of Psychiatry,* **129,** 532–8.

Corbett, J. (1979). Psychiatric morbidity and mental retardation. In *Psychiatric Illness and Mental Handicap,* ed. P. Snaith & F. E. James, pp. 11–25. Ashford: Headley Brothers.

Crow, T. J., Macmillan, J. F., Johnson, A. L. & Johnstone, E. C. (1986). A randomised controlled trial of prophylactic neuroleptic treatment. *British Journal of Psychiatry,* **148,** 120–7.

Cutting, J. (1987). The phenomenology of acute organic psychosis. *British Journal of Psychiatry,* **151,** 324–32.

Davison, K. & Bagley, C. R. (1969). Schizophrenia-like psychoses associated with organic disorders of the nervous system: a review of the literature. In *Current problems in Neuropsychiatry,* ed. R. N. Herrington, pp. 113–84. Ashford: Headley Brothers.

Denmark, J. C. (1973). The education of deaf children. *Hearing. The Journal of the Royal National Institute for the Deaf.* September 1973.

Denmark, J. C. (1985). A study of 250 patients referred to a department of psychiatry for the deaf. *British Journal of Psychiatry,* **146,** 282–6.

Denmark, J. C. & Eldridge, R. W. (1969). Psychiatric services for the deaf. *Lancet,* **ii,** 259–62.

Denmark, J. C. & Warren, J. (1972). A psychiatric unit for the deaf. *British Journal of Psychiatry,* **120,** 423–8.

Doody, G. A., Owens, D. G. C. & Johnstone, E. C. (1995). The relevance of premorbid cognitive deficit to the concept of neurodevelopmental schizophrenia. *Schizophrenia Research,* **14,** 115.

Doody, G. A., Johnstone, E. C., Sanderson, T. L., Owens, D. G. C. & Muir, W. J. (1998). 'Pfropfschizophrenie' revisited. Schizophrenia in people with mild learning disability. *British Journal of Psychiatry*, **173**, 145–53.

Drake, R. E. & Wallach, M. A. (1989). Substance abuse among the chronically mentally ill. *Hospital and Community Psychiatry*, **40**, 1041–6.

Drake, R. E., McHugo, G. J. & Noordsy, D. L. (1993). A pilot study of outpatient treatment of alcoholism in schizophrenia: four year outcomes. *American Journal of Psychiatry*, **150**, 328–9.

Feinstein, A. & Ron, M. A. (1990). Psychosis associated with demonstrable brain disease. *Psychological Medicine*, **20**, 793–803.

Forrest, A. D. & Ogunremi, O. O. (1984). The prevalence of psychiatric illness in a hospital for the mentally handicapped. *Health Bulletin*, **32**, 198–202.

Fraser, W. I., Lendar, I., Gray, J. & Campbell, I. (1986). Psychiatric and behaviour disturbance in mental handicaps. *Journal of Mental Deficiency Research*, **30**, 49–57.

Geddes,. J., Mercer, G., Frith, C. D., Macmillan, J. F., Owens, D. G. C. & Johnstone, E. C. (1994). Predictors of outcome following a first episode of schizophrenia. *British Journal of Psychiatry*, **165**, 564–8.

Glass, I. B. (1989). Alcholic hallucinosis: a psychiatric enigma. I. The development of an idea. *British Journal of Addiction*, **84**, 29–41.

Grahame, P. S. (1982). Late paraphrenia. *British Journal of Hospital Medicine*, **27**, 522–7.

Greene, R. A. (1930). Psychoses and mental deficiencies, comparisons and relationship. *Journal of Psychoasthenics*, **35**, 128–47.

Griffiths, J. D., Cavanagh, J. & Oates, J. (1972). Paranoid episodes induced by drugs. *Journal of the American Medical Assocation*, **205**, 39–46.

Harrison, G., Owens, D., Holton, A., Neilson, D. & Boot, D. (1988). A prospective study of severe mental disorder in Afro Caribbean patients. *Psychological Medicine*, **18**, 643–57.

Hassett, A. M., Keks, N. A., Jackson, H. J. & Copolov, D. L. (1992). The diagnostic validity of paraphrenia. *Australian & New Zealand Journal of Psychiatry*, **26**, 18–29.

Herrman, H. E., Baldwin, J. A. & Christie, D. (1983). A record linkage study of mortality and general hospital discharge in patients diagnosed as schizophrenic. *Psychological Medicine*, **13**, 581–93.

Hirsch, S. R., Jolley, A. G., Barnes, T. R. E. et al. (1989). Dysphoric and depressive symptoms in chronic schizophrenia. *Schizophrenia Research*, **2**, 259–64.

Hodges, A., Byrne, M., Grant, E. & Johnstone, E. (1999). Subjects at risk of schizophrenia *British Journal of Psychiatry*, **173**, (in press).

Horowitz, M. J. (1969). Flashbacks: recurrent intrusive images after the use of LSD. *American Journal of Psychiatry*, **126**, 565–9.

Humphreys, M., Johnstone, E. C. & Macmillan, J. F. (1994). Offending among first episode schizophrenics. *Journal of Forensic Psychiatry*, **5**, 51–61.

Imade, A. G. T. & Ebie, J. C. (1991). A retrospective study of symptom patterns of cannabis induced psychosis. *Acta Psychiatrica Scandinavica*, **83**, 134–6.

Johnson, S., Ramsay, R., Thornicroft, G. et al. (1997). *London's Mental Health*. London: King's Fund.

Johnstone, E. C., Crow, T. J., Johnson, A. L. & Macmillan, J. F. (1986). The Northwick Park study of first episodes of schizophrenia. 1. Presentation of the illness and problems relating to admission. *British Journal of Psychiatry*, **148**, 115–20.

Johnstone, E. C., Macmillan, J. F. & Crow, T. J. (1987). The occurrence of organic disease of possible aetiological significance in a population of 268 cases of first episode schizophrenia. *Psychological Medicine*, **17**, 371–9.

Johnstone, E. C., Cooling, N. J. & Frith, C. D. (1988). Phenomenology of organic and functional psychoses and the overlap between them. *British Journal of Psychiatry*, **153**, 770–6.

Kane, J. M., Honigfeld, G., Singer, J. & Meltzer, H. (1988). Clozapine for the treatment resistant schizophrenic: a double blind comparison versus chlorpromazine/benztropine. *Archives of General Psychiatry*, **45**, 789–96.

Lewis, N. & Pietrowski, Z. (1954). Clinical diagnosis of manic depressive psychosis. In *Depression*, ed. P. M. Hoch & J. Zubin, pp. 25–38. New York: Greene and Stratton.

Lewis, S. (1995). The secondary schizophrenias. In *Schizophrenia*, ed. S. R. Hirsch & D. R. Weinberger, pp. 324–40. Oxford: Blackwell.

Linszen, D. H., Dingemans, P. M. & Lenior, M. E. (1994). Cannabis abuse and the course of recent onset schizophrenic disorders. *Archives of General Psychiatry*, **51**, 273–9.

Lipsedge, M. & Littlewood, R. (1979). Transcultural psychiatry. In *Recent Advances in Clinical Psychiatry*, ed. K. Granville-Grossman, pp. 91–134. Edinburgh: Churchill Livingstone.

McGlashan, T. H. & Carpenter, W. I. (1976). Post-psychotic depression in schizophrenia. *Archives of General Psychiatry*, **33**, 231–9.

Mackay, R. & Wright, R. (1984). Schizophrenia and anti-social (criminal) behaviour – some responses from sufferers and relatives. *Medicine, Science and the Law*, **24**, 192–8.

Macmillan, J. F. & Johnson, A. L. (1987). Contact with the police in early schizophrenia: its nature, frequency and relevance to the outcome of treatment. *Medicine, Science and the Law*, **27**, 191–200.

Martinez-Arevalo, M. J., Calcedo-Ordonez, A. & Varo-Prieto, J. R. (1994). Cannabis consumption as a prognostic factor in schizophrenia. *British Journal of Psychiatry*, **164**, 679–81.

Mayer-Gross, W. (1920). Uber die stellungsnahme auf abgelanfenen akuten psychose. *Z. Gesamte Neurol Psychiatr.*, **60**, 160–212.

Meadows, G., Turner, T., Campbell, L., Lewis, S. W., Reveley, M. S. & Murray, R. M. (1991). Assessing schizophrenia in adults with mental retardation: a comparative study. *British Journal of Psychiatry*, **158**, 103–5.

Menezes, P., Johnson, S., Thornicroft, G. et al. (1996). Drug and alcohol problems among individuals with severe mental illness in South London. *British Journal of Psychiatry*, **168**, 612–19.

Mercer, G., Finlayson, A., Johnstone, E. C., Murray, C. & Owens, D. G. C. (1997). A study of enhanced management in patients with treatment-resistant schizophrenia. *Journal of Psychopharmacology*, **11**, 349–56.

Odegaard, O. (1932). Emigration and insanity. *Acta Psychiatrica et Neurologica*, Supplement 4.

O'Gorman, G. (1954). Psychosis as a cause of mental deficit. *Journal of Mental Science*, **100**, 934–43.

Post, F. (1966). *Persistent Persecutory State in the Elderly*. Oxford: Pergamon.

Regier, D. A., Farmer, M. E., Rae, D. S. et al. (1990). Comorbidity of mental disorders with alcohol and other drug abuse: results from the Epidemiological Catchment Area (ECA) study. *Journal of the American Medical Association*, **264**, 2511–18.

Reid, A. H. (1972). Psychoses in adult mental defectives. I. Manic depressive psychoses. II. Schizophrenia and paranoid psychoses. *British Journal of Psychiatry*, **120**, 205–18.

Sheldrick, C., Jablensky, A., Sartorius, N. & Shepherd, M. (1977). Schizophrenia succeeded by affective illness: catamnestic study and statistical enquiry. *Psychological Medicine*, **7**, 619–24.

Siris, S. G. (1991). Diagnosis of secondary depression in schizophrenia: implications for DSM IV. *Schizophrenia Bulletin*, **17**, 75–98.

Siris, S. G., Adam, F., Cohen, M., Mandeli, J., Aronson, E. & Casey, E. (1988). Postpsychotic depression and negative symptoms: an investigation of syndromal overlap. *American Journal of Psychiatry*, **145**, 1532–7.

Tennant, F. S. & Groesbeck, C. J. (1972). Psychiatric effects of hashish. *Archives of General Psychiatry*, **27**, 133.

Thacker, A. J. (1994). Formal Communication Disorder – sign language in deaf people with schizophrenia. *British Journal of Psychiatry*, **165**, 818–23.

Turner, T. H. (1989). Schizophrenia and mental handicap: an historical review with implications for further research. *Psychological Medicine*, **19**, 301–14.

Victor, M. (1966). Treatment of alchol intoxication and the withdrawal syndrome. *Psychosomatic Medicine*, **28**, 636–50.

Victor, M. & Hope, J. M. (1958). The phenomenon of auditory hallucinations in chronic alcoholism. A critical evaluation of the status of alcoholic hallucinosis. *Journal of Nervous & Mental Disease*, **126**, 451–81.

Wessely, S., Castle, D., Der, G. & Murray, R. (1991). Schizophrenia and Afro Caribbeans: a case control study. *British Journal of Psychiatry*, **159**, 795–801.

Will, R. G., Ironside, J. W., Zeidler, M. et al. (1996). A new variant of Creutzfeldt–Jakob disease in the UK. *Lancet*, **347**, 921–5.

World Health Organization (1973). *Report of the International Pilot Study of Schizophrenia.* Geneva: WHO.

World Health Organization (1992). *Manual of the International Statistical Classification of Diseases, Injuries and Causes of Death (I.C.D. 10).* Geneva: WHO.

Wyatt, R. J., Green, M. F. & Tuma, A. H. (1997). Long term morbidity associated with delayed treatment of first admission schizophrenic patients: a re-analysis of the Camarillo State Hospital data. *Psychological Medicine*, **27**, 261–8.

Zeidler, M., Johnstone, E. C., Bamber, R. W. K. et al. (1997). New Variant Creutzfeldt–Jakob disease: psychiatric features. *Lancet*, **350**, 908–10.

4

The pharmacological basis of schizophrenia

The pharmacological treatment of schizophrenia, like most pharmacological treatments in medicine, began with empirical discovery of drugs that alleviated symptoms of psychosis. The root of the plant *Rauwolfia serpentina* had been used to treat insanity for several centuries. In 1952 the alkaloid reserpine was identified as the active substance in extracts from *Rauwolfia serpentina* (Frankenburg, 1994). The first synthetic antipsychotic drug was the phenothiazine, chlorpromazine (Delay & Deniker, 1952). The development of the phenothiazines was not based on an understanding of their pharmacological actions or an understanding of the mechanism of production of psychotic symptoms. The fact that the drugs were clinically effective provided the drive to better understand their pharmacological action. This has in turn led to the development of hypotheses relating to the mechanism of production of symptoms. More recent advances in neuroscience have enhanced our knowledge of neurotransmission in the brain. This has allowed the refining of hypotheses regarding drug action and the pharmacological mechanism of schizophrenia as well as providing a theoretical basis for the development of new pharmacological agents.

A further source of hypotheses regarding the pharmacological basis of schizophrenia comes from the elucidation of the pharmacology of drugs that induce psychotic symptoms. Compounds that are known to induce psychosis include lysergic acid diethylamide (LSD), L-dihydroxyphenylalanine (L-DOPA), cocaine, amphetamine and phencyclidine (PCP). The drug-induced psychoses do not exactly mimic the entire clinical picture of schizophrenia, but do produce individual symptoms that are clinically the same as those occurring in schizophrenia.

The demonstration of a biochemical disturbance in the brain that would provide a pharmacological explanation of the symptoms of schizophrenia remains an elusive goal.

The relevance of different neurotransmitter systems to schizophrenia will be discussed. Discussion will focus on hypotheses derived from the understanding of the pharmacology of antipsychotics and psycho-tomimetic drugs as well as investigations of the transmitters themselves in patients with schizophrenia.

Dopamine

The antipsychotic mechanism of typical neuroleptics

The phenothiazines, butyrophenones and thioxanthines share similar pharmacological properties and are referred to as typical neuroleptics. The newer generation of antipsychotics (including drugs such as clozapine and risperidone) are referred to as atypical neuroleptics. They are effective in some patients with schizophrenia whose symptoms have proved resistant to typical neuroleptics. Atypical neuroleptics also have different side-effects and different pharmacological actions from the typical neuroleptics. All of these drugs have effects on a range of different neurotransmitter systems.

It was the side-effect of parkinsonism induced by the typical neuroleptics that gave the first clue to their mechanism of action (Flugel, 1953). Hor-nykiewicz (1973) had related parkinsonism to depletion of dopamine from the basal ganglia. Carlsson & Lindqvist (1963) demonstrated the selective effects of antipsychotic drugs on central dopamine turnover. Furthermore, the antipsychotic drugs are able to reverse amphetamine-induced abnormal behaviours in laboratory animals that are dependent upon central dopamine release (Randrup & Munkvad, 1965). The significance of dopamine was also suggested by the action of reserpine which depletes stores of monoamines, including dopamine, in nerve terminals (Rang & Dale, 1991). The relevance of dopaminergic mechanisms to the therapeutic action of the typical neuro-leptic drugs was supported by the finding that there is a strong correlation between the clinical potency of these drugs and their ability to block dopamine D_2 receptors in vitro assays (Seeman et al., 1976; Burt et al., 1977; Peroutka & Snyder, 1980).

Dopamine receptors have been sub-typed into D_1, D_2, D_3, D_4 and D_5 (Kandel, 1991). The D_1 and D_5 receptors are expressed in neurones of the cortex and hippocampus and are coupled to a G-protein that activates adenylate cyclase. Dopamine D_2 receptors are expressed in neurones of the caudate and limbic systems and parts of the cerebral cortex. They are further subtyped into D_{2a} and D_{2b}. The D_{2a} receptors are linked to an inhibitory G-protein that increases phospoinositide turnover. D_3 and D_4

receptors are expressed in the limbic system and cortex and only weakly expressed in the basal ganglia.

Understanding of the pharmacology of the neuroleptics in alleviating psychotic symptoms led to the formulation of the 'dopamine hypothesis' of schizophrenia – that schizophrenia is a manifestation of a hyper-dopaminergic state. Since dopamine D_2 receptors seemed to be the important site of action of antipsychotic drugs, new drug development was targeted towards compounds that blocked D_2 receptors.

Much of the testing of the dopamine hypothesis has been laboratory based. A clinical study was carried out involving a comparison of the antipsychotic efficacy of stereoisomers of flupenthixol (Johnstone et al., 1978), since it had been shown that only the cis-isomer possesses significant activity in blocking dopamine receptors (Miller et al., 1974; Enna et al., 1976). The study blindly compared three groups of patients with acute schizophrenia, one receiving cis-flupenthixol, one trans-flupenthixol and one an inactive placebo. All patients showed a significant ($p < 0.05$) improvement. Improvement was significantly greater in the patients on cis-flupenthixol than those in the placebo and trans-flupenthixol groups, who showed similar improvement to one another. The result is consistent with the hypothesis that antipsychotic efficacy is dependent upon dopamine receptor blockade. However, it did not rule out serotonin receptor antagonism as being of at least some relevance (the cis-isomer being significantly more effective as a serotonin antagonist).

Psychosis induced by drugs that increase dopaminergic activity

The fact that several drugs that induce schizophrenia-like psychoses have actions which increase dopaminergic activity has lent support to hypotheses of the involvement of dopaminergic systems in schizophrenia. Examples of such drugs include the following:

Amphetamine

In 1958 a syndrome closely resembling paranoid schizophrenia was described in subjects who had taken large doses of amphetamine (Green & Costain, 1981). This psychosis usually resolves over a few days as the drug is excreted. In low doses the major effect of amphetamines is to release dopamine. At high doses amphetamines also release serotonin and noradrenaline. Amphetamine can also inhibit reuptake of monoamines by nerve terminals, thus potentiating dopamine mediated behaviours. As described above, the antipsychotic drugs are able to reverse amphetamine-induced abnormal behaviours in animals (Randrup & Munkvad, 1965).

Cocaine

In large doses, cocaine may induce a paranoid psychosis, often with tactile hallucinations. The pharmacological action of cocaine is to inhibit neuronal uptake of noradrenaline and dopamine (Green & Costain, 1981).

L-DOPA

L-DOPA, a dopamine precursor used in the treatment of Parkinson's disease, can induce a paranoid psychosis similar to schizophrenia.

Dopamine in the brain

Though dopamine blockade is important in the antipsychotic action of typical neuroleptic drugs, evidence to suggest an increase of dopamine in the brains of patients with schizophrenia is lacking. Measurement of homovanillic acid (HVA), a metabolite of dopamine, in the cerebrospinal fluid (CSF) has shown no consistent difference between unmedicated patients with schizophrenia and controls (Lieberman & Koreen, 1993). Treatment with antipsychotic medication increases the level of HVA in the CSF. Post-mortem studies have also shown no differences in synthesis and degradation of dopamine between schizophrenic and control samples (Cooper et al., 1991).

Current status of the dopamine hypothesis

Though dopamine mechanisms are involved in the therapeutic actions of the typical neuroleptic drugs, the symptoms of many patients with schizophrenia are not relieved by these drugs. Furthermore, the drugs are able to alleviate the symptoms of other psychoses, e.g. manic psychoses and drug-induced psychoses. This suggests that the antipsychotic effect of dopamine blockade is not specific for schizophrenia. The symptoms of some patients with schizophrenia who have failed to respond to the typical neuroleptics are responsive to the atypical neuroleptics. These drugs act on several neurotransmitter systems. It has been hypothesized that their antipsychotic action is due to effects other than on the dopamine system or due to combined neurotransmitter effects. Though a primary abnormality of dopamine neurotransmission alone cannot be excluded as being the basis for the symptoms of some patients, it does not appear to provide the pharmacological basis of symptoms for all patients with schizophrenia.

Serotonin

Serotonin, also known as 5-hydroxytryptamine (5HT), has long been hypothesized to be associated with mental illness.

Psychotomimetic drugs and serotonin

Lysergic acid diethylamide (LSD) is a potent hallucinogen, active at microgram doses. Though the psychological phenomena of the acute state of intoxication differ from schizophrenia, there seems to be a risk of a more prolonged schizophrenia-like reaction in some individuals. The major pharmacological property of LSD is its propensity for 5-HT receptors. It is similar in structure to 5-HT and can act at different locations as a 5-HT agonist and as an antagonist (Green & Costain, 1981). It also has actions on dopaminergic systems (Kelly & Iversen, 1975). It is not clear whether the hallucinogenic properties of LSD are related to its 5-HT or dopaminergic effects.

Antipsychotic drugs and serotonin

There has been renewed interest in the 5-HT system in schizophrenia because of the development of the atypical neuroleptics, many of which have potent activity at 5-HT receptors. It has been hypothesized that the combination of activities at dopamine and 5-HT receptors accounts for the antipsychotic activity of atypical neuroleptics. There is an interaction between serotonin and dopamine such that serotonin systems inhibit dopaminergic systems in the midbrain as well as in the terminal dopaminergic fields in the forebrain (Kapur & Remington, 1996).

Serotonin in the brain

Direct neurochemical evidence of dysfunction of the 5-HT system in the brain of patients with schizophrenia is lacking (Lieberman & Koreen, 1993).

Noradrenaline

It has been hypothesized that noradrenaline plays an important role in the pathophysiology of schizophrenia (Hornykiewicz, 1982; van Kammen, 1991). These hypotheses are based on the relationship of the synthetic pathways of dopamine and noradrenaline, empirical data on noradrenergic measures in other neuropsychiatric disease and experimentally demonstrated interactions between dopaminergic and noradrenergic systems in the central nervous system. As with other neurotransmitters, there has been no clear demonstration of abnormal noradrenergic activity in patients with schizophrenia (Lieberman & Koreen, 1993). Noradrenergic neurones may be suppressed by antipsychotic drug treatment and activated upon drug withdrawal and immediately before symptom exacerbations. Clozapine has potent effects on the noradrenergic system which may be related to its antipsychotic properties.

Excitatory amino acids

Interest in the role of excitatory amino acids in the pathogenesis of schizophrenia was stimulated by the finding that phencyclidine (PCP), a potent psychotomimetic which causes symptoms similar to those of schizophrenia, was a non-competitive antagonist of the N-methyl-D-aspartate subtype of glutamate receptors (Javitt & Zukin, 1991). Unlike amphetamine-induced psychosis, PCP-induced psychosis incorporates both positive and negative schizophrenic symptoms. There is as yet little data regarding excitatory amino acid activity in schizophrenia. Findings reported include decreased glutamate binding in medial temporal cortical areas of post-mortem brains of schizophrenic patients (Kerwin et al., 1988; Deakin et al., 1989) and increased glutamate binding in the frontal cortex (Deakin et al., 1989).

Gamma-amino-butyric acid (GABA)

GABA is the most abundant inhibitory neurotransmitter in the brain. It has long been hypothesized to play a role in the pathophysiology of schizophrenia. Post-mortem studies have tended to find a reduction of GABA in the brains of patients with schizophrenia, though there has not been consistency in the results and the confounding effects of antipsychotic medication cannot be excluded (Lieberman & Koreen, 1993). A decrease in GABA uptake sites has been found in hippocampus in post-mortem brains of schizophrenic subjects (Reynolds et al., 1990). This probably reflects decreased neuronal numbers in patients with schizophrenia.

Peptides

Since neuropeptides were demonstrated to act as neurotransmitters, co-transmitters and neuromodulators, their possible significance in schizophrenia has been of interest. Amongst the most studied neuropeptides are cholesystokinin (CCK), neurotensin, substance P and somatostatin.

CCK

The report of the coexistence of CCK and dopamine in a subset of mesencephalic dopaminergic neurones (Hökfelt et al., 1980) suggested that it may be of some relevance to schizophrenia. CCK has been found to display characteristics of a neuromodulator or neurotransmitter. Dopamine and CCK have been found to interact at pre and post-synaptic levels in the nucleus accumbens. In animal studies, CCK antagonists reduced the activity of dopaminergic neurones in the midbrain (Rasmussen et al., 1991). Measurement of CCK in cerebrospinal fluid (CSF) and post-mortem brains has shown no consistent increase or decrease in schizophrenic subjects compared with controls (Lieberman & Koreen, 1993). CCK has been tried as a treatment for schizophrenia, but no significant antipsychotic effect has been found (Montgomery & Green, 1988).

Neurotensin

Neurotensin has also been shown to be co-localized with dopamine in hypothalamic and midbrain neurones and mimics the action of antipsychotic drugs when administered centrally (Lieberman & Koreen, 1993). In patients with schizophrenia CSF levels of neurotensin are lowered (Nemeroff et al., 1989). A low CSF neurotensin has been found to be associated with a therapeutic response to drug treatment (Garver et al., 1991).

Substance P

Substance P has a widespread distribution in the central nervous system and interacts with the dopamine system. Measurements of substance P in the post-mortem brains of patients with schizophrenia have been inconsistent (Takeuchi et al., 1988). No differences in CSF substance P have been found between schizophrenics and controls (Heikkila et al., 1990).

Somatostatin

Somatostatin has a widespread distribution throughout the CNS. Somatostatin stimulates dopamine release in the striatum and dopamine release in the striatum and dopamine in turn stimulates somatostatin release from various regions. In post-mortem studies of schizophrenic brains, decreased somatostatin concentrations have been found in the hippocampus (Ferrier et al., 1983) and frontal cortex (Nemeroff et al., 1983). The results of studies of somatostatin in the CSF have been less consistent (Lieberman & Koreen, 1993).

Phospholipids

As well as their importance in membrane structure, fatty acids or their metabolites are involved in a wide range of actions in intracellular second messenger systems. The behaviour of receptors may differ quite markedly depending on the composition of the membrane in which they are embedded. A single change in membrane structure could produce changes in the behaviour of all the receptor types associated with that membrane (Horrobin et al., 1994). Abnormalities have been found in the fatty acid composition of plasma phospholipids in patients with schizophrenia. The most consistent finding has been a reduction in linoleic acid (Lieberman & Koreen, 1993). Levels of 20 and 22 carbon unsaturated fatty acids have been shown to be lower in patients with schizophrenia who manifest mainly negative symptoms (Glen et al., 1994).

Conclusion

The development of antipsychotic medication has led to a greater understanding of neuropharmacology and spawned many hypotheses about the pharmacological basis of schizophrenia. Developments in basic neuroscience have independently led to further hypotheses and means of testing them either in the laboratory or clinically. With further advances, pharmacological mechanisms appear to be ever more complex, with proliferation of molecules that act as transmitters and modulators, burgeoning receptor subtypes, and more diverse second messenger systems. As yet there is no single pharmacological explanation for schizophrenia. A possible reason for this is that the clinical manifestations of schizophrenia represent a final common pathway of symptoms due to heterogeneous causes. However, current understanding has yet to explain the subtlety of interplay of transmitter and receptor systems, how they function in health and how they might be perturbed when mental functioning is disturbed.

References

Burt, D. R., Creese, I. & Snyder, S. H. (1977). Antischizophrenic drugs: chronic treatment elevates dopamine receptor binding in the brain. *Science*, **196**, 326–8.

Carlsson, A. & Lindqvist, M. (1963). Effect of chlorpromazine and haloperidol on formation of 3-methoxy-tyramine and normetanephrine in mouse brain. *Acta Pharmacologica Toxicologica*, **20**, 140–4.

Cooper, J. R., Bloom, F. E. & Roth, R. H. (1991). *The Biochemical Basis of Neuropharmacology*. Oxford University Press: Oxford.

Deakin, J. F. W., Slater, P., Simpson, M. D. C., et al. (1989). Frontal cortical and left temporal glutamatergic dysfunction in schizophrenia. *Journal of Neurochemistry*, **52**, 1781–6.

Delay, J. & Deniker, P. (1952). Le traitment des psychoses par une methode neurolyptique derive de l'hibernotherapie. In *Neurologistes de France*, ed. P. Cossa, pp. 497–502. Paris & Luxembourg. Masson et cie, Librares de L'academie de medicine.

Enna, S. J., Bennett, J. P., Burt, D. R., Cresse, I. & Snyder, S. H. (1976). Stereospecificity of interaction of neuroleptic drugs with neurotransmitters and correlation with clinical potency. *Nature (London)*, **263**, 338–47.

Ferrier, I. N., Roberts, G. W., Crow, T. J., et al. (1983). Reduced cholecystokinin-like and somatostatin-like immuno-reactivity in limbic lobe is associated with negative symptoms in schizophrenia. *Life Sciences*, **33**, 475–82.

Flugel, F. (1953). Therapeutique par medication neuroleptique obtenue en realisant systematiquement des etats parkinsoniformes. *L'Encephale*, **45**, 1090–2.

Frankenburg, F. R. (1994). History of the development of antipsychotic medication. *Psychiatric Clinics of North America*, **17**, 531–40.

Garver, D. L., Bisette, G., Yao, J. K. & Nemeroff, C. B. (1991). Relation of CSF neurotensin concentrations to symptoms and drug response of psychotic patients. *American Journal of Psychiatry*, **148**, 484–8.

Glen, A. I. M., Glen, E. M. T., Horrobin, D. F., et al. (1994). A red cell membrane abnormality in a subgroup of schizophrenic patients: evidence for two diseases. *Schizophrenia Research*, **12**, 53–61.

Green, A. R. & Costain, D. W. (1981). *Pharmacology and Biochemistry of Psychiatric Disorders*. London: John Wiley & Sons.

Heikkila, L., Rimon, R. & Terenius, L. (1990). Dynorphin A and substance P in the cerebrospinal fluid of schizophrenic patients. *Psychiatry Research*, **34**, 229–36.

Hökfelt, T., Rehfeld, J. F., Skirboll, L., Ivemark, B., Goldstein, M. & Markey, K. (1980). Evidence for co-existence of dopamine and CCK in mesolimbic neurons. *Nature*, **285**, 476–8.

Hornykiewicz, O. (1973). Dopamine in the basal ganglia. Its role and therapeutic implications. *British Medical Bulletin*, **29**, 172–8.

Hornykiewicz, O. (1982). Brain catecholamines in schizophrenia: a good case for noradrenaline. *Nature*, **229**, 484–6.

Horrobin, D. F., Glen, A. I. M. & Vaddad, K. (1994). The membrane hypothesis of schizophrenia. *Schizophrenia Research*, **13**, 195–207.

Javitt, D. C. & Zukin, S. R. (1991). Recent advances in the phencyclidine model of schizophrenia. *American Journal of Psychiatry*, **148**, 1301–8.

Johnstone, E. C., Crow, T. J., Frith, C. D., Carney, M. W. P. & Price, J. S. (1978).

References

Mechanism of the antipsychotic effect in the treatment of acute schizophrenia. *Lancet*, **i**, 848–51.

Kandel, E. (1991). Disorders of thought: schizophrenia. In *Principles of Neural Science*, ed. E. R. Kandel, J. H. Schwartz & T. M. Jessel, pp. 853–68. Elsevier: New York.

Kapur, S. & Remington, G. (1996). Serotonin-dopamine interaction and its relevance to schizophrenia. *American Journal of Psychiatry*, **153**, 466–76.

Kelly, P. H. & Iversen, L. L. (1975). LSD as an agonist at mesolimbic dopamine receptors. *Psychopharmacologia*, **45**, 221.

Kerwin, R. W., Patel, S., Meldrum, B. S., Czudek, D. & Reynolds, G. P. (1988). Asymmetrical loss of a glutamate receptor subtype in left hippocampus in schizophrenia. *Lancet*, **1**, 583–4.

Lieberman, J. A. & Koreen, A. R. (1993). Neurochemistry and neuroendocrinology of schizophrenia: a selective review. *Schizophrenia Bulletin*, **19**, 371–429.

Miller, R. J., Horn, A. S. & Iversen, L. L. (1947). The action of neuroleptic drugs on dopamine stimulated adenosine cyclic $3'5'$ monophosphate production in neostriatum and limbic forebrain. *Molecular Pharmacology*, **10**, 759–66.

Montgomery, S. A. & Green, M. (1988). The use of cholecystokinin in schizophrenia: a review. *Psychological Medicine*, **18**, 593–603.

Nemeroff, C. B., Youngblood, W. W., Manberg, P. J., Prange, A. L. & Kizer, J. S. (1983). Regional brain concentrations of neuropeptides in Huntington's chorea and schizophrenia. *Science*, **221**, 972–5.

Nemeroff, C. B., Bisette, G., Widerlov, E., et al. (1989). Neurotensin-like immunoreactivity in cerebrospinal fluid in patients with schizophrenia, depression, anorexia nervosa, bulimia, and premenstrual syndrome. *Journal of Neuropsychiatry*, **1**, 16–20.

Peroutka, S. J. & Snyder, S. H. (1980). Relationship of neuroleptic drug effects at brain dopamine serotonin adrenergic and histamine receptors to clinical potency. *American Journal of Psychiatry*, **137**, 1518–22.

Randrup, A. & Munkvad, I. (1965). Special antagonism of amphetamine-induced abnormal behaviours. *Psychopharmacologica*, **7**, 416–22.

Rang, H. P. & Dale, M. M. (1991). *Pharmacology*. Churchill Livingstone: Edinburgh.

Rasmussen, K., Stockton, M., Czachura, J. & Howbert, J. (1991). Cholecystokinin and schizophrenia: the selective CCKb antagonist LY26691 decreased midbrain dopamine unit activity. *European Journal of Pharmacology*, **9**, 515–24.

Reynolds, G. P., Czudek, C. & Andrews, H. B. (1990). Deficit and hemispheric asymmetry of GABA uptake sites in the hippocampus in schizophrenia. *Biological Psychiatry*, **27**, 1308–44.

Seeman, P., Lee, T., Chau-Wong, M. & Wong, K. (1976). Antipsychotic drug doses and neuroleptic/dopamine receptors. *Nature*, **261**, 717–19.

Takeuchi, K., Uematsu, M., Ofuji, M., Morikiyo, M. & Kaiya, H. (1988). Substance P involved in mental disorders. *Progress in Neuro-Psychopharmcology and Biological Psychiatry*, **12**, 5157–64.

Van Kammen, D. P. (1991). The biochemical basis of relapse and drug response in schizophrenia: review and hypothesis. *Psychological Medicine*, **21**, 881–95.

athology and brain imaging in
irenia

Introduction

The resurgence of interest in the neuropathology and neuropsychology of schizophrenia over the past decade parallels the development of sensitive tools for in vivo imaging of the structure and function of the brain. These approaches have secured definite advances in our understanding of the pathophysiology of the disorder and are among the first pieces of evidence cited in any account of schizophrenia as a brain disease. Indeed, the current proliferation of imaging studies during cognitive or pharmacological activation and the increasing availability of non-invasive techniques such as functional magnetic resonance imaging is, in this author's opinion, as likely as any area of study to lead to further advances in the relatively near future.

This chapter covers a large body of work in a relatively limited space. This is achieved by focusing on well replicated findings and the most plausible recent developments – particularly those that can be integrated with other results. Macroscopic and microscopic neuropathology will be discussed first (post-mortem neurochemistry being part of the previous chapter). Structural imaging will then be reviewed, with a brief summary of the methodology and possible artifacts of each technique, the main findings in schizophrenia and their relation to key clinical characteristics, and a consideration of disease specificity. The section on functional imaging will follow a similar pattern. Finally, an attempt will be made to integrate the results from these various disciplines, before finishing with a consideration of future experimental directions.

Neuropathology

The history of neuropathology in schizophrenia has been discussed in Chapter 1 and will not be repeated here. Suffice it to say that very little work was done for 50 years, until the demonstration of gross morphological abnormalities on computerized tomography. Since then, however, a host of researchers have examined the size of various parts of the brain (macroscopic neuropathology) and looked for putative reductions in cell numbers or abnormal patterns of neuronal organization (microscopic neuropathology).

Macroscopic neuropathology

Bogerts et al. (1985) were among the first of the new generation of neuro-pathologists to complete a study. They examined the brains of 13 patients (three male) and nine controls (six male) with a similarly acute cause of death but no neuropsychiatric disease, although the controls were on average ten years older at the time of death. All the brains had been collected between 1928 and 1953, before the advent of neuroleptics, and none of the patients had been exposed to any form of convulsive therapy. Three regions in the striatum (caudate, putamen, accumbens) and in the temporal lobe (hippocampus, parahippocampus, amygdala), as well as the pallidum and the inferior horn of the lateral ventricle, were outlined on projected enlargements. A planimeter was used to calculate outlined areas and volumes were derived by taking account of the brain slice thickness and the distance between slices. Although the researchers attempted to remain blind to diagnosis, in practice this was difficult as most of the schizophrenics could be recognized by their unusually small hippocampi. Several statistically significant volume reductions were found in the schizo-phrenic brains – of the parahippocampus (by 44%), hippocampus (32%), amygdala (22%), pallidium (20%) – while the lateral ventricle horn was non-significantly 24% larger. The mean fresh brain weight was similar in patients and controls (2% smaller), basal ganglia structures were only 2–5% smaller in schizophrenic patients, and none of the above structures showed any apparent sex difference. The post-mortem delays and his-tological processing were apparently similar in all subjects and therefore an unlikely cause of the observed differences. However, only the left hemi-sphere was available for examination and no nutritional information was available – although previous studies of institutionalized Huntingdon's patients had not shown similar changes.

Subsequent studies have used similar techniques but generally in larger samples. Brown et al. (1986) obtained the brains of all those with psychosis who died in one institution over 22 years. After excluding those without typical schizophrenia or affective disorder, and those with neurological disease, they were left with the brains of 41 schizophrenics and 29 affectives.

Fixed brain weight was 6% lighter in the schizophrenics, who also had substantially increased temporal horn areas (97%) and thinner parahippocampi (11%) bilaterally but particularly on the left side. Pakkenberg (1987) reported a brain weight reduction of 8% in 29 schizophrenics as compared with 30 controls, accompanied by a 33% increased volume of the ventricular system, that was apparently attributable to a loss of cortical (12%) and central grey (6%) matter, as white matter volumes were no different. Jeste & Lohr (1989) replicated the findings of volume reductions in the hippocampus and found them to be most marked anteriorly on the left side. In a new series of brains, collected between 1985 and 1988, Bogerts et al. (1990a,b) again found large reductions of hippocampal and pallidal volumes that were bilateral but most marked in males. This group have since also found some evidence for abnormalities of temporal lobe asymmetry in schizophrenia – with reduced Sylvian fissure lengths on the left side and larger planum temporale on the right side (rather than the left as in controls) particularly in male patients (Falkai et al., 1995).

One final report merits particular mention as the brains were collected prospectively as part of a series of clinical studies. Bruton et al. (1990) compared the brains of 56 schizophrenic patients and 56 age- and sex-matched controls. They reported reduced fixed brain weight (by 4.5%) and length (4%), and an increased ventricular size on inspection. In keeping with one previous report (Stevens, 1982), there was a high rate (43%) of pathological changes such as infarcts, but there was no evidence of a link between these abnormalities and gliosis (that would suggest an acquired inflammatory process). Rather, the findings generally correlate with measures of pre-morbid functioning, as described in a previous study (Pakkenberg, 1987), suggesting a developmental disruption that may also confer a vulnerability to other neuropathology.

In summary, there is good evidence from gross post-mortem studies that the brain is generally smaller in schizophrenics, particularly in limbic structures such as the (para)hippocampus, that the ventricles are enlarged, and that these changes are developmental rather than acquired. In recent years, there has been less interest in macroscopic abnormalities but there has been a much greater amount of research attempting to establish their microscopic associations.

Microscopic neuropathology

These studies have focused on the temporal and frontal lobes. Kovelman & Scheibel (1984) reported pyramidal cell disorganization in the hippocampus, particularly in the anterior and middle portions, the pattern of which they considered to be indicative of abnormal neuronal migration. Hippocampal disorganization as such has only been partially replicated (Luts et al., 1998). However, some groups have reported a reduction of pyramidal cell numbers in the hippocampus (Falkai & Bogerts, 1986; Jeste & Lohr, 1989), and others have found smaller cells but normal cell density (Arnold et al., 1995) or smaller cells of abnormal shape (Zaidel et al., 1997).

In a series of studies, Benes and colleagues have concentrated on the frontal lobe and particularly the cingulate gyrus. They first described a reduction in the number of neurones in pre-frontal (layer VI), cingulate (V) and motor (III) cortex (Benes et al., 1986). This was followed by findings of smaller, more dispersed cells in layer II of the cingulate (Benes & Bird, 1987) and an increase in the amount of vertical (association) axons (Benes et al., 1987) – suggesting a loss of local inter-neurones rather than a loss of pyramidal projections. They were subsequently able to confirm these reductions of cells in layer II of pre-frontal and anterior cingulate cortex (Benes et al., 1991). Hypothesizing that this reduction was of inhibitory basket cells, they predicted that a compensatory upregulation of Gamma-aminobutyric acid-A (GABA-A) receptors would lead to increased binding of bicuilline in layers II and III but not V or VI of the cingulate gyrus – a prediction they confirmed in a comparison of six schizophrenics with 'affective disturbance' and eight healthy control brains (Benes et al., 1992). As methodical and interesting as these findings are, they have yet to be replicated. Selemon et al. (1995) reported an increased density of pyramidal neurones in layers III–VI of the prefrontal area 9 in 16 schizophrenics, but they also found an increase in the occipital lobe and thinner cortex (suggesting either confounding by differential fixation time or generalized cellular atrophy), and others have failed to find reduced interneurone densities (Akbarian et al., 1995). Indeed, some researchers have studied GABA-A receptor binding with functional imaging techniques in vivo and generally failed to find abnormalities (see below).

Akbarian et al. (1993a,b) have also used immunocytochemistry to focus on neurones containing nicotinamide-adenine dinecleotide phosphate-dia-phorase (NADPH-d). This enzyme is a crucial component of the oxidative phosphorylation, energy generating, cell machinery and cells expressing it are curiously resistant to degenerative diseases. In five schizophrenics, the researchers found reduced numbers of NADPH-d immunoreactive neur-ones in the cortical grey matter and superficial white matter of the frontal lobes, but an increase in deep white matter numbers (Akarian et al., 1993a). Similarly, numbers were reduced in the hippocampus and temporal neocortex, but increased in lateral temporal white matter and parahip-pocampus (Akbarian et al., 1993b). Not only do these findings suggest a pervasive and generalized developmental (second trimester) defect of neur-onal migration, but they could also be a means whereby other migrating cells may not be able to establish normal cortical connections and disturb fronto-temporal functioning. However, external replication is awaited and abnormally positioned cells do not necessarily cause malfunction.

Unfortunately, all this microscopic work is encouraging rather than definitive. The current consensus is that neuronal numbers are essentially normal in schizophrenia but that neuronal connections and circuitary are disturbed. It may be, as Shapiro (1993) suggested after a comprehensive review of neuropathology findings in schizophrenia, that little further progress will be made until researchers start to work more closely together, particularly obtaining and sharing larger samples.

Computed tomography (CT)

CT images are obtained by reconstructing multiple projections of X-ray attenuations by the object of interest – accurate measurement of trans-missions depending on the sensitivity of photomultiplier tubes and a sodium iodide detector. The independent realization of this possibility earned Cormack & Hounsfield the 1979 Nobel prize for medicine and physiology.

Limitations of the technique

The technique is limited to imaging a single 'slice' of brain in one (axial) plane, and can only generate area measurements. The main potential artifacts in CT scanning, given that X-ray source and detection are correct-ly aligned and calibrated, arise from 'beam hardening' and 'partial volume effects'. Beam hardening refers to effects of the absorption of lower energy X-ray photons as they pass through dense structures such as bone, so that the beam becomes composed of higher energy rays and attentuation values are lowered. In general, therefore, peripheral structures are assigned rela-tively less dense CT values; specifically, CT is an unreliable technique for imaging the posterior fossa and temporal lobes. Partial volume effects are common to all imaging methods, arising from the fitting of non-linear anatomy to linear geometry and leading to a loss of resolu-tion.

As a result, boundary tissues tend to be assigned the average characteris-tics of adjacent tissues. It is for these reasons that comparing absolute CT or Hounsfield numbers, as measures of 'cerebral density', can be highly misleading. Moreover, partial volume effects are greater with low resolution methods such as CT, where comparatively thick slices are used, such that most researchers have concluded that CT cannot give reliable information on regional abnormalities (Pearlson et al., 1989).

Main findings

CT scanning in schizophrenia has however, been able to reliably demonstrate an increase in the size of the ventricular system and of cortical sulci. It has also been used to study the clinical associations and course of such abnormalities, although few firm conclusions can be made from this work. The first study in schizophrenia, in which the outline of the lateral ventricles and the brain were traced by planimetry and a ventricle: brain ratio (VBR) was calculated, showed a relative ventriculomegaly that was most pronounced in those with cognitive impairment (Johnstone et al., 1976). The finding of ventriculomegaly in (chronic) schizophrenia was soon replicated (Weinberger et al., 1979) and has been since in more than 50 controlled studies (see Lewis, 1990). An immediate concern was whether certain treatments or institutionalization could account for these findings, but treatment exposure and length of hospitalization have not been found to correlate with the VBR (e.g. Johnstone et al., 1976; Weinberger et al., 1979; Owens et al., 1985; Lewis, 1990). More convincingly, ventriculomegaly has been described at onset in first episode cases (e.g. Weinberger et al., 1982; Turner et al., 1986), and individual studies have generally not been able to detect any progression of the abnormalities beyond that expected from aging (Nasrallah et al., 1986; Illowsky et al., 1988; Vita et al., 1988; Kemali et al., 1989; Jaskiw et al., 1994).

Indeed, it has been remarkably difficult to find any consistent clinical associations of ventriculomegaly in schizophrenia. Although some studies have reported relationships with positive or negative symptoms severity, many more have not; and there are about equal numbers of reports finding and refuting associations with poor pre-morbid adjustment, treatment resistance or worse overall illness outcome (see Lewis, 1990). It has also proved difficult to relate the increased VBR to putative risk factors such as family history and obstetric complications (the theory being – after Crow (1980) – that those schizophrenics with ventriculomegaly would be less genetically mediated and more environmentally caused than those without). Although very few studies have found an inverse correlation between family history and ventriculomegaly (e.g. Turner et al., 1986), many more have not (e.g. Nimgaonkar et al., 1988; Pearlson et al., 1989) and high risk studies have even suggested a positive correlation – in that the degree of ventriculomegaly runs with the level of genetic risk (Cannon et al., 1989). Only a couple of papers have suggested a positive correlation with obstetric complications (e.g. Turner et al., 1986; Pearlson et al., 1989) and most have not (e.g. Nimgaonkar et al., 1988). However, cognitive impairment has been found to correlate with the VBR in almost every study to date (e.g. Johnstone et al., 1976, 1978; Donnelly et al., 1980; Golden et al., 1980, 1982; Owens et al., 1985) and there are several possible reasons for a failure to find other consistent associations. These include methodological factors such as slice positioning, small study size (possible type II errors), varying assessment scales, natural variations in brain size and expecting simple dichotomies in risk factors that are probably continuously distributed.

Slice positioning effects are a particularly important consideration in follow-up studies. Woods and colleagues – who are alone in finding some progression in the VBR over time (1990) – have shown that a 1 mm change in positioning can alter the VBR by as much as 10% (1991). This experimental 'noise' could hide subtle progression, as could the regression to the mean demonstrated by Nasrallah et al. (1986) and Kemali et al. (1989), and small study sizes. Type II errors in particular studies can be overcome in meta-analyses of the literature – of which some relevant examples have recently been published. Indeed, two meta-analyses have reported a correlation between the VBR and cumulative length of hospitalization (Raz & Raz, 1990) or illness duration (Van Horn & McManus, 1992), suggesting some progression and/or that an increased VBR is a marker for a poor prognosis. Friedman et al. (1992), however, found a weak but non-significant relationship between the VBR and treatment response in their overview. Vita et al. (1994) have also described an association between negative family history and the VBR, limited to males, but were rather selective in the studies they included. Unfortunately, therefore, none of these issues has been finally resolved.

CT studies have also shown increases in the size of the third ventricle relative to the whole brain (see Lewis, 1990). Indeed, Raz & Raz (1990) actually found a greater effect than for the VBR once the measurement methods was taken into account. It is intriguing, therefore, that illness duration has more often shown an assocation with third ventricle size and shows a stronger overall relationship (Raz & Raz, 1990).

As already mentioned, CT studies in schizophrenia have also consistently reported increases in the width of cortical sulci – despite the use of many different measurement techniques and the fact that beam hardening is a greater concern than when estimating ventricular size. Such 'atrophy' – better referred to widened sulci or as a loss of cerebral substance – is only noticeable (more than two standard deviations outside a control mean) in about one-third of patients and is not as large an effect as ventriculomegaly (Raz & Raz, 1990). Again, consistent clinical correlations are rare, other than with cognitive impairment (e.g. Johnstone et al., 1978; Weinberger et al., 1979; Raz & Raz, 1990). One potentially very important observation, however, is that VBR and sulcal size usually do not show a significant correlation (e.g. Weinberger et al., 1979) and any relationship is at most weak (Vita et al., 1988), suggesting that two or more relatively distinct disease processes may be operating in schizophrenia (Cannon et al., 1989). The failure of Vita et al. (1994) to find any relationship between family history and sulcal enlargement, in contrast to the VBR, is also compatible with this suggestion. This raises the possibility that the VBR measurement may confound two separate variables, which may in turn partially account for the difficulties in finding consistent correlates of ventriculomegaly. Unfortunately, the importance of this was not realized until late in the CT research effort (Pearlson et al., 1989); since then some workers have advocated using multivariate statistical techniques to control for the effect of brain area on ventricle size (Harvey et al., 1990), but these are important considerations for MRI studies.

Other findings

A variety of other interesting findings has been reported in schizophrenia on CT, albeit with little consistency. Gross lesions are found in up to 11% of patients, but these are mainly of developmental and acquired types, are generally more common in most psychiatric disorders and do not usually alter clinical management (see Lewis, 1990 and Lawrie et al., 1997). Studies of putatively abnormal cerebral asymmetry (in contrast to the normal pattern of larger right frontal and left occipital lobes or 'brain torque') are about equally divided into positive and negative findings and uncorrected head tilt in the scanner could be responsible for false positive results (Zipursky et al., 1991). However, a recent study of multiply affected families found that the Sylvian fissure was larger on the left in schizophrenics, larger on the right on normals and intermediate in those 'obligate carriers' who were presumed to carry but not express the gene that is believed to be relevant (Honer et al., 1995). Arguably the most important aetiological finding is that the affected sib in discordant monozygotic twin pairs shows ventriculomegaly (Reveley et al., 1982), which suggests an enviromental

rather than a genetic cause, but this may not generalize to all schizophrenics and does not exclude gene–environment interaction. Indeed, studies of high risk subjects (Cannon et al., 1989) and multiply affected families
(DeLisi et al., 1986) suggest that both genetic risk and obstetric complications have additive effects on ventricular size.

A final consideration is the extent to which ventriculomegaly and sulcul
enlargement are found in other psychiatric or medical conditions. It is
sobering to note that these are well documented in the affective disorders,
although usually to a lesser extent (e.g. Pearlson et al., 1989), and have also
been described in eating disorders, hypercortisolaemia, malnutrition and
alcoholism (e.g. Heinz et al., 1977). A recent meta-analysis has confirmed
that these changes are less pronounced in mood disorders than in schizophrenia (Elkis et al., 1995), but the difference is small. This, together with
the lack of a bimodal distribution of the VBR in schizophrenia (Daniel et
al., 1991a), strongly argues against a specific structural brain change in
schizophrenia – at least as detectable on CT.

Summary

CT studies have provided good evidence for ventricular and sulcal enlargement in schizophrenia. This is essentially developmental but a progressive
component has not been excluded. The general absence of reliable clinical
correlations, other than with cognitive impairment, suggests that these
abnormalities are trait markers for schizophrenia distributed on a continuum with normality. The studies have not directly implicated any specific
aetiological factors; rather, they suggest that more than one disease process
may be at work. However, family studies have shown that the VBR is under
genetic control and risk factors may additively interact, suggesting that the
variability in the size of brain components may obscure meaningful correlations unless this is somehow controlled for. Some workers continue to
publish the results of CT studies but, given the substantial advantages of
MRI, the only definite remaining value of further CT work is in long-term
follow-up studies of large numbers of patients.

Magnetic resonance imaging (MRI)

MRI has considerable advantages over CT imaging. Using magnetic fields
and radio waves rather than X-rays, it poses no risks to patients (unless
they have metal aneurism clips or pacemakers) and can be safely repeated.
MRI has greater resolution than CT, gives reliable images of the whole

brain/head and can therefore generate tissue volumes rather than just areas. For these reasons it is the technique of choice for structural imaging studies in schizophrenia and other neuropsychiatric disorders.

Methodology

Bloch and Purcell received the Nobel prize for physics in 1952 for their observation that tissue structure could be inferred from the changes in magnetic fields when they were applied to atomic nuclei. However, it was 30 years before the necessary technological developments – of static and gradient magnets, radio frequency transmitters and receivers, and computerized analysis – allowed clinical applications.

The physical basis of the MRI signal is complex and incompletely understood (see Schild, 1990). Briefly, protons (in tissue water) in the scanner magnetic field align themselves longitudinally and spin or 'precess'. An emitted radio frequency pulse, 'resonant' with the precession rate, is used to increase proton energy – reducing longitudinal magnetization (LM) and stimulating transverse magnetization (TM). When the pulse is switched off, LM returns as the protons return energy to their field ('spin-lattice' or T1 relaxation) and TM is reduced as protons lose phase coherence ('spin–spin' or T2 relaxation). Brain tissues differ in T1 and T2 values depending on their water and fat content, so that brain, CSF and skull can be distinguished by particular pulse sequences. Spin-echo sequences use repeated pulses to generate images that are useful for lesion detection, but generally take a few minutes to image the whole brain. Fast imaging, in seconds, can be done by inducing additional magnetic gradients to speed proton dephasing and by imaging several brain slices simultaneously, but tends to cause intense blood flow signals that can degrade images. The anatomical position of particular proton species is determined by gradient read-out magnets and images are constructed by computerized Fourier transformation of the signals. The numerical value of each volume element or 'voxel' is determined by the T1, T2 and proton density and gives images on a grey scale.

Provided the magnets and pulse generator are regularly calibrated, by scanning a 'phantom' object of known composition to prevent 'signal drift', artifacts with MRI are relatively few (but see Plante & Turkstra, 1991). The inevitable coil inhomogeneities will result in lesser signals from tissues further from the centre of the coil unless all images are 'phantom corrected'. Partial volume effects are less than with CT but remain a problem, particularly if slice thickness exceeds the volume of the structure of interest, and any head tilt needs to be corrected at the image analysis stage. The usual method of volume derivation is extremely labour intensive – generally raters trace structures on successive brain slices, which may be as many as e.g. 100 for the whole brain and 50 for the temporal lobes – so that considerable attention has been and is being given to various automated techniques.

Main findings

Early MRI studies in schizophrenia inevitably reported areas rather than volumes and focused on midline structures that were prominent on mid-saggital localizing scans (e.g. Figure 5.1). These have limited value and will only be briefly discussed. Consistent findings are rare (Waddington et al., 1990), and reports of various abnormalities of the corpus callosum are matched in number by negative studies – such that a recent meta-analysis found no reduction in size after controlling for brain size (Woodruff et al., 1995). However, an important methodological consideration became evident after workers in Iowa first produced evidence for reductions in frontal lobe, brain and cranial areas (Andreasen et al., 1986) that were subsequently shown to be attributable to educational and economic advantages in the hospital staff controls (Andreasen et al., 1990).

   Volumetric studies give much more reliable information and have generated a much greater degree of consensus. Over 50 such studies have been published, since the first in 1988, allowing both narrative and quantitative reviews of them. This account will therefore describe important individual studies, region by region, as well as giving median differences between cases and controls derived from all relevant papers published by June 1997 (after Lawrie & Abukmeil, 1998).

Cranium and whole brain

Ten MRI studies have reported volumes of the cranium. Most have found no significant differences between schizophrenic patients and normal controls and although they point towards volume reductions (as suggested in the single largest study to date by Flaum et al., 1995, and a recent meta-analysis by Ward et al., 1996), four actually suggest an increased cranial volume in male schizophrenics (Shenton et al., 1991, 1992; Zipursky et al., 1994; Lauriello et al., 1997). The 20 studies of the whole brain and cerebral hemispheres are more consistent. Although few report significant differences, all show volume reductions and the Ward (1996) meta-analysis and the

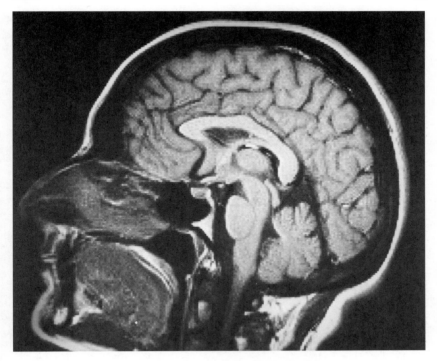

Figure 5.1. A midline sagittal section through the brain on MRI.

authors' median calculations (see Table 5.1 and Lawrie & Abukmeil, 1998) agree in overall and bilateral reductions of about 3% in schizophrenia. Segmentation studies, where grey and white matter volumes are separated automatically, suggest that this deficit is largely attributable to a loss of grey matter (Shenton et al., 1992; Zipursky et al., 1992; Harvey et al., 1993; Schlaepfer et al., 1994; Woods et al., 1996; Lim et al., 1996a,b,c; Lauriello et al., 1997; Pearlson et al., 1997). These cranium and brain results are not apparently influenced by whether the entire structure was imaged or if small portions were missed (e.g. Harvey et al., 1993; Flaum et al., 1995); and most have controlled for possible age and sex effects – albeit by often studying only men (e.g. Shenton et al., 1992).

CSF and the ventricular system
Statistically significant increases in the amount of cerebro-spinal fluid (CSF) are generally reported regardless of technique – but see Gur et al. (1991, 1994a) – and the median increases are about 14–18%. The few

Table 5.1. *Median percentage differences in MRI volumes from studies (N of studies, range of results) in patients with DSM–III(R) schizophrenia and normal controls*

Region	Both sexes	Men	Women
Cranium	−2 (3, −3 to −1.5)	−0.5 (7, −3 to +4)	−2.5 (4, −3.5 to −1)
Whole Brain	−3 (9, −9.5 to −0.5)	−3 (7, −5.5 to −1.5)	−2.5 (5, −4 to −2.5)
Left Hemisphere	−2 (2, −3.5 to −0.5)	−3 (4, −4.5 to −1.5)	−2.5 (2, −2 to −3)
Right Hemisphere	−2.5 (2, −4.5 to −0.5)	−3.5 (4, −4.5 to −2)	−2.5 (2, −2 to −2.5)
Cerebro-Spinal Fluid	+18 (4, 0 to +26)	+14 (4, −7.5 to +35)	+14 (3, +12 to +19)
Lateral Ventricle (LV)	+22 (9, +14 to +67)	+24 (7, 0 to +43)	+12 (5, +10 to +30)
Left LV	+44 (7, +31 to +66)	+2 (3, 0 −2.5 to +65)	+30 (3, +25 to +76)
Right LV	+28 (7, +12 to +67)	−2 (3, −6 to +29)	+23 (3, +22 to +29)
LV body – Left side	+50 (2, +40 to +49)	+50 (3, −2 to +58)	—
LV body – Right side	+47 (2, +33 to +61)	+68 (3, −0.5 to +75)	—
Frontal horn – Left	+15 (3, −8.5 to +35)	—	—
Frontal horn – Right	+2.5 (3, +2 to +24)	—	—
Temporal horn – Left	+20 (4, +2 to +300)	+13 (8, −7.5 to +200)	+22 (4, +10 to +32)
Temporal horn – Right	+14 (4, −1 to +65)	+10 (8, +2.5 to +74)	+10 (4, +5 to +12)
Occipital horn – Left	+31 (2, +30 to +32)	—	—

Occipital horn – Right	+ 28 (2, + 14 to + 41)	—	—
Third Ventricle	+ 17 (6, − 6 to + 52)	+ 20 (8, − 5 to + 29)	+ 8.5 (4, 0 to + 17)
Pre-frontal lobe – Left	− 5.5 (6, − 10 to + 2.5)	− 3 (3, − 15 to − 2)	− 1 (2, − 2 to + 0.5)
Pre-frontal lobe – Right	− 7 (6, − 10 to + 2)	− 5.5 (3, − 9.5 to − 3.5)	− 4 (2, − 5 to − 3)
Temporal lobe – Left	− 3.5 (6, − 13 to + 3.5)	− 3 (9, − 5.5 to + 3.5)	− 3 (6, − 4.5 to + 5)
Temporal lobe – Right	− 4.5 (6, − 15 to + 2.5)	− 3.5 (9, − 9 to + 3.5)	− 4 (6, − 3.5 to + 5)
Amyg. & Hipp. – Left	− 6.5 (4, − 12 to + 2.5)	− 7.5 (4, − 11 to + 0.5)	+ 3.5 (2, + 2 to + 4.5)
Amyg. & Hipp. – Right	− 5.5 (4, − 15 to + 2.5)	− 6.5 (4, − 12 to + 1.5)	+ 0.5 (2, − 1 to + 2)
Amygdala – Left	− 16 (2, − 19 to − 12)	− 9 (7, − 21 to + 15)	+ 4 (2, + 1.5 to + 5)
Amygdala – Right	− 16 (2, − 18 to − 14)	− 9 (6, − 10 to − 3)	− 7 (2, − 11 to − 4.5)
Hippocampus – Left	− 8 (3, − 19 to 0)	− 3.5 (10, − 20 to + 5.5)	− 2 (4, − 7.5 to + 1.5)
Hippocampus – Right	− 5 (3, − 24 to − 3)	− 8.5 (10, − 15 to + 10)	− 8 (4, − 12 to + 7)
Parahippocampus – Left	− 20 (2, − 30 to − 10)	− 9 (4, − 15 to + 5)	—
Parahippocampus – Right	− 16 (2, − 22 to − 10)	− 9 (4, − 10 to − 1)	—

Note: Figures are only given where at least two comparable studies are available for a given structure in a particular subject group.

relevant reports suggest that these increases are most apparent in frontal (Andreasen et al., 1994a; Lim et al., 1996a) and temporal (Harvey et al., 1993; Turetsky et al., 1995) regions.

Following the CT findings, the ventricular system has been the most intensively studied part of the brain with MRI and additional information about ventricular sub-divisions has also been generated. The entire system, with the exception of the fourth ventricle, has been shown to be enlarged. One study which focused on the ventricles and their sub-divisions described large increases in the volumes of the lateral and third ventricles, as well as the body, frontal, temporal and occipital horns – differences that were generally greater on the left side and in men (Degreef et al., 1992). Others have also reported similar increases, but with less clear side or sex effects (e.g. Dauphinais et al., 1990; DeLisi et al., 1991; Jernigan et al., 1991; O'Callaghan et al., 1992; Kawasaki et al., 1993a; Zipursky et al., 1994; Vita et al., 1995a). The medians across all relevant studies show convincingly larger increases in men for the lateral (24%) and third ventricles (20%), and in the left temporal horn in both sexes (13% men and 22% women) but there are insufficient studies of the other sub-divisions to confidently answer whether abnormalities are generally greatest in men and on the left side or not (see Table 5.1).

Prefrontal lobes

Most of the 11 studies examining this structure have used serial slice counting from the frontal pole to the genu of the corpus callosum. Three studies report statistically significant volume reductions of 5–10% (Breier et al., 1992; Andreasen et al., 1994a; Nopoulos et al., 1995), but two of these are from one group and the overall median reductions of 1–7% are at most only slightly greater than those for the whole brain. Segmentation studies again suggest that this is largely attributable to a loss of grey rather than white matter (Suddath et al., 1989; Breier et al., 1992; Wible et al., 1995; Woods et al., 1996; Ohnuma et al., 1997).

Temporal lobes

Although some studies have suggested that frontal lobe reductions are similar to or larger than temporal lobe deficits, the balance of MRI evidence points towards some of the constituent parts of the temporal lobes as the regions of the brain that are most abnormal in schizophrenia. The first two published volumetric MRI studies, from NIMH (Kelsoe et al., 1988; Suddath et al., 1989), reported large (6–15%) but non-significant decreases in temporal volume that were most pronounced in the amygdala and hippocampus (12–23%). They followed this with a demonstration that the affected twin in a discordant monozygotic pair almost always had larger ventricles and hippocampi that could be seen with the naked eye (Suddath et al., 1990). Subsequent studies of the temporal lobes, which matched subjects for age and sex, have rarely found such large differences, such that the median reductions by sex are no larger than those for the whole brain (see Table 5.1). Reductions are however most pronounced in grey matter, as white matter volume may actually be increased (Suddath et al., 1989; Harvey et al., 1993; Zipursky et al., 1994; Woods et al., 1996; Ohnuma et al., 1997), i.e. in the amygdala, hippocampus and parahippocampal gyrus.

Indeed, studies of the amygdala and hippocampus together or individually have fairly consistently found significant volume reductions, particularly in men and on the left side (e.g. Bogerts et al., 1990b, 1993; Breier et al., 1992; Shenton et al., 1992; Rossi et al., 1994; Becker et al., 1996; Fukuzako et al., 1996). The median volume reductions are between 4–16% overall and in men, but less in women. However, there are few studies giving figures for women and the largest published study reports greater reductions in women than men (Flaum et al., 1995). Fukuzako et al. (1996) have reported that the hippocampus volume deficit may be largely attributable to a reduction in length. A recent meta-analysis of these studies found bilateral volume reductions of 4% in both sexes (Nelson et al., 1988).

The parahippocampal gyrus has only been examined, at least in published reports, in six studies. Three have examined men only and generally found significant reductions of up to 15%, particularly on the left side (Becker et al., 1990; Shenton et al., 1992; Kawasaki et al., 1993a). The median reductions in both sexes together (DeLisi et al., 1991; Ohnuma et al., 1997) and in men are among the largest cortical reductions in the literature and accord with post-mortem findings and some functional imaging studies (see below). Pearlson et al. (1997) also studied the entorhinal cortex for the first time on MRI and reported large volume reductions in this region as well as in the superior temporal gyrus.

Superior temporal gyrus (STG)

Barta et al. (1990) were the first to report volumes of this part of the temporal lobe, which were substantially reduced, by about 12%, in their male sample. Subsequent studies have produced a bewildering array of results as they have often examined different portions of the gyrus or the same part with different boundaries that give raw volumes that vary by as much as a factor of three. However, several groups have replicated Barta's finding of a significant volume reduction in the anterior portion of the STG (Shenton et al., 1992; DeLisi et al., 1994; Pearlson et al., 1997). Non-significant reductions have also been reported in the middle (Menon et al., 1995) and posterior (Kulynych et al., 1996) portions, and for the whole gyrus (Flaum et al., 1995), but consensus has not been achieved. The importance of methodological factors was demonstrated by Kulynych et al. (1996), who found no reduction in whole gyral volume with standard serial slice measurement but a 12% reduction on the left side with surface rendering (i.e. isolating the structure by cortical gyral anatomy first). This group have also reported non-significant reductions in the surface area of the planum temporale and Heschl's gyrus, in the middle and posterior parts of the STG respectively, with surface rendering (Kulynych et al., 1995).

Cerebral asymmetry

The STG has been most studied in the search for anomalous asymmetry in the brains of schizophrenics as it is the location of the primary auditory cortex (normally larger on the left side) and may be involved in the pathogenesis of hallucinations. The planum temporale has been reported to show less asymmetry (e.g. Rossi et al., 1994; DeLisi et al., 1994) or even reversed asymmetry (Petty et al., 1995) by some, but not by others (Klein-schmidt et al., 1994; Barta et al., 1995). Results are similarly conflicting for the whole or posterior STG (Zipursky et al., 1994; Kulynych et al., 1995; Pearlson et al., 1997). More generally, many groups have reported diag-nosis by side interactions, but in different regions and in different directions (e.g. Suddath et al., 1989; Flaum et al., 1995). These discrepancies are likely to be attributable to a failure to control for handedness and gender effects on laterality and any head tilt in the scanner. Even in those studies which meet these criteria, which have described greater reductions in the right than the left frontal lobe (Bilder et al., 1994; Turetsky et al., 1995) but not in the temporal lobe (Zipursky et al., 1994; Turetsky et al., 1995), image analysis has not been conducted blind to side. Moreover, in most of these studies, data analysis has not adequately controlled for whole brain vol-ume reductions as 'asymmetry quotients' tend to be used rather than regression techniques (Bullmore et al., 1995).

Other regions

Volume reductions have also been reported in the occipital lobes (An-dreasen et al., 1994a), the parieto-occipital and pre-motor cortex (Bilder et al., 1994), the cerebellum (Andreasen et al., 1994a; Flaum et al., 1995), the cingulate gyrus (Noga et al., 1995) and the thalamus (Andreasen et al., 1994b; Flaum et al., 1995) but these are rarely greater than 3% and have not been widely studied. In contrast to these results, the most consistent and persuasive evidence for abnormalities in subcortical nuclei is for volume increases (e.g. Kelsoe et al., 1988; DeLisi et al., 1991; Swayze et al., 1992; Buchanan et al., 1993) which evolve over 12–18 months of anti-psychotic drug treatment (Chakos et al., 1994; Keshavan et al., 1994) and reverse when patients are switched to clozapine (Chakos et al., 1995; Frazier et al., 1996a).

Clinical correlations

These observations are all the more important when one considers that no study has ever reported a correlation between medication and cortical volumes, and that the vast majority of studies have not found correlations between illness duration and volumes (e.g. Kelsoe et al., 1988; Marsh et al., 1994; Zipursky et al., 1994), with only two weak exceptions (Gur et al., 1991; DeLisi et al., 1991). Similarly, studies of first episode subjects have reported abnormalities of whole brain and ventricular volumes (Lim et al., 1996c; Ohnuma et al., 1997), CSF and frontal lobe volumes (Nopoulos et al., 1995) or temporal lobe volumes (Bogerts et al., 1990b; Bilder et al., 1994) that are generally of a similar extent to those in chronic patients. Two published follow-up studies have suggested some slight loss of cerebral volume (DeLisi et al., 1997) or frontal volume (Gur et al, 1988), but patient drop-out and substance abuse mean that further studies are required to settle this issue.

As with CT, it has been difficult to link MRI abnormalities with symptoms of psychosis. Some groups have reported correlations between negative symptoms and parts of the ventricular system (Degreef et al., 1992; Kawasaki et al., 1993a; Zipursky et al., 1994) or frontal lobe (Zipursky et al., 1992; Wible et al., 1995; Chua et al., 1997); or between positive symptoms and the temporal lobes (Bogerts et al., 1993; Chua et al., 1997) – but many have not and it is not known how many researchers do not report negative findings. More success has been had in trying to tie particular psychotic features to parts of the STG – e.g. hallucinations (Barta et al., 1990; Flaum et al., 1995) and thought disorder (Shenton et al., 1992; Rossi et al., 1994; Menon et al., 1995; Vita et al., 1995a) – but there are some negative studies (DeLisi et al., 1994; Zipursky et al., 1994) and the exact region of the STG and (more concerningly) the sign of the correlation coefficient vary from study to study. Attempt to find greater degrees of structural abnormality in deficit (Buchanan et al., 1993) or treatment resistant patients (Lawrie et al., 1995) have not found large differences. Similar considerations as with the CT studies probably apply, particularly as studies which have looked for correlations between volumes and neuro-psychological test performance generally find them. For example, parahippocampal gyrus and STG lobe volume reductions have been linked to language test deficits (DeLisi et al., 1991; Nestor et al., 1993; Vita et al., 1995a), and temporal lobe volumes to performance on tests usually considered sensitive to the integrity of the frontal lobes (Bilder et al., 1995; Lawrie et al., 1995).

The latter finding is relevant to considerations of pathophysiology, as are three reports that fronto-temporal volume correlations are stronger in schizophrenia than in controls (Suddath et al., 1990; Breier et al., 1992; Wible et al., 1995). Integrated fronto-temporal anatomy (and function – see below) therefore appears to be disturbed in schizophrenia. Together with recurrent suggestions that volume losses are largely limited to grey matter, while white matter volumes may actually be increased, this suggests that this disintegration may be associated with excessive connectivity between small neuronal populations. The other pathophysiologically relevant evidence from MRI studies is the generally weak or absent correlations between ventricular and cortical volumes (Kelsoe et al., 1988; Suddath et al., 1989) – suggesting, as do CT findings, that they may reflect two relatively distinct disease processes. Relatively few MRI studies have examined the relationship between volume reductions and aetiological factors such as family history – with familial cases showing small brains (Schwartzkopf et al., 1991) or more ventricular asymmetry (Roy et al., 1994) – but an interesting preliminary study has shown cerebral asymmetry in cases and 'obligate carriers' but not controls (Sharma et al., 1996). Reduced brain volumes have also been reported in childhood onset schizophrenia (Frazier et al., 1996b) and ventricular enlargement in adults has been associated with childhood motor deficits and negative affect rated from old home movies (Walker et al., 1996). Our own work (Lawrie et al., in press) has found temporal lobe abnormalities in subjects at high risk of developing schizophrenia for genetic reasons suggesting that volumetric differences are evident before the onset of symptoms and are genetically mediated.

Other findings

MRI signal intensity values attracted some early attention from researchers, but findings of T1 and T2 prolongation have not been replicated,

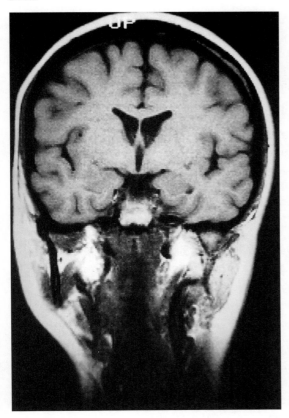

Figure 5.2. A coronal section on MRI in a patient with schizophrenia highlighting some mild qualitative abnormalities. Note the slightly asymmetrical lateral ventricles, dilated temporal horns of the lateral ventricles, enlarged third ventricle and widened cortical sulci ('mild atrophy'). The mesial temporal lobe structures of most interest in schizophrenia are seen on the most medial and superior aspect of the temporal lobes.

could be artifactual and have no definite meaning (Waddington et al., 1990). Recently, two groups have studied the surface pattern of brain sulci and gyri in schizophrenia: Kikinis et al. (1994) reported an abnormal configuration of the temporal lobes, but the only other published report failed to find any differences between discordant monozygotic twins (Noga et al., 1996).

Qualitative MRI scan appearances can provide useful information that may supplement that from quantitative studies (see Figure 5.2). Atrophy has been described in 4–40% of schizophrenics, depending on definition;

high intensity signal (HIS) foci are reported in 5–22% of patients and gross lesions in 0–4%. Although these figures are higher than those in controls, they are often found in other psychiatric patients, HIS foci are closely related to blood pressure and age, and gross lesions are non-specific and rarely clinically important (Lawrie et al., 1997). However, Lieberman et al. (1992) devised a clinically orientated scale of such abnormalities and found a greater number of them in chronic than acute cases, and we have recently reported a tendency to more 'atrophy' in treatment resistant than responsive patients (Lawrie et al., 1997).

Finally, turning to disease specificity, it appears that similar volume reductions as those described above can be found in affective disorder although these are not as marked (e.g. Pearlson et al., 1997). Intriguingly, given that some patients with temporal lobe epilepsy (TLE) can present with schizophreniform psychosis, some recent reports suggest that TLE patients may have similar abnormalities of the temporal lobes to those reported in schizophrenia that are only found on the side of the epileptic focus (e.g. Barr et al., 1997).

Summary

In summary, volumetric MRI studies in schizophrenia have convincingly shown that the whole brain, amygdala and hippocampus are smaller in schizophrenia than in groups of controls. The same may be true of the cranium and parahippocampal gyrus, and abnormalities may be most marked in men and on the left side. Further work is required to clarify these potential findings, and to examine possible changes over time, aetiological associations, clinical correlations and potential anomalies of asymmetry. Methodological refinements will help in these regards but, as with post-mortem studies, it is clear that larger samples will be required – including more women – with a greater amount of multi-centre collaboration.

Single photon emission (computed) tomography (SPET)

Although structural imaging has shown which parts of the brain are anatomically abnormal, it has provided limited information as to how these may produce the characteristic symptoms and signs of the disorder. Greater insights have been expected and to some extent realized from functional imaging studies with SPET (and PET), both at rest and after cognitive or pharmacological activation. These techniques use administered radio-isotope tracers to measure regional cerebral blood flow (rCBF) or metabolism, and assume that the tracers are linearly distributed with blood flow to active parts of the brain (Raichle et al., 1976). Kety and colleagues (1948) were the first to use a SPET scanner in schizophrenia, but could only generate a measure of global blood flow and oxygen consumption by subtracting venous from arterial concentrations of nitrous oxide and could detect no abnormalities in schizophrenia. Many years were to pass before technological advances allowed less invasive and more detailed examinations.

Methodology

The essential developments have been in gamma cameras, with gamma photon focussing collimators and sodium iodide scintillation detectors and tomographic methods to generate two and three dimensional images (Van Heertum & Tikofsky, 1995). After a tracer is administered, the subject is required to rest (sometimes with eyes and ears patched to minimize stimulation) to allow the isotope to be distributed in the brain according to a reliable neuronal activity baseline. The head is relatively immobilized during scanning and positioned with reference to the orbito-meatal line. Early studies used a single gamma camera detector that spun around the head to acquire information on the whole brain, but some current scanners use multiple detectors to enhance resolution and speed image acquisition. The photons emitted by the radiotracer are focused by passing through parallel holes in a lead collimator, scintillate on contact with the sodium iodide crystal, and are concentrated by photomultiplier tubes before computerized image reconstruction. The origin of a particular photon is determined by its trajectory through the collimator and the strength of scintillation.

A number of radiotracers have been used over the years (Morretti et al., 1995). Initially, radioactive Krypton was used but required surgical brain exposure. The discovery that radioactive Xenon (Xe^{133}) emitted gamma rays that could be detected through the intact skull led to research possibilities. As a diffusible or dynamic tracer, inhaled Xe^{133} could quickly generate quantitative rCBF values (sometimes called D-SPECT) if input was also measured by e.g. scintillation over the lungs. However, Xe^{133} emits relatively soft radiation, so that D-SPECT has relatively poor resolution and cannot image deep structures. It also tends to overestimate perfusion in low flow (white matter) areas and is insensitive to small rCBF differences at high perfusion. Subsequently, static or fixed tracers, which only generate relative rCBF values and require longer imaging time but give better resolution, have been developed. Radioactive Iodine (I^{123}) labelled lipo-philic compounds, such as IMP (n-isopropul p-iodoamphetamine), give good resolution but need a cyclotron for manufacture, require 20 minutes for equilibration and only measure rCBF reliably for up to one hour. Technetium (Tc^{99m}) labelled lipophilics, such as HMPAO (hexa-methyl propylamineoxime), are now most commonly used as they are relatively cheap, widely available, and require only five minutes equilibration; their main problem being that HMPAO has poorer contrast than IMP as it back-diffuses from high flow regions and has higher extraction in low flow areas. The final tracer category, of I^{123} labelled neuroreceptor ligands, such as Iomazenil (for GABA) and Iodobenzamide (for dopamine D_2), are expensive but are increasingly used. There is no current SPET tracer for metabolism, but one is apparently under development.

After an image is acquired and is assessed for adequacy – to exclude for example 'ring images' from detector non-uniformity – it is processed ('by filtered back-projection') or 'smoothed' to reduce noise and then recon-structed with an attenuation correction. Artifacts can arise from excessive or inadequate filtering, which reduce resolution. Image picture elements (or 'pixels') are then sized, ideally so that their width equals the brain slice width to avoid distortion. Quantitative image analysis requires the fitting of a standardized template to the images, to count the total tracer count and pixels in a given region of interest (ROI) – see Figure 5.3 for example. These ROI values, of average pixel tracer count, must then be 'normalized' to control for global or whole slice rCBF, before a true comparison can be made between subject groups. A number of normalization procedures have been devised, with differing results, but the standard approach of calculat-ing a ratio of ROI values to a reference region appears to be the most reliable (Gullion et al., 1996). The reference region may be the whole brain or whole slice (although this may obscure some effects), or regions which are not thought to be involved in the disorder under study – such as the occipital cortex or (less reliably) the cerebellum. Finally, some sort of multivariate statistical procedure is used to examine potential differences in the ROIs. These may number 12 or more per slice analysed so true hypothesis testing should only examine one or two specific regions to avoid high false positive rates.

Main findings

Functional imaging in schizophrenia has concentrated on whether or not patients have a relatively reduced rCBF in frontal regions ('hypofrontality')

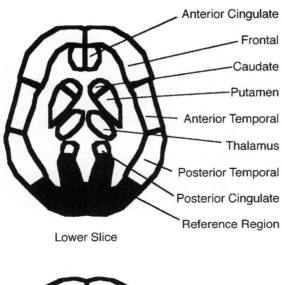

Lower Slice

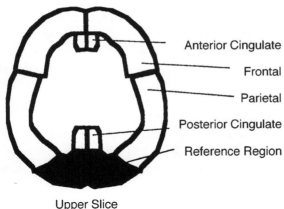

Upper Slice

Figure 5.3. An example of region of interest templates for SPET scan analysis (the reference region is the occipital cortex). A PET scan, with its better resolution, allows for more precise and detailed anatomical localization.

(see Figure 5.4). This was first reported, using arterial injection of Xe^{133}, in chronic patients by Ingvar & Franzen (1974a,b), who also demonstrated that negative symptom severity (but not medication dose) was negatively correlated with frontal perfusion and that the most 'autistic' patients failed to increase frontal rCBF on cognitive activation. Later studies are best considered by whether they used Xe^{133} or other tracers, and whether they scanned subjects at rest or during some activation procedure.

Xenon inhalation studies

Subsequent Xe[133] studies have used the less invasive inhalation method, with cortical probes or SPECT, although this has a lower regional resolution. Mathew and collagues (1982) found no hypofrontality, but generalized rCBF reductions in patients with schizophrenia, regardless of whether they were on medication or had been withdrawn for one week, and hallucination severity was inversely correlated with postcentral blood flow. Ariel et al. (1983) did find reduced grey matter rCBF values in frontal areas bilaterally, although this was only significant in the left hemisphere. No significant reductions in resting rCBF were found by Pennsylvania researchers in either medicated or unmedicated patients (Gur et al., 1983, 1985), but these experiments were conducted on only 15 and 19 subjects respectively and there is only one other Xe study (also in small numbers) to find no such effect (Dousse et al., 1988). In contrast, hypofrontality at rest has been reported in several other studies in medicated (Kurachi et al., 1985; Mathew et al., 1988; Paulman et al., 1990) and unmedicated patients (Weinberger et al., 1986; Berman et al., 1986; Geraud et al., 1987; Sagawa et al., 1990). It has also been demonstrated in the same patients before and after medication (Warkentin et al., 1990), and Matsuda et al. (1991) found that medication appeared if anything to normalize rather than worsen frontal perfusion. Kurachi et al. (1985) also found a 'hyper-temporality' that was greatest on the left in patients with auditory hallucinations, while Mathew et al. (1988) reported left temporal rCBF reductions and that illness duration was related to hypofrontality. Paulman and colleagues (1990) also found that reduced left frontal rCBF was associated with neuropsychological impairment on the Wisconsin Card Sort Test (WCST) and that increased hemispheric blood flow was correlated with positive symptoms.

Even more consistent differences between patients with schizophrenia and normal controls have been found on various cognitive activations. In Philadelphia, medicated schizophrenics had aberrant hemispheric activation patterns, with left sided rCBF increases on a spatial task and bilateral increases for a verbal task (Gur et al., 1983), a pattern that was not substantially different in unmedicated patients (Gur et al., 1985). These workers have replicated this finding and extended it by showing that their patients' greatest deficit was in specific verbal recognition and that this correlated with the severity of hallucinations and delusions (Gur et al., 1994b). Wood & Flowers (1990) have also reported hypofrontality and reduced activation of language areas on verbal memory tasks in patients as compared with normal controls.

In the first of an influential series of studies, workers at NIMH showed that medication-free schizophrenic patients had smaller relative and absolute increases in dorso-lateral pre-frontal cortex (DLPFC) flow than controls while performing a slightly modified version of the WCST, but not during a number-matching task, and that DLPFC rCBF correlated with performance (Weinberger et al., 1986). They confirmed these findings in medicated patients and established that DLPFC rCBF was not reduced on a visual continuous performance test (Berman et al., 1986). This was employed as a baseline reference to reduce resting rCBF variability and suggests that rCBF deficits were not simply attributable to a generally poor performance or lack of attention to the task. Weinberger et al. (1988) then reported a correlation between monoamine metabolite concentration and activated DLPFC rCBF, and Berman et al. (1988) showed that activations with Raven's progressive matrices were post-central and not different between cases and controls. Some support for the WCST related DLPFC deficit has been forthcoming (Sagawa et al., 1990; Kawasaki et al., 1993b; Steinberg et al., 1996). Daniel et al. (1991b) have provided a link between such findings and the dopamine hypothesis of schizophrenia by showing that giving amphetamine to schizophrenics improved both WCST performance and DLPFC rCBF. The NIMH researchers have also refuted suggestions of abnormal lateralization in schizophrenia beyond any task dependent increases in left anterior and right posterior regions (Berman & Weinberger, 1990); and reported WCST related DLPFC deficits in schizophrenics, but not their unaffected co-twins, that were related to hippocampal volume (Berman et al., 1992; Weinberger et al., 1992). Finally, Andreasen et al. (1992) studied never medicated and currently unmedicated patients performing another executive task, the Tower of London test. Activations were reduced in the left mesial frontal cortex in both groups, particularly in those with negative symptoms, although neither medication nor task performance were significantly associated with rCBF.

HMPAO studies

There are fewer studies using HMPAO as it has only been widely available for less than ten years. However, the enhanced resolution of grey/white matter and ability to image subcortical structures with HMPAO has definite advantages. Some small studies have failed to detect hypofrontality (Kawasaki et al., 1992; Rubin et al., 1991, 1994), but power issues are paramount here as a combined analysis of the Rubin studies did find relative hypofrontality (Rubin et al., 1994). Only a few other studies have detected resting hypofrontality with HMPAO (Erbas et al., 1990; Dupont et al., 1994; Vita et al., 1995b) and some have actually reported 'hyperfrontality' in unmedicated patients with acute illness (Ebmeier et al., 1992; Catafau et al., 1994). However, all the studies which have differentiated medial and lateral frontal rCBF have reported medial hypofrontality (Kawasaki et al., 1992; Lewis et al., 1992; Ebmeier et al., 1995), sometimes even co-existent with lateral increases in activity (Ebmeier et al., 1993).

The main advantage of HMPAO has been in imaging specific anatomical regions and thereby allowing meaningful clinical correlational analyses. Ebmeier et al. (1993) found that negative symptoms were associated with resting reduced prefrontal rCBF and that disorganization was positively correlated with cingulate tracer uptake. Some studies have reported 'hypotemporality' in medicated patients (Catafau et al., 1994; Dupont et al., 1994), but Kawasaki and colleagues (1992) found increases in resting relative left hippocampal and basal ganglia blood flow that were inversely correlated with negative symptoms. This apparent discrepancy may be related to the levels of particular drugs (Miller et al., 1997) or clinical features in different patient groups – in a within-subjects follow-up study McGuire et al. (1993) found that auditory hallucinations were associated with increased blood flow in inferior frontal (Broca's area) and anterior cingulate cortex. However, as recently shown (Sabri et al., 1997), it is probably too simplistic to expect neat correlations between rCBF and complex experiences such as positive and negative symptoms.

Two groups have studied HMPAO distributions as a possible predictor of treatment response, but from different perspectives. Lawrie et al. (1995) found no differences in rCBF between neuroleptic responders and non-responders, while Rodriguez et al. (1996) reported that treatment resistant patients who subsequently responded to clozapine showed higher thalamic, left basal ganglia and right pre-frontal perfusion than those who did not respond.

Activation experiments with HMPAO-SPECT have at least confirmed earlier reports of hypofrontality. Lewis et al. (1992) found reduced lateral and medial frontal perfusion on a word fluency test, with negative symptoms being correlated with mesial blood flow and performance with lateral rCBF. A failure of (usually left sided) lateral and medial pre-frontal cortex activation with the WCST has been replicated in unmedicated and neuroleptic-naive subjects (Rubin et al., 1991 & 1994; Kawasaki et al., 1993b; Catafau et al., 1994). Other workers have tried to shed light on medial temporal lobe functioning in schizophrenia with verbal memory testing. The first study identified generally greater rCBF increases in the left medial temporal and anterior cingulate cortices (Busatto et al., 1994), while the second showed left basal ganglia hyperactivity in hallucinating patients that was not related to medication levels (Busatto et al., 1995). A previous resting study found a similar association between hallucinations and sub-cortical blood flow (Musalek et al., 1989), as has another in which a failure of striatal suppression was evident during the WCST in never medicated patients (Rubin et al., 1991). Such a failure to deactivate the left striatum might conceivably be related to postulated internal monitoring deficits in schizophrenia (see below).

Other tracers

There are a handful of SPET reports using the tracers IMP, IBZM or Iomazenil in patients with schizophrenia. Resting IMP studies have shown both hypofrontality (Suga et al., 1994) and hypotemporality (Cohen et al., 1989a), while two reports have described increased IMP uptake in left superior temporal regions during active hallucinating (Matsuda et al., 1988; Suzuki et al., 1993) and factor analysis has related negative symptoms to hypofrontality, disorganization to the anterior cingulate cortex and hallucinations to right sided rCBF increases (Yuasa et al., 1995).

IBZM is a highly specific D_2-receptor ligand with relatively specific striatal uptake and a long radioactive half-life, making it suitable for in vivo ligand studies. Pilowsky and colleagues compared IBZM binding in patients on standard and atypical neuroleptics and found that therapeutic response was not dependent upon D_2 blockade (1992); they went on to establish that there was no difference in striatal D_2 receptor availability in typical antipsychotic responders and non-responders (1993). Other resear-chers have replicated these findings (Klemm et al., 1996; Pickar et al., 1996), and Sherer et al. (1994) found that striatal receptor occupancy was related to extra-pyramidal side-effects. These studies not only suggest that such techniques could improve drug monitoring in clinical practice, but also challenge a simple dopamine model of schizophrenia. However, a recent study reported that amphetamine induced reduction in IBZM binding was greater in schizophrenics than controls and was associated with a wor-sening of positive symptoms (Laruelle et al., 1996). Taken together with Daniel et al. (1991b), this supports the importance of dopaminergic neuro-transmission in having at least some role in producing the symptoms and cognitive deficits of schizophrenia.

Finally, to the authors' knowledge, there are three reports of Iomazenil binding in schizophrenia. All have failed to find simple resting differences between patients and controls (Schroder et al., 1995a; Lawrie et al., 1996), but Busatto and colleagues (1997) did find positive symptom correlations with binding and have suggested a modulatory role for GABA in schizophrenia.

Summary

It is apparent that an 'absolute' hypofrontality, as measured with Xenon inhalation, is a relatively robust finding in schizophrenia and that it does not appear to be an artifact of medication exposure. The results are much less consistent with the tracer HMPAO, but these studies do consistently suggest a medial hypofrontality. Activation experiments with both techniques reliably show hypofrontality – particularly with the WCST – which is, if anything, improved with treatment. Although such impairment could simply reflect a worse performance on the task, it can be seen that frontal lobe function is disturbed in schizophrenia. The majority of clinical correlation studies show that such frontal rCBF deficits are related to negative symptoms, while acute episodes tend to be associated with increases in frontal perfusion. Auditory hallucinations appear to result from a dysregulated neuronal circuit that includes cingulate, temporal and subcortical regions; and whether perfusion is increased or decreased may depend on methodological factors such as the reference region.

However, similar abnormalities of general hypoperfusion, hypofrontality (Austin et al., 1992) and hypertemporality (Zohar et al., 1989), have been reported in the affective disorders. Berman et al. (1993) reported that WCST activated hypofrontality was not found in depression, but they only included ten patients in the study. Future research should therefore concentrate on using larger samples of patients and novel activation paradigms to try and identify differences between schizophrenia and affective disorders. Another crucial and unresolved issue is whether hypofrontality is attributable to structural tissue loss. Some such progress will also be made with PET and other functional imaging techniques.

Positron emission tomography (PET)

PET has several advantages over SPET, in having better resolution, less (Compton) scatter and therefore less need for attenuation correction, and being able to give absolute values of rCBF or metabolism as well as measures of neuroreceptor density or occupancy.

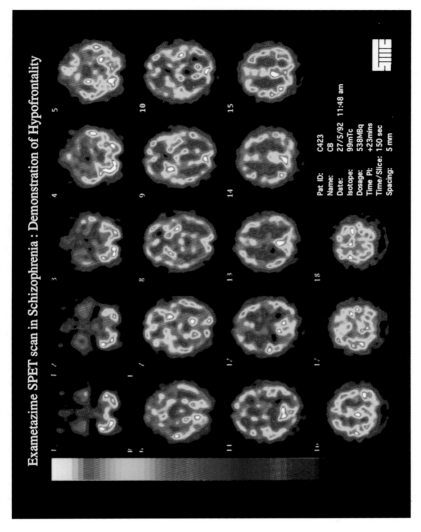

Exametazime SPET scan in Schizophrenia : Demonstration of Hypofrontality

Pat ID:	C423
Name:	CB
Date:	27/5/92 11:48 am
Isotope:	99mTc
Dosage:	538MBq
Time PI:	+23mins
Time/Slice:	150 sec
Spacing:	5 mm

Figure 5.4. Example of a SPET scan in a patient with schizophrenia suggestive of hypofrontality. Note that such qualitative impressions can be highly misleading – group averaging is required for reliable results. A PET scan would give a very similar but sharper image.

Methodology

The principles of image determination and analysis are similar for PET and SPET, but there are some notable differences. The PET scanner uses a ring of radiation detectors to image the distribution of radio-isotopes in the brain. The isotopes are labelled with a radio-nuclide – usually ^{11}C, ^{15}O or ^{18}F – which are unstable and emit positrons as they decay. The positrons travel 1–3 mm before colliding with an electron, leading to the emission of two gamma ray photons at 180 degrees to each other. The gamma cameras scintillate in response to two 'simultaneous' (5–20 nanoseconds apart) photons – giving better spatial resolution than SPET. The image is reconstructed by a filtered back projection algorithm of all these coincidences. For quantitative analysis, the photon count must be converted into true radioactivity readings and compared with substrate concentration in the blood. Together with a mathematical model of neuronal metabolism, the metabolic rate of each pixel is then calculated.

Particular nuclides, as incorporated into specific tracers, have certain advantages and disadvantages. Most early work was done with ^{11}C or ^{18}F labelled 2-deoxy-glucose (2DG and FDG respectively), but 2DG has a half-life of only fifteen minutes and FDG requires activations that do not cause habituation in the 30–45 minute uptake period. Water labelled with ^{15}O, with a very short life of 2–3 minutes, is now most commonly used as it is ideal for activations although these have to be done within the scanner. PET can also be used to measure neurotransmitter turnover (with e.g. ^{18}F-L-dopa) and receptor quantification (with e.g. ^{11}C-raclopride), with a variety of complex techniques that cannot be briefly summarized (see Sedvall et al., 1986).

Statistical analysis, as with SPET, faces the problem of numerous highly correlated measures in an even smaller numbers of subjects (as PET is more expensive). Possible scanning artefacts are similar in nature but less of a problem, due to enhanced resolution. An activated within-subject test–retest and subtraction design has therefore proved to be the most effective use of the technique. Early studies used ROI ratio calculations, but Friston et al. (1990, 1992a) have devised a Statistical Parametric Programme (SPM) which can cover the whole brain – activated areas being identified with a conservative test of significance, with co-variance for global blood flow and a principal components analysis to detect 'functional connectivity' between discrete regions – and this approach has now become the norm. SPM has recently been adapted for SPET and even structural MRI analysis (Wright et al., 1995).

A final methodological issue, for both PET and SPET, is subject selection. Inevitably, subjects who are willing and able to consent to such procedures may not be typical of all patients with schizophrenia. Differences in age, sex, anxiety or habitual drug consumption can systematically confound results. Increasing age is associated with reduced grey matter perfusion (and dopamine receptor numbers), and females have increased perfusion – perhaps particularly in frontal regions (Mathew et al., 1986; Baxter et al., 1987). Low levels of arousal or anxiety and the acute effects of many drugs (including nicotine and caffeine) tend to increase rCBF, and vice versa (Mathew & Wilson, 1990 & 1991). These effects are however probably more likely to cause false negative (due to increased measurement variation) than false positive results.

Main findings

PET studies can be conveniently divided into resting, activated and receptor binding studies as these are more distinct than the results using particular tracers.

Resting studies

The first replicated finding with PET studies in schizophrenia was the demonstration of 'hypofrontality' and most subsequent studies have focused on this issue. Buchsbaum and colleagues (1982) at NIMH were the first to demonstrate this, reporting that the relative frontal: occipital glucose metabolism (and left central grey matter utilization) at rest was significantly reduced in eight unmedicated patients as compared with six normal controls. Subsequent resting FDG studies have reported relative (Farkas et al., 1984; DeLisi et al., 1985a) or absolute (Wolkin et al., 1985) reductions in frontal: occipital metabolism, or both (Wolkin et al., 1988; Siegel et al., 1993), and most of those that find neither have still found non-significant reductions (Kling et al., 1986; Gur et al., 1987a; Tamminga et al., 1992). Although the subjects in these studies have either been medicated or only off medication for about two weeks, medicated and unmedicated patients were no different in one study (Farkas et al., 1984), and prospective studies have found that relative hypofrontality persists after treatment despite a general improvement in glucose utilization (Farkas et al., 1984; DeLisi et al., 1985b; Wolkin et al., 1985) – although a few workers have found hypofrontality to be compounded in patients with prominent negative symptoms (Buchsbaum et al., 1992a,b; Wolkin et al.,

1996). However, workers in Ontario have reported relative hyper-frontality in both medicated (Szechtman et al., 1988) and drug-naive patients with schizophrenia (Cleghorn et al., 1989); and Gur et al. (1995) also reported non-significant tendencies to increased frontal metabolism in first episode and medication free patients.

FDG studies have also tended to report some extent of absolute or relatively reduced glucose metabolism in the temporal lobes (Buchsbaum et al., 1982; Wolkin et al., 1985; Gur et al., 1987a; Cohen et al., 1989b; Tamminga et al., 1992; Siegel et al., 1993), although some have found 'hyper-temporality' (DeLisi et al., 1985b,c; Gur et al., 1995) particularly on the left side. The other brain region to receive extensive study, the basal ganglia, has been shown to have generally reduced absolute metabolism but less consistently reduced relative glucose use (Buchsbaum et al., 1982, 1987; Wolkin et al., 1985; Gur et al., 1987b; Resnick et al., 1988; Szechtman et al., 1988; Cohen et al., 1989b; Tamminga et al., 1992; Siegel et al., 1993; Gur et al., 1995). A possible explanation of these inconsistencies is that metabolism is habitually increased in both temporal lobes and the basal ganglia by antipsychotic medication (Wolkin et al., 1985; DeLisi et al., 1985b; Buchsbaum et al., 1987; Holcolmb et al., 1996), so that the medication status of patients is particularly important when studying these regions. Other statistically significant results of interest to be reported with FDG-PET include 'hypo-parietality' (Cleghorn et al., 1989), and an increased sub-cortical/cortical gradient as well as greater left–right asymmetry in unmedicated patients (Gur et al., 1987a).

Some of these findings have been replicated by researchers using other radio-isotopes, such as carbon-11 labelled DG (CDG). Volkow et al. reported general hypermetabolism in unmedicated patients that did not alter substantially after treatment (1986), and widespread hypometabolism but hyper-subcorticality in medicated patients (1987). Other 'CDG' findings include hypofrontality and hypoparietality in sub-groups of medicated patients (Kishimoto et al., 1987), and left sided hypofrontality and hypotemporality in unmedicated patients (Wiesel et al., 1987a). Two studies using the oxygen steady-state technique have failed to demonstrate hypofrontality (Sheppard et al., 1983; Early et al., 1987). The former study included medicated patients and found reduced basal ganglia activity and diminished left–right asymmetry, while the latter reported increased left globus pallidus metabolism in never medicated patients. However, as with SPET studies, schizophrenia more probably reflects distributed dysfunctional circuits than any specific regional abnormalities (Andreasen et al., 1997); those studies which have isolated medial frontal lobe/anterior cingulate have consistently reported reductions in metabolism (Tamminga et al., 1992; Siegel et al., 1993; Haznedar et al., 1997), and more consistent results have been forthcoming in activation experiments.

Activation experiments

The main advantage of activated measures of metabolism is that this is a relatively straightforward method of controlling for inter-individual behavioural and physiological differences. The first such study reported that patients with schizophrenia (and bipolar affective disorder) showed a lower anteroposterior gradient and lesser lateralization than controls after unpleasant electrical stimulation to the right arm. However, an increased posterior utilization (rather than reduced frontal) was responsible for the reduced gradient (Buchsbaum et al., 1984). On auditory vigilance tasks, schizophrenics have shown non-significant hypofrontality and significant hypertemporality in one study where only six patients were examined (Jernigan et al., 1985), and significantly reduced metabolism in the middle frontal and anterior temporal lobes in a larger study of drug-free subjects (Cohen et al., 1987). Other FDG activation experiments, employing visual continuous performance tests (CPT), have reported relative hypofrontality, hypotemporality and diminished subcortical metabolism in both ex-medicated and never medicated patients (Buchsbaum et al., 1992a), and in a large series of 83 subjects (Schroder et al., 1994), although these results have still to be independently replicated. The one FDG activated experiment found evidence of significantly reduced left temporal metabolism on amphetamine challenge, although this was associated with negative rather than positive symptoms (Wolkin et al., 1994).

Various researchers have also used other PET techniques to measure activation. Guenther et al. (1994), using ^{11}C, reported results suggestive of an abnormal (hypofrontal-hypersubcortical) pattern on motor tasks that was in keeping with their previous study (Guenther et al., 1989). The only other ^{11}C study examined the effects of an eye-tracking task in 18 medicated schizophrenics and revealed marked hypofrontality both at rest and on activation (Volkow et al., 1987). Nakashima et al. (1994) also found a frontal activation in medicated and unmedicated patients whilst performing visually and memory guided saccades, although $H_2^{15}O$-rCBF was actually higher in all conditions in the patients.

Workers in London, using the $H_2^{15}O$ technique, have particularly focused on the functional anatomy of auditory hallucinations as one of the central features of the disorder. Following their demonstration of increased rCBF in Broca's area during hallucinations (McGuire et al., 1993), they asked hallucinators and non-hallucinators to imagine being spoken to in another persons's voice. All groups, including controls, exhibited a normal left frontal response but only the hallucinators had reduced activation in the left middle temporal gyrus and rostral supplementary motor area – suggesting that a predisposition to such phenomena is associated with a failure to activate areas concerned with the monitoring of internal speech (McGuire et al., 1995). In another experiment, with paced verbal fluency that matched for performance, chronic patients showed a greater spatial extent of activation in the DLPFC and a convincing lack of rCBF reductions in the left superior temporal cortex was found in simple word repetition (Frith et al., 1995). These workers have also recently examined the effect of dopaminergic (apomorphine) modulation of the neural response to paced verbal fluency and found that the impaired activation of anterior cingulate was reversed into a significantly augmented response as compared with normal controls – although task performance did not improve (Dolan et al., 1995). These findings, together with those of an association between ketamine-induced psychosis and fronto-temporal activity (Lahti et al., 1995; Breier et al., 1997) and abnormal fronto-temporal activations on verbal memory tasks (Mozley et al., 1996; Ganguli et al., 1997), not only provide a bridge between the putative neuropharmacological and cognitive abnormalities in schizophrenia, but have also been seen as evidence against simple hypofrontality and for hypotheses of abnormal fronto-temporal connectivity. The latter, in particular, has also been supported by some of the findings from clinical correlational analyses of PET data.

Clinical and biological correlations

Many workers have attempted to relate abnormalities of metabolism to the clinical features of schizophrenia. There are, in particular, strong suggestions that hypofrontality may be related to the presence of negative symptoms (Volkow et al., 1987; Wiesel et al., 1987a; Tamminga et al., 1992; Wolkin et al., 1992; Schroder et al., 1996) or total symptomatology (Siegel et al., 1993). Hypertemporality may be associated with both positive and negative symptoms (Gur et al., 1995; Schroder et al., 1996), but Wiesel et al. (1987a) found the relationship was with reduced temporal metabolism. The severity of hallucinations has been positively correlated with anterior cingulate metabolism and associated with reduced metabolism in the auditory cortex and Broca's area (Cleghorn et al., 1990, 1992). Others have reported that auditory hallucinations were associated with activation in limbic (hippocampus), paralimbic (parahippocampus) and subcortical (thalamus) structures, as well as the right anterior cingulate, and also found that the association cortices were activated in a single case with both visual and auditory hallucinations (Silbersweig et al., 1996).

Following the lead of Liddle et al. (1992), others have shown a negative symptoms factor ('psychomotor poverty') to be related to left DLPFC metabolism, positive symptoms ('reality distortion') with right medial prefrontal cortex (and left temporal) metabolism, and disorganization with left superior temporal activity (Kaplan et al., 1993; Schroder et al., 1996). Although the sign of these correlations, and their precise location, differs in some of these studies this could be attributable to whether the patients are fundamentally hypo- or hyper-frontal, and to activation or medication status differences. Differences are also evident, for example, in the common symptom cluster in medicated resting (Liddle et al., 1992) or unmedicated activated (Schroder et al., 1996) patients, which has been located in the left parahippocampal gyrus (Friston et al., 1992b) and the anterior cingulate respectively. Two groups have also examined the pattern of inter-regional correlations in unmedicated patients; the first reporting more positive inter-correlations of metabolism between neo-, sub- and limbo-cortical regions in patients than in controls at rest (Wiesel et al., 1987b), and the second finding fewer positive inter-correlations between frontal and temporal cortex and subcortical structures whilst performing the CPT (Katz et al., 1996). Finally, three interesting studies have suggested that hypofrontality is related to underlying structural change (Chua et al., 1997), that passivity phenomena may be attributable to hyperactivation of parietal cortex (Spence et al., 1997) and that thought disorder maps onto limbic cortex circuits (McGuire et al., 1998), but each of these findings requires replication.

Receptor binding studies

As already described, these studies can be used to quantify receptor numbers and to image the effects of drugs in the brain. Seminal work in the 1970s had shown that the potency of a drug in binding to dopamine receptors was very strongly correlated with the dosage required in clinical practice (see Sedvall et al., 1986) – one of the main pillars of the 'dopamine hypothesis of schizophrenia'. Subsequent PET studies have shown that conventional doses of typical neuroleptics result in 70–90% D_2 blockade, with higher occupancy in those with extra-pyramidal side effects, while the atypical neuroleptic clozapine is associated with only 40–60% occupancy (Farde et al., 1992). Others have shown that non-response to neuroleptics is not simply attributable to a lack of dopamine receptor blockade (Wolkin et al., 1989; Coppen et al., 1991). With the development of more receptor ligands such studies may help in the rational development of new treatments for schizophrenia, but they have already begun to shed light on the pathophysiology of the disorder.

Post-mortem studies described increased densities of dopamine receptors in decreased patients with schizophrenia (see previous chapter) but these changes could have been attributable to antipsychotic medication effects and in vivo PET studies have been able to examine this possibility. The ideal ligand needs to be selective, saturable and bind with high affinity so as to give anatomical and neurochemical specificity (Sedvall et al., 1986); such as the relatively selective (labelled) dopamine binding drugs ^{11}C-raclopride and ^{11}C-3N-methylspiperone (NMSP). Wong et al. (1986) reported two to three fold higher D_2 receptor densities in the caudate nucleus of both treated and untreated patient groups using NMSP. However, workers at the Karolinska institute in Sweden used the much more selective dopamine blocker raclopride (Farde et al., 1985) in a larger number of never medicated patients and found no significant difference in D_2 receptor density on PET (Farde et al., 1990). Subsequent studies have failed to resolve these discrepancies. Although an independent raclopride study also failed to find significant differences in schizophrenia (Hietala et al., 1994), and the NMSP results have only been internally replicated – by Tune et al. (1993), but not by Nordstrom et al. (1995) – the Johns Hopkins group have suggested that Type II errors have hidden an overall increase of 65% in dopamine receptor numbers across the five studies (Gjedde et al., 1995). A recent meta-analysis of post-mortem and PET studies suggests the latter conclusion (Zakzanis & Hansen, 1998). It has also been suggested that raclopride underestimates changes in D_2 receptor density (Seeman et al., 1990) and that the NMSP studies may reflect an increase in the recently discovered D_4 receptors rather than D_2 activity (Seeman et al., 1993). Two other studies have widened this research agenda by reporting pre-synaptic abnormalities of increased fluorodopa uptake (Hietala et al., 1995) and elevated dopa decarboxylase activity (Reith et al., 1994) in schizophrenia that suggest increased dopamine turnover.

Disease specificity

Similar results (and inconsistencies) to those described above are apparent in the neuro-imaging literature in other psychiatric disorders. Most work has been done on the affective disorders, where hypofrontality has been reported in unipolar depression (Buchsbaum et al., 1984; Cohen et al.,

1989b), bipolar affective disorder (Baxter et al., 1985) or both (Baxter et al., 1989), and reduced metabolism in the caudate nucleus is a fairly consistent finding in studies of depressed patients (Buchsbaum et al., 1984; Baxter et al., 1985). Furthermore, increased D_2 binding may also be found in bipolar affective disorder (Pearlson et al., 1995). In addition, increases in subcortical metabolism have been repeatedly demonstrated in obsessive–compulsive disorders, which normalize after successful behavioural treatment (Schwartz et al., 1996). Anxiety states are also associated with PET scan changes with, for example, parahippocampal gyrus abnormalities in panic disorder (Reiman et al., 1984) and perfusion increases in limbic regions on symptom provocation in phobias and post-traumatic stress disorder (Rauch et al., 1995, 1996).

Although these findings are nothing like as well replicated as in schizophrenia, there are far fewer relevant studies. As well as questioning disease specificity, they raise important methodological issues – such as the necessity to exclude co-morbid patients. Finally, intriguing evidence for possible similarities in the neurobiology underlying sub-types of the major psychoses has come from a study where poverty of speech was associated with left sided hypofrontality independent of diagnosis in 40 patients with depression and 30 with schizophrenia (Dolan et al., 1993).

Summary

The resting PET studies, therefore, do generally report a hypofrontality in schizophrenia that does not appear to be attributable to the effects of medication, while putative abnormalities in other regions are less well replicated and more influenced by medication status. Activation experiments, as with SPET, provide almost unanimous support for functional abnormalities, although the exact direction and location of these appears to critically depend on methodological factors such as the task employed, scanning technique and clinical status of the subjects. Whether hypofrontality is a state (Spence et al., 1988) or trait variable (Scottish Schizophrenia Research Group, 1998) remains controversial. Deficits in frontal and temporal perfusion or metabolism seem to be linked to negative and positive symptoms respectively, but there is a gradually increasing awareness that such neuroanatomical localization is simplistic and ignores likely abnormalities in the connectivity between these and other brain regions. Receptor binding studies not only promise a clear clinical application of neuroimaging – in drug development and monitoring – but also suggest a possible pathophysiological mechanism of increased dopamine receptor numbers and/or activity in schizophrenia. The potential lack of specificity of these findings is somewhat concerning, but simple anatomical localization of putative abnormalities has limited exploratory power. Future PET and other functional imaging studies will have to develop inventive cognitive and pharmacological activation paradigms to try and tease the functional psychoses apart.

Other functional imaging techniques

A variety of other methods are increasingly available for studying the brain at work in schizophrenia and other neuropsychiatric disorders, although most are still in the development stage and have largely been applied to the study of mental processes in healthy subjects. Functional MRI (fMRI) is arguably the most promising of these, as it measures activation related increases in perfusion through reductions in blood deoxyhaemoglobin content, without the need for exogenous contrast agents and can therefore be employed in multiple scans over time and conveniently co-registered with structural images obtained in the same scanning session. A lot of work in normal subjects has largely replicated PET findings (Roland, 1993), confirming the validity of results, and preliminary studies in schizophrenia have suggested reduced and/or less lateralized responses to motor tasks (e.g. Schroder et al., 1995b) and reduced left frontal but increased left temporal or parietal activation during verbal fluency testing (Yurgelun-Todd et al., 1996; Curtis et al., 1998). Another adaptation of MRI, in Magnetic Resonance Spectroscopy (MRS), has been used to study biochemical processes in vivo. MRS can measure the concentration of some neuronal metabolites and has largely overcome initial problems with poor spatial resolution. There is some emerging consensus that patients with schizophrenia may have reduced concentrations of phosphomonoesters and inorganic phosphate in the frontal cortex (Deicken et al., 1994; Stanley et al., 1995), and reduced N-acetyl-aspartate in temporal structures (Renshaw et al., 1995; Maier et al., 1995), which may reflect increased neuronal membrane breakdown. Some workers have also reported similar abnormalities to be present before illness onset, in those with a family history and in those with disturbances in another putative trait marker measured electrophysiologically.

Electrophysiological methods, such as the EEG and event-related potentials (ERP), have been available for many years but have not delivered many consistent findings in schizophrenia that are not also present in a variety of other conditions. Their main advantage is in high temporal resolution (milliseconds), but they suffer from very poor spatial resolution. However, some interesting correlations of abnormal ERP amplitude or latency with regional brain structure and function have been reported (e.g. Blackwood et al., 1994), and such 'multimodal imaging' has exciting possibilities. Finally, two recent developments, combining the functional imaging potential of magnetic and electrical forces, show promise. Magnetoencephalography (MEG) is a non-invasive way of measuring magnetic fields induced by synaptic currents and can therefore map cortical changes due to experience, while Transcranial Magnetic Stimulations (TMS) can induce or inhibit cortical activity and may have an application as an effective antidepressant. As yet, however, it is too early to say whether or not these techniques will deliver consistent findings in the study of schizophrenia.

Integration

Several research groups have tried to tie known aetiological factors for schizophrenia (genes, obstetric complications, drugs) with brain imaging findings of putative pathophysiological importance and the symptoms and signs of the disorder. As described above, particularly in the CT literature, such studies have delivered inconsistent results apart from links between structural (and to a lesser extent functional) abnormalities and neuro-psychological deficits. Even tying the imaging results together has been difficult – 'hypofrontality' was not associated with CT measured 'cortical atrophy' in two studies (DeLisi et al., 1985a; Wiesel et al., 1987a), although has been related to ventriculomegaly and sylvian fissure enlargement in another two (Kling et al., 1986; Berman et al., 1987). There are many possible reasons for these failures – including insensitive measures, the variance in collected data, clinical differences between patients and the likelihood that more than one disease process is responsible. However, workers in two research groups in particular have dealt with some of these problems and provided insight into the pathophysiology of the disease.

In a series of studies from NIMH on discordant monozygotic twin pairs, it was shown that hippocampal size reductions were associated with schizophrenia (Suddath et al., 1990) and that this deficit was associated with a failure to activate the DLPFC on the WCST (Weinberger et al., 1992) and impaired verbal memory performance (Goldberg et al., 1994). Workers in London have focused on auditory hallucinations – finding evidence for abnormalities of fronto-temporal interaction that could underlie misattributing internal speech or thought as external stimuli (e.g. Frith et al., 1995; McGuire et al., 1995). The present review has already described important abnormalities in schizophrenia that can be integrated with this work in Washington and London and will now attempt to construct a coherent integrative summary of the current consensus.

Patients with schizophrenia, as a group, have smaller brains and limbic structures and larger ventricles than healthy controls. This appears to be mediated by an interaction between family history and obstetric complications (Cannon et al., 1989; Sharma et al., 1996). Such developmental anomalies disrupt the usual pattern of connections within and between the frontal and temporal lobes. Generally, frontal abnormalities are associated with negative symptoms and attentional/executive impairments – which are at least partly mediated by dopaminergic mechanisms as amphetamine or apomorphine can go some way to normalization (Daniel et al., 1991b; Dolan et al., 1995). Similarly, temporal lobe abnormalities are usually associated with positive symptoms and memory impairment. The functional imaging literature most consistently implicates the anterior cingulate (AC) and DLPFC regions in schizophrenia, while PM and MRI studies strongly suggest that the parahippocampal gyrus (PHG) is most reduced in volume. The PHG has also been shown to be a common component to all the three syndromes described by Liddle et al. (1992). The AC and PHG are richly connected and play a role in the integration of internal and external information in conscious processing, and in monitoring intended actions – failures of integration or monitoring could lead to misattributions of internal processes (as hallucinations). AC and DLPFC dysfunction may be associated with working memory problems and cognitive rigidity, leading to a failure to initiate various actions (negative symptoms) or to consider alternative interpretations of perceptions (delusions and hallucinations) – see Silbersweig & Stern (1996) and Silbersweig et al. (1996). Obviously, more than one or two brain regions (or neurotransmitters) are involved, but it may be that these structures and the circuits between them are of particular importance – as suggested by the verbal fluency studies. These findings of abnormal frontal decreases and temporal increases on word production suggest that the frontal lobe fails to suppress temporal activity in schizophrenia (or vice versa) and thus produces the characteristic symptoms of the disorder.

Future directions

After reviewing this extensive literature, there can be little doubt that the intense research activity over the past 20 years has demonstrated numerous abnormalities of brain structure and function in schizophrenia. However, greater attention will have to be paid to overcoming the difficulties in establishing the aetiological and clinical associations of these findings. Patient and disease heterogeneity is often blamed for this but can and should be specifically addressed by, for example, studying particular symptoms or sub-syndromes. If diagnostic groups within the 'functional psychosis' spectrum are to be differentiated, future studies must concentrate on the basis of their original separation, i.e. differing longitudinal course. Long term follow-up studies with structural MRI should be able to confirm or refute the possibility of degenerative change. Functional MRI and the other relatively safe and less invasive functional imaging methods, which are currently finding their earliest applications in neuropsychiatric research, are more suitable than PET/SPET for monitoring changes over time. There is a general need for large multi-centre collaborations, but these are difficult to coordinate and confer less prestige on individual researchers or departments. Post-mortem binding studies of various neurotransmitter systems, such as glutamate (see Chapter 4), will augment these in vivo approaches. In this author's opinion, however, the greatest advances are likely to be realized from cognitive and particularly pharmacological activation experiments on functional imaging that test specific hypotheses about pathophysiological mechanisms. There is good reason to be optimistic that all these approaches will continue to slowly but steadily deliver further insight into schizophrenia.

References

Akbarian, S., Bunney, W. E., Potkin, S. G., et al. (1993a). Altered distribution of NADPH-d cells in frontal lobe of schizophrenics implies disturbances of cortical development. *Archives of General Psychiatry*, **50**, 169–77.

Akbarian, S., Vinuela, A., Kim, J. J., Potkin, S. G., Bunney, W. E. & Jones, E. G. (1993b). Altered distribution of NADPH-d cells in temporal lobe of schizophrenics implies anomalous cortical development. *Archives of General Psychiatry*, **50**, 178–87.

Akbarian, S., Kim, J. J., Potkin, S. G., et al. (1995). Gene expression for Glutamic Acid Decarboxylase is reduced without loss of neurons in prefrontal cortex of schizophrenics. *Archives of General Psychiatry*, **52**, 258–66.

Andreasen, N. C., Nasrallah, H. A., Dunn, V., et al. (1986). Structural abnormalities in the frontal system in schizophrenia: a MRI study. *Archives of General Psychiatry*, **43**, 136–44.

Andreasen, N. C., Ehrhardt, J. C., Swayze, V. W., et al. (1990). Magnetic resonance imaging of the brain in schizophrenia. The pathophysiological significance of structural abnormalities. *Archives of General Psychiatry*, **47**, 35–44.

Andreasen, N. C., Rezai, K., Allinger, R., et al. (1992). Hypofrontality in neuroleptic-naive patients and in patients with chronic schizophrenia. *Archives of General Psychiatry*, **49**, 943–58.

Andreasen, N. C., Flashman, L., Flaum, M., et al. (1994a). Regional brain abnormalities in schizophrenia measured with magnetic resonance imaging. *Journal of the American Medical Association*, **272**, 1763–9.

Andreasen, N. C., Arndt, S., Swayze, V., et al. (1994b). Thalamic abnormalities in schizophrenia visualized through magnetic resonance image averaging. *Science*, **226**, 294–8.

Andreasen, N. C., O'Leary, D. S., Flaum, M., et al. (1997). Hypofrontality in schizophrenia: distributed dysfunctional circuits in neuroleptic-naive patients. *Lancet*, **349**, 1730–4.

Ariel, R. N., Golden, C. H., Berg, R. A., et al. (1983). Regional cerebral blood flow in schizophrenics: tests using the Xenon-133 inhalation method. *Archives of General Psychiatry*, **40**, 258–63.

Arnold, S. E., Franz, B. R., Gur, R. C., et al. (1995). Smaller neuronal size in schizophrenia in hippocampal subfields that mediate cortical–hippocampal interactions. *American Journal of Psychiatry*, **152**, 738–48.

Austin, M. P., Dougall, N., Ross, M., et al. (1992). SPET with 99mTc-Exametazime in major depression and the pattern of brain activity underlying the psychotic/neurotic continuum. *Journal of Affective Disorders*, **25**, 31–44.

Barr, W. B., Ashtari, M., Bilder, R. M., Degreef, G. & Lieberman, J. A. (1997). Brain morphometric comparison of first-episode schizophrenia and temporal lobe epilepsy. *British Journal of Psychiatry*, **170**, 515–19.

Barta, P. E., Pearlson, G. D., Powers, R. E., Richards, S. S. & Tune, L. E. (1990). Auditory hallucinations and smaller superior temporal gyral volume in schizophrenia. *American Journal of Psychiatry*, **147**, 1457–62.

Barta, P. E., Petty, R. G., McGilchrist, I., et al. (1995). Asymmetry of the planum temporale: methodological considerations and clinical associations. *Psychiatry Research: Neuroimaging*, **61**, 137–50.

Baxter, L. R., Phelps, M. E., Mazziotta, J. C., et al. (1985). Cerebral metabolic rates for glucose in mood disorders. *Archives of General Psychiatry*, **42**, 441–7.

Baxter, L. R., Mazziotta, J. C., Phelps, M. E., et al. (1987). Cerebral glucose metabolic rates in normal human females versus human males. *Psychiatry Research*, **21**, 237–45.

Baxter, L. R., Schwartz, J. M., Phelps, M. E., et al. (1989). Reduction of prefrontal cortex glucose metabolism common to three types of depression. *Archives of General Psychiatry*, **46**, 243–50.

Becker, T., Elmer, K., Mechla, B., et al. (1990). MRI findings in medial lobe structures in schizophrenia. *European Neuropsychopharmacology*, **1**, 83–6.

Becker, T., Elmer, K., Schneider, F., et al. (1996). Confirmation of reduced temporal limbic structure volume on magnetic resonance imaging in male patients with schizophrenia. *Psychiatry Research*, **67**, 135–43.

Benes, F. M. & Bird, E. D. (1987). An analysis of the arrangement of neurons in the cingulate cortex of schizophrenic patients. *Archives of General Psychiatry*,

44, 608–16.

Benes, F. M., Davidson, J. & Bird, E. D. (1986). Quantitative cytoarchitectural studies of cerebral cortex of schizophrenics. *Archives of General Psychiatry*, **43**, 31–5.

Benes, F. M., Majocha, R., Bird, E. D. & Marrotta, C. A. (1987). Increased vertical axon numbers in cingulate cortex of schizophrenics. *Archives of General Psychiatry*, **44**, 1017–21.

Benes, F. M., McSparren, J., Bird, E. D., SanGiovanni, J. P. & Vincent, S. L. (1991). Deficits in small interneurons in prefrontal and cingulate cortices of schizophrenic and schizoaffective patients. *Archives of General Psychiatry*, **48**, 996–1001.

Benes, F. M., Vincent, S. L., Aisterberg, G., Bird, E. D. & SanGiovanni, J. P. (1992). Increased GABA-A receptor binding in superficial layers of cingulate cortex in schizophrenics. *Journal of Neuroscience*, **12**, 924–9.

Berman, K. F. & Weinberger, D. R. (1990). Lateralisation of cortical function during cognitive tasks: regional cerebral blood flow studies of normal individuals and patients with schizophrenia. *Journal of Neurology, Neurosurgery and Psychiatry*, **53**, 150–60.

Berman, K. F., Zec, R. F. & Weinberger, D. R. (1986). Physiologic dysfunction of dorsolateral pre-frontal cortex in schizophrenia, II: role of neuroleptic treatment, attention, and mental effort. *Archives of General Psychiatry*, **43**, 126–35.

Berman, K. F., Weinberger, D. R., Shelton, R. C. & Zec, R. F. (1987). A relationship between anatomical and physiological brain pathology in schizophrenia: lateral cerebral ventricular size predicts cortical blood flow. *American Journal of Psychiatry*, **144**, 1277–82.

Berman, K. F., Illowsky, B. P. & Weinberger, D. R. (1988). Physiologic dysfunction of dorsolateral pre-frontal cortex in schizophrenia, IV: further evidence for regional and behavioural specificity. *Archives of General Psychiatry*, **45**, 616–22.

Berman, K. F., Torrey, E. F., Daniel, D. G. & Weinberger, D. R. (1992). Regional cerebral blood flow in monozygotic twins discordant and concordant for schizophrenia. *Archives of General Psychiatry*, **49**, 927–34.

Berman, K. F., Doran, A. R., Pickar, D. & Weinberger, D. R. (1993). Is the mechanism of prefrontal hypofunction in depression the same as in schizophrenia? *British Journal of Psychiatry*, **162**, 183–92.

Bilder, R. M., Wu, H., Bogerts, B., et al. (1994). Absence of regional hemispheric volumes of asymmetries in first-episode schizophrenia. *American Journal of Psychiatry*, **151**, 1437–47.

Bilder, R. M., Bogerts, B., Ashtari, M., et al. (1995). Anterior hippocampal volume reductions predict frontal lobe dysfunction in first episode schizophrenia. *Schizophrenia Research*, **17**, 47–58.

Blackwood, D. H. R., Ebmeier, K. P., Muir, W. J., et al. (1994). Correlation of regional CBF equivalents measured by SPECT with P300 latency and eye movement abnormality in schizophrenia. *Acta Psychiatrica Scandanavica*, **90**, 157–66.

Bogerts, B., Meertz, E. & Schonfeldt-Bausch, R. (1985). Basal ganglia and limbic system pathology in schizophrenia. *Archives of General Psychiatry*, **42**, 784–91.

Bogerts, B., Falkai, P., Haupts, M., et al. (1990a). Post-mortem measurements of limbic system and basal ganglia structures in chronic schizophrenics.

Schizophrenia Research, **3**, 295–301.

Bogerts, B., Ashtari, M., Degreef, G., et al. (1990b). Reduced temporal limbic structure volumes on magnetic resonance images in first episode schizophrenia. *Psychiatric Research: Neuroimaging*, **35**, 1–13.

Bogerts, B., Lieberman, J. A., Ashtari, M., et al. (1993). Hippocampus–amygdala volumes and psychopathology in chronic schizophrenia. *Biological Psychiatry*, **33**, 236–46.

Breier, A., Buchanan, R. W. Elkashef, A., et al. (1992). A magnetic resonance imaging study of limbic, prefrontal cortex, and caudate structures. *Archives of General Psychiatry*, **49**, 921–6.

Breier, A., Malhotra, A. K., Pinals, D. A., Weisenfeld, N. I. & Pickar, D. (1997). Association of ketamine-induced psychosis with focal activation of the prefrontal cortex in healthy volunteers. *American Journal of Psychiatry*, **154**, 805–11.

Brown, R., Colter, N., Corsellis, N., et al. (1986). Postmortem evidence of structural brain changes in schizophrenia. *Archives of General Psychiatry*, **43**, 36–42.

Bruton, C. J., Crow, T. J., Frith, C. D., Johnstone, E. C., Owens, D. G. C. & Roberts, G. W. (1990). Schizophrenia and the brain: a prospective clinico-neuropathological study. *Psychological Medicine*, **20**, 285–304.

Buchanan, R. W., Breier, A., Kirkpatrick, B., et al. (1993). Structural abnormalities in deficit and nondeficit schizophrenia. *Archives of General Psychiatry*, **150**, 59–65.

Buchsbaum, M. S., Ingvar D. H., Kessler, R., et al. (1982). Cerebral glucography with positron tomography: use in normal subjects and in patients with schizophrenia. *Archives of General Psychiatry*, **39**, 251–9.

Buchsbaum, M. S., DeLisi, L. E., Holcomb, H. H., et al. (1984). Anteroposterior gradients in cerebral glucose use in schizophrenia and affective disorders. *Archives of General Psychiatry*, **41**, 1159–66.

Buchsbaum, M. S., Wu, J. C., DeLisi, L. E., et al. (1987). PET studies of basal ganglia and somatosensory cortex neuroleptic drug effects. *Biological Psychiatry*, **22**, 479–94.

Buchsbaum, M. S., Potkin, S. G., Siegel, B. V., et al. (1992a). Striatal metabolic rate and clinical response to neuroleptics in schizophrenia. *Archives of General Psychiatry*, **49**, 966–74.

Buchsbaum, M. S., Haier, R. J., Potkin, S. G., et al. (1992b). Frontostriatal disorder of cerebral metabolism in never-medicated schizophrenics. *Archives of General Psychiatry*, **49**, 935–42.

Bullmore, E., Brammer, E., Harvey, I. & Ron, M. (1995). Against the laterality index as a measure of cerebral asymmetry. *Psychiatry Research: Neuroimaging*, **61**, 121–4.

Busatto, G. F., Costa, D. C., Ell, P. J., Pilowsky, L. S., David, A. S. & Kerwin, R. W. (1994). Regional cerebral blood flow in schizophrenia during verbal memory activation: a HMPAO-SPET study. *Psychological Medicine*, **24**, 463–72.

Busatto, G. F., David, A. S., Costa, D. C., et al. (1995). Schizophrenic auditory hallucinations are associated with increased regional cerebral blood flow during verbal memory activation in a SPET study. *Psychiatric Research: Neuroimaging*, **24**, 463–72.

Busatto, G. F., Pilowsky, L. S., Costa, D. C., et al. (1997). Correlation between reduced in vivo benzodiazepine receptor binding and severity of psychotic symptoms in schizophrenia. *American Journal of Psychiatry*, **154**, 56–63.

Cannon, T. D., Mednick, S. A. & Parnas, J. (1989). Genetic and perinatal determinants of structural brain deficits in schizophrenia. *Archives of General Psychiatry*, **46**, 883–9.

Catafau, A. M., Parallada, E., Lomena, F. J., et al. (1994). Prefrontal and temporal blood flow in schizophrenia: resting and activation Technetium-99m-HMPAO SPECT patterns in young acute neuroleptic-naive patients. *Journal of Nuclear Medicine*, **35**, 935–41.

Chakos, M. H., Lieberman, J. A., Bilder, R. M., et al. (1994). Increase in caudate nuclei volumes of first-episode schizophrenic patients taking antipsychotic drugs. *American Journal of Psychiatry*, **151**, 1430–6.

Chakos, M. H., Lieberman, J. A., Alvir, J., Bilder, R. & Ashtari, M. (1995). Caudate nuclei volumes in schizophrenic patients treated with typical antipsychotics or clozapine. *Lancet*, **345**, 456–7.

Chua, S. E., Wright, I. C., Poline, J-B., et al. (1997). Grey matter correlates of syndromes in schizophrenia. *British Journal of Psychiatry*, **170**, 406–10.

Cleghorn, J. M., Garnett, E. S., Nahmias, C., et al. (1989). Increased frontal and reduced parietal glucose metabolism in acute untreated schizophrenia. *Psychiatry Research*, **28**, 119–33.

Cleghorn, J. M., Garnett, E. S., Nahmias, C., et al. (1990). Regional brain metabolism during auditory hallucinations in chronic schizophrenia. *British Journal of Psychiatry*, **157**, 562–70.

Cleghorn, J. M., Franco, S., Szechtman, B., et al. (1992). Towards a brain map of auditory hallucinations. *American Journal of Psychiatry*, **149**, 1062–9.

Cohen, M. B., Lake, R. R., Graham, L. S., et al. (1989a). Quantitative Iodine-123 IMP imaging of brain perfusion in schizophrenia. *Journal of Nuclear Medicine*, **30**, 1616–20.

Cohen, R. M., Semple, W. E., Gross, M., et al. (1987). Dysfunction in a prefrontal substrate of sustained attention in schizophrenia. *Life Sciences*, **40**, 2031–9.

Cohen, R. M., Semple, W. E., Gross, M., et al. (1989b). Evidence for common alterations in cerebral glucose metabolism in major affective disorders and schizophrenia. *Neuropsychopharmacology*, **2**, 241–54.

Coppen, H. J., Slooff, C. J., Paans, A. M. J., et al. (1991). High central D2-dopamine receptor occupancy as assessed with PET in medicated but therapy-resistant schizophrenic patients. *Biological Psychiatry*, **29**, 629–34.

Crow, T. J. (1980). Molecular pathology of schizophrenia: more than one disease process? *British Medical Journal*, **280**, 66–8.

Curtis, V. A., Bullmore, E. T. & Brammer, M. J. (1998). Attenuated frontal activation during a verbal fluency task in patients with schizophrenia. *American Journal of Psychiatry*, **155**, 1056–63.

Daniel, D. G., Goldberg, T. E., Gibbons, R. D. & Weinberger, D. R. (1991a). Lack of a bimodal distribution of ventricular size in schizophrenia: a gaussian mixture analysis of 1056 cases and controls. *Biological Psychiatry*, **30**, 887–903.

Daniel, D. G., Weinberger, D. R., Jones, D. W., et al. (1991b). The effect of amphetamine on regional cerebral blood flow during cognitive activation in schizophrenia. *Journal of Neuroscience*, **11**, 1907–17.

Dauphinais, D., DeLisi, L. E., Crow, T. J., et al. (1990). Reduction in temporal size in siblings with schizophrenia: A magnetic resonance imaging study. *Psychiatric Research: Neuroimaging*, **35**, 137–47.

Degreef, G., Ashtari, M., Bogerts, B., et al. (1992). Volumes of ventricular system subdivisions measured from magnetic resonance images in first-episode schizophrenic patients. *Archives of General Psychiatry*, **49**, 531–7.

Deicken, R. E., Calabrese, G., Merrin, E. L., et al. (1994). 31-Phosphurus MRS of the frontal and parietal lobes in chronic schizophrenia. *Biological Psychiatry*, **36**, 503–10.

DeLisi, L. E., Buchsbaum, M. S., Holcomb, H. H., et al. (1985a). Clinical correlates of relative hypofrontality in PET of schizophrenic patients. *American Journal of Psychiatry*, **142**, 78–81.

DeLisi, L. E., Holcomb, H. H., Cohen, R. M., et al. (1985b). PET in schizophrenic patients with and without neuroleptic medication. *Journal of Cerebral Blood Flow and Metabolism*, **5**, 201–6.

DeLisi, L. E., Buchsbaum, M. S., Holcomb, H. H., et al. (1985c). Increased temporal lobe glucose activity with PET in schizophrenic patients. *Biological Psychiatry*, **25**, 835–51.

DeLisi, L. E., Goldin, L. R., Hamovit, J. R., Maxwell, E., Kurtz, D. & Gershon, E. S. (1986). A family study of the association of increased ventricular size with schizophrenia. *Archives of General Psychiatry*, **43**, 148–53.

DeLisi, L. E., Hoff, A. L., Schwartz, J. E., et al. (1991). Brain morphology in first-episode schizophrenia-like psychotic patients: A quantitative magnetic resonance imaging study. *Biological Psychiatry*, **29**, 159–75.

DeLisi, L. E., Hoff, A. L., Neale, C. & Kushner, M. (1994). Asymmetries in the superior temporal lobe in male and female first-episode schizophrenic patients: measures of the planum temporale and superior temporal gyrus by MRI. *Schizophrenia Research*, **12**, 19–28.

DeLisi, L. E., Sakuma, M., Tew, W., Kushner, M., Hoff, A. L. & Grimson, R. (1997). Schizophrenia as a chronic active brain process: a study of progressive brain structural change subsequent to the onset of schizophrenia. *Psychiatry Research: Neuroimaging*, **74**, 129–40.

Dolan, R. J., Bench, C. J., Liddle, P. F., et al. (1993). Dorsolateral prefrontal cortex dysfunction in the major psychoses; symptom or disease specificity? *Journal of Neurology, Neurosurgery and Psychiatry*, **56**, 1290–4.

Dolan, R. J., Fletcher, P., Frith, C. D., et al. (1995). Dopaminergic modulation of impaired cognitive activation in the anterior cingulate cortex in schizophrenia. *Nature*, **378**, 180–2.

Donnelly, E. F., Weinberger, D. R., Waldman, I. N., et al. (1980). Cognitive impairment associated with morphological brain abnormalities. *Journal of Nervous and Mental Disease*, **168**, 305–8.

Dousse, M., Mamo, H., Ponsin, J. C. & Dinh, Y. T. (1988). Cerebral blood flow in schizophrenia. *Experimental Neurology*, **199**, 98–111.

Dupont, R. M., Lehr, P. P., Lamoureux, G., et al. (1994). Preliminary report: cerebral blood flow abnormalities in older schizophrenic patients. *Psychiatric Research: Neuroimaging*, **55**, 121–30.

Early, T. S., Reiman, E. M., Raichle, M. E. & Spitznagal, E. L. (1987). Left globus pallidus abnormality in never-medicated patients with schizophrenia. *Proceedings of the National Academy of Sciences*, **84**, 561–3.

Ebmeier, K. P., Blackwood, D. H. R., Murray, C., et al. (1993). Single-photon emission computed tomography with 99mTc-exametazime in unmedicated schizophrenic patients. *Biological Psychiatry*, **33**, 487–95.

Ebmeier, K. P., Lawrie, S. M., Blackwood, D. H. R., Johnstone, E. C. & Goodwin, G. M. (1995). Hypofrontality revisited: a high resolution SPECT study in schizophrenia. *Journal of Neurology, Neurosurgery and Psychiatry*, **58**, 452–6.

Elkis, E., Friedman, L., Wise, A. & Meltzer, H. Y. (1995). Meta-analysis of studies of ventricular enlargement and cortical sulcal prominence in mood disorders. Comparisons with controls or patients with schizophrenia. *Archives of General Psychiatry*, **52**, 735–46.

Erbas, B., Kumbasser, H., Erbengi, G. & Bekdik, C. (1990). Tc-99m-HMPAO/SPECT determination of regional cerebral blood flow changes in schizophrenics. *Clinical Nuclear Medicine*, **12**, 904–7.

Falkai, P. & Bogerts, B. (1986). Cell loss in the hippocampus of schizophrenics. *European Archives of Psychiatry and Neuroscience*, **236**, 154–61.

Falkai, P., Bogerts, B., Schneider, T., et al. (1995). Disturbed planum temporale asymmetry in schizophrenia. A quantitative post-mortem study. *Schizophrenia Research*, **14**, 161–76.

Farde, L., Ehrin, E., Eriksson, L., et al. (1985). Substituted benzamides as ligands for visualisation of dopamine receptor binding in the human brain by PET. *Proceedings of the National Academy of Sciences*, **82**, 3863–7.

Farde, L., Wiesel, F. A., Stone–Elander, S., et al. (1990). D_2-Dopamine receptors in neuroleptic-naive schizophrenic patients. *Archives of General Psychiatry*, **47**, 213–19.

Farde, L., Nordstrtom, A-L., Wiesel, F. A., Pauli, S., Halldin, C. & Sedvall, G. (1992). PET analysis of central D_1 and D_2 dopamine receptor occupancy in patients treated with classical neuroleptics and clozapine. *Archives of General Psychiatry*, **49**, 538–44.

Farkas, T., Wolfe, A. P., Jaeger, J., et al. (1984). Regional brain glucose metabolism in chronic schizophrenia: a positron emission transaxial tomographic study. *Archives of General Psychiatry*, **41**, 293–300.

Flaum, M., Swayze, V. W., O'Leary, D. S., et al. (1995). Effects of laterality, and gender on brain morphology in schizophrenia. *American Journal of Psychiatry*, **152**, 704–14.

Frazier, J. A., Giedd, J. N., Kaysen, D., et al. (1996a). Childhood-onset schizophrenia: brain MRI rescan after 2 years of clozapine maintenance treatment. *American Journal of Psychiatry*, **153**, 564–6.

Frazier, J. A., Giedd, J. N., Hamburger, S. D., et al. (1996b). Brain anatomic MRI in childhood-onset schizophrenia. *Archives of General Psychiatry*, **53**, 617–24.

Friedman, L., Lys, C. & Schulz, S. C. (1992). The relationship of structural brain imaging parameters to antipsychotic treatment response: a review. *Journal of Psychiatry and Neuroscience*, **17**, 42–54.

Friston, K. J., Frith, C. D., Liddle, P. F., et al. (1990). The relationship between global and local changes in PET scans. *Journal of Cerebral Blood Flow and Metabolism*, **10**, 458–66.

Friston, K. J., Frith, C. D., Liddle, P. F. & Frackowiak, R. S. J. (1992a). Functional connectivity: the principal component analysis of large PET data sets. *Journal of Cerebral Blood Flow and Metabolism*, **13**, 5–14.

Friston, K. J., Liddle, P. F., Frith, C. D., Hirsch, S. R. & Frackowiak, R. S. J. (1992b). The left medial temporal region and schizophrenia. *Brain*, **115**, 367–82.

Frith, C. D., Friston, K. J., Herold, S., et al. (1995). Regional brain activity in chronic schizophrenic patients during the performance of a verbal fluency task. *British Journal of Psychiatry*, **167**, 343–9.

Fukuzako, H., Fukuzako, T., Hashiguchi, T., et al. (1996). Reduction in hippocampal formation volume is caused mainly by its shortening in chronic schizophrenia: assessment by MRI. *Biological Psychiatry*, **39**, 938–45.

Ganguli, R., Carter, C., Mintum, M., et al. (1997). PET brain mapping study of auditory verbal supraspan memory versus visual fixation in schizophrenia. *Biological Psychiatry*, **41**, 33–42.

Geraud, G., Arne-Bes, M. C., Guell, A. & Bes, A. (1987). Reversibility of haemodynamically measured hypofrontality in schizophrenia. *Journal of Cerebral Blood Flow and Metabolism*, **7**, 9–12.

Gjedde, A., Reith, J. & Wong, D. (1995). Dopamine receptors in schizophrenia. *Lancet*, **346**, 1302–3 (and further details from the authors).

Goldberg, T. E., Torrey, E. F., Berman, K. F. & Weinberger, D. R. (1994). Relations between neuropsychological performance and brain morphological and physiological measures in monozygotic twins discordant for schizophrenia. *Psychiatry Research: Neuroimaging*, **55**, 51–61.

Golden, C. J., Moses, J. A., Zelazowski, R., et al. (1980). Cerebral ventricular size and neuropsychological impairment in young chronic schizophrenics: measurement by the standardised Luria–Nebraska neuropsychological battery. *Archives of General Psychiatry*, **37**, 619–23.

Golden, C. J., MacInnes, W. D., Ariel, R. N., et al. (1982). Cross-validation of the Luria–Nebraska Neuropsychological battery to differentiate chronic schizophrenics with and without ventricular enlargement. *Journal of Consulting and Clinical Psychology*, **50**, 87–95.

Guenther, W., Moser, E., Petsch, R., et al. (1989). Pathological cerebral blood flow and corpus callosum abnormalities in schizophrenia: relations to EEG mapping and PET data. *Psychiatry Research*, **29**, 453–5.

Guenther, W., Brodie, J. D., Bartlett, E. J., et al. (1994). Diminished cerebral metabolic response to motor stimulation in schizophrenics: a PET study. *European Archives of Psychiatry and Clinical Neuroscience*, **244**, 115–25.

Gullion, C. M., Devous, M. D. & Rush, A. J. (1996). Effects of four normalising methods on data analytic results in functional brain imaging. *Biological Psychiatry*, **40**, 1106–21.

Gur, R. E., Skolnick, B. E., Gur, R. C., et al. (1983). Brain function in psychiatric disorders, I: regional cerebral blood flow in medicated schizophrenics. *Archives of General Psychiatry*, **40**, 1250–4.

Gur, R. E., Gur, R. C., Skolnick, B. E., et al. (1985). Brain function in psychiatric disorders, III: regional cerebral blood flow in unmedicated schizophrenics. *Archives of General Psychiatry*, **42**, 329–34.

Gur, R. E., Resnick, S. M., Alavi, A., et al. (1987a). Regional brain function in schizophrenia I. A PET study. *Archives of General Psychiatry*, **44**, 119–25.

Gur, R. E., Resnick, S. M., Gur, R. C., et al. (1987b). Regional brain function in schizophrenia II. Repeated evaluation with PET. *Archives of General Psychiatry*, **44**, 126–9.

Gur, R. E., Mozley, P. D., Resnick, S. M., et al. (1991). Magnetic resonance imaging in schizophrenia. Volumetric analysis of brain and cerebrospinal fluid. *Archives of General Psychiatry*, **48**, 407–12.

Gur, R. E., Mozley, P. D., Shatsel, D. L., et al. (1994a). Clinical subtypes of schizophrenia: differences in brain and CSF volume. *American Journal of Psychiatry*, **151**, 343–50.

Gur, R. E., Jaggi, J. L., Shatsel, D. L., Ragland, J. D. & Gur, R. C. (1994b). Cerebral blood flow in schizophrenia: effects of memory processing on regional activation. *Biological Psychiatry*, **35**, 3–15.

Gur, R. E., Mozley, P. D., Resnick, S. M., et al. (1995). Resting cerebral glucose metabolism in first-episode and previously treated patients with schizophrenia relates to clinical features. *Archives of General Psychiatry*, **52**, 657–67.

Gur, R. E., Cowell, P. & Turetsky, B. I. (1998). A follow-up MRI study of schizophrenia. *Archives of General Psychiatry*, **55**, 145–52.

Harvey, I., Williams, M., Toone, B. K., Lewis, S. W., Turner, S. W. & McGuffin, P. (1990). The VBR in functional psychoses: the relationship of lateral ventricular and total intracranial area. *Psychological Medicine*, **20**, 55–62.

Harvey, I., Ron, M. A., Du Boulay, G., et al. (1993). Reduction of cortical volume in schizophrenia on magnetic resonance imaging. *Psychological Medicine*, **23**, 591–604.

Haznedar, M. M., Buchsbaum, M. S., Luu, C., et al. (1997). Decreased anterior cingulate gyrus metabolic rate in schizophrenia. *American Journal of Psychiatry*, **154**, 682–4.

Heinz, E. R., Martinex, J. & Haenggell, A. (1977). Reversibility of cerebral atrophy in anorexia nervosa and Cushing's syndrome. *Journal of Computer Assisted Tomography*, **1**, 415–17.

Hietala, J., Syvalahti, E., Vuorio, K., et al. (1994). Striatal D_2 dopamine receptor characteristics in neuroleptic-naive schizophrenic patients studies with PET. *Archives of General Psychiatry*, **51**, 116–23.

Hietala, J., Syvalahti, E., Vuorio, K., et al. (1995). Presynaptic dopamine function in striatum of neuroleptic-naive schizophrenic patients. *Lancet*, **346**, 1130–1.

Holcomb, H. H., Cascella, N. G., Thaker, G. K., et al. (1996). Functional sites of neuroleptic drug action in the human brain: PET/FDG studies with and without haloperidol. *American Journal of Psychiatry*, **153**, 41–9.

Honer, W. G., Bassett, A. S., Squires-Wheeler, E., et al. (1995). The temporal lobes, reversed asymmetry and the genetics of schizophrenia. *Neuroreport*, **7**, 221–4.

Illowsky, B., Juliano, D. M., Bigelow, L. B., et al. (1988). Stability of CT scan findings in schizophrenia. *Journal of Neurology, Neurosurgery and Psychiatry*, **51**, 209–12.

Ingvar, D. H. & Franzen, G. (1974a). Abnormalities of cerebral blood flow distribution in patients with chronic schizophrenia. *Acta Psychiatrica Scandinavica*, **50**, 425–62.

Ingvar, D. H. & Franzen, G. (1974b). Distribution of cerebral activity in chronic schizophrenia. *Lancet*, **i**, 1484–6.

Jaskiw, G. E., Juliano, D. M., Goldber, T. E., Hertzman, M., Urow-Hamell, E. & Weinberger, D. R. (1994). Cerebral ventricular enlargement in schizophreniform disorder does not progress: a seven year follow-up study. *Schizophrenia Research*, **14**, 23–8.

Jernigan, T. L., Sargent, T., Pfefferbaum, A., et al. (1985). 18FDG PET in schizophrenia. *Psychiatry Research*, **16**, 317–29.

Jernigan, T. L., Zisook, S., Heaton, R. K., et al. (1991). Magnetic resonance imaging abnormalities in lenticular nuclei and cerebral cortex in schizophrenia. *Archives of General Psychiatry*, **48**, 881–90.

Jeste, D. & Lohr, J. B. (1989). Hippocampal pathologic findings in schizophrenia. A morphometric study. *Archives of General Psychiatry*, **46**, 1019–24.

Johnstone, E. C., Crow, T. J., Frith, C. D., Husband, J. & Kreel, L. (1976). Cerebral ventricular size and cognitive impairment in chronic schizophrenia. *Lancet*, **ii**, 924–6.

Johnstone, E. C., Crow, T. J., Frith, C. D., et al. (1978). The dementia of dementia praecox. *Acta Psychiatrica Scandinavica*, **57**, 305–24.

Kaplan, R. D., Sczechtman, H., Franco, S., et al. (1993). Three clinical syndromes of schizophrenia in untreated subjects: relation to brain glucose activity by PET. *Schizophrenia Research*, **11**, 47–54.

Katz, M., Buchsbaum, M. S., Siegel, B. V., et al. (1996). Correlational patterns of cerebral glucose metabolism in never-medicated schizophrenics. *Neuropsychobiology*, **33**, 1–11.

Kawasaki, Y., Suzuki, M., Maeda, Y., et al. (1992). Regional cerebral blood flow in patients with schizophrenia. *European Archives of Psychiatry and Clinical Neuroscience*, **241**, 195–200.

Kawasaki, K. Y., Maeda, Y., Urata, K., et al. (1993a). A quantative magnetic resonance imaging study of patients with schizophrenia. *European Archives of Psychiatry and Clinical Neurosciences*, **242**, 268–72.

Kawasaki, Y., Maeda, Y., Suzuki, M., et al. (1993b). SPECT analysis of regional cerebral blood flow changes in patients with schizophrenia during the Wisconsin Card Sorting Test. *Schizophrenia Research*, **10**, 109–16.

Kelsoe, J. R., Cadet, J. L., Picard, D. & Weinberger, D. R. (1988). Quantitative neuroanatomy in schizophrenia. *Archives of General Psychiatry*, **45**, 533–41.

Kemali, D., Maj, M., Galderisi, S., et al. (1989). VBR in schizophrenia: a controlled follow-up study. *Biological Psychiatry*, **26**, 756–62.

Keshavan, M. S., Bagwell, W. W., Haas, G. L., Sweeney, J. A., Schooler, N. R. & Pettegrew, J. W. (1994). Changes in caudata volume with neuroleptic treatment. *Lancet*, **344**, 1434.

Kety, S. S., Woodford, R. B., Harmel, M. H., Freyhan, F. A., Appel, K. E. & Schmidt, C. F. (1948). Cerebral blood flow and metabolism in schizophrenia. *American Journal of Psychiatry*, **104**, 765–70.

Kikinis, R., Shenton, M. E., Gerig, G., et al. (1994). Temporal lobe sulco-gyral pattern anomalies in schizophrenia: an in vivo MR three-dimensional surface rendering study. *Neuroscience Letters*, **182**, 7–12.

Kishimoto, H., Kuwahara, H., Ohno, S., et al. (1987). Three sub-types of chronic schizophrenia identified using ^{11}C-glucose PET. *Psychiatry Research*, **21**, 285–92.

Kleinschmidt, A., Falkai, P., Huang, Y., et al. (1994). In vivo morphometry of planum temporale asymmetry in first-episode schizophrenia. *Schizophrenia Research*, **12**, 9–18.

Klemm, E., Grunwald, F., Kaspar, S., et al. (1996). IBZM SPECT for imaging of striatal D2 receptors in 56 schizophrenic patients taking various neuroleptics. *American Journal of Psychiatry*, **153**, 183–90.

Kling, A. S., Metter, E. J., Riege, W. H. & Kuhl, D. E. (1986). Comparison of PET measurement of local brain glucose metabolism and CAT measurement of brain atrophy in chronic schizophrenia and depression. *American Journal of Psychiatry*, **14**, 175–80.

Kovelman, J. A. & Scheibel, A. B. (1984). A neurohistological correlate of schizophrenia. *Biological Psychiatry*, **191**, 1601–21.

Kulynych, J. J., Vladar, K., Fantie, B., Jones, D. W. & Weinberger, D. R. (1995). Normal asymmetry of the planum temporale in patients with schizophrenia. *British Journal of Psychiatry*, **166**, 742–9.

Kulynych, J. J., Vladar, K., Jones, D. W. & Weinberger, D. R. (1996). Superior temporal gyrus volume of schizophrenia: a study using MRI morphometry assisted by surface rendering. *American Journal of Psychiatry*, **153**, 50–6.

Kurachi, M., Kobayashi, K., Matsubara, R., et al. (1985). Regional cerebral blood flow in schizophrenic disorders. *European Neurology*, **24**, 176–81.

Lahti, A. C., Holcomb, H. H., Medoff, D. R. & Tamminga, C. A. (1995). Ketamine activates psychosis and alters limbic blood flow in schizophrenia. *Neuroreport*, **6**, 869–72.

Laruelle, M., Abi-Dargham, A., Van Dyck, C. H., et al. (1996). Single photon emission computerised tomography imaging of amphetamine-induced dopamine release in drug-free schizophrenic subjects. *Proceedings of the National Academy of Sciences*, **93**, 9235–40.

Lauriello, J., Hoff, A., Wieneke, M. H., et al. (1997). Similar extent of brain dysmorphology in severely ill women and men with schizophrenia. *American Journal of Psychiatry*, **154**, 819–25.

Lawrie, S. M. & Abukmeil, S. A. (1998). How abnormal is the brain in schizophrenia? A systematic and quantitative review of volumetric MRI studies. *British Journal of Psychiatry*, **172**, 110–20.

Lawrie, S. M., Ingle, G. T., Santosh, C. G., et al. (1995). MRI and SPET in treatment responsive and treatment resistant schizophrenia. *British Journal of Psychiatry*, **167**, 202–10.

Lawrie, S. M., Ebmeier, K. P., Vernhoef, N. P. L. G., Van Royen, E. A., Johnstone, E. C. & Goodwin, G. M. (1996). Benzodiazepine GABA-A receptor binding in schizophrenia – a study with Single Photon Emission Tomography and 123I-Iomazenil. *Schizophrenia Research*, **18**, 199 (abstract).

Lawrie, S. M., Abukmeil, S., Santosh, C., Chiswick, A., Rimmington, J. E. & Best J. J. K. (1997). Qualitative morphological abnormalities in schizophrenia: an MRI study and systematic literature review. *Schizophrenia Research*, **25**, 155–66.

Lawrie, S. M., Whalley, H., Kestelman, J., et al. (in press). MRI of the brain in subjects at high risk of developing schizophrenics. *Lancet* (in press).

Lewis, S. W. (1990). Computerised tomography in schizophrenia: 15 years on. *British Journal of Psychiatry*, **157 (supplement 9)**, 16–24.

Lewis, S. W., Ford, R. A., Syed, G. M., Reveley, A. M. & Toone, B. K. (1992). A controlled study of HMPAO-SPET in chronic schizophrenia. *Psychological Medicine*, **22**, 27–35.

Liddle, P. F., Friston, K. J., Frith, C. D., et al. (1992). Patterns of cerebral blood flow in schizophrenia. *British Journal of Psychiatry*, **160**, 179–86.

Lieberman, J., Bogerts, B., Degreef, G. Ashtari, M., Lantos, G. & Alvir, J. (1992). Qualitative assessment of brain morphology in acute and chronic schizophrenia. *American Journal of Psychiatry*, **149**, 784–94.

Lim, K. O., Sullivan, E. V., Zipursky, R. B., Pfefferbaum, A. (1996a). Cortical gray matter volume deficits in schizophrenia: a replication. *Schizophrenia Research*, **20**, 157–64.

Lim, K. O., Harris, D., Beal, M., et al. (1996b). Gray matter deficits in young onset schizophrenia are independent of age of onset. *Biological Psychiatry*, **40**, 4–13.

Lim, K. O., Tew, W., Kushner, M., Chow, K., Matsumoto, B. & DeLisi, L. E. (1996c). Cortical gray matter volume deficit in patients with first-episode schizophrenia. *American Journal of Psychiatry*, **153**, 1548–53.

Luts, A, Jonsson, S., Guldberg, A. T., Kjaar, M. & Brun, A. (1998). Uniform abnormalities in the hippocampus of five chronic schizophrenic men compared with age-matched controls. *Acta Psychiatrica Scandinavica*, **98**, 60–4.

Maier, M., Ron, M. A., Barker, G. J. & Tofts, P. S. (1995). Proton MRS: an in vivo method of estimating hippocampal neuronal depletion in schizophrenia. *Psychological Medicine*, **25**, 1201–9.

Marsh, L., Suddath, R. L., Higgins, N., et al. (1994). Medial temporal lobe structures in schizophrenia: relationship of size to duration of illness. *Schizophrenia Research*, **11**, 225–38.

Mathew, R. J., Duncan, G. C., Weinman, M. L., et al. (1982). Regional cerebral blood flow in schizophrenia. *Archives of General Psychiatry*, **39**, 1121–4.

Mathew, R. J., Wilson, W. H. & Tant, S. R. (1986). Determinants of resting regional cerebral blood flow in normal subjects. *Biological Psychiatry*, **21**, 907–14.

Mathew, R. J., Wilson, W. H., Tant, S. R., Robinson, L. & Prakash, R. (1988). Abnormal resting regional cerebral blood flow patterns and their correlates in schizophrenia. *Archives of General Psychiatry*, **45**, 542–9.

Mathew, R. J. & Wilson, W. H. (1990). Anxiety and cerebral blood flow. *American Journal of Psychiatry*, **147**, 838–49.

Mathew, R. J. & Wilson, W. H. (1991). Substance abuse and cerebral blood flow. *American Journal of Psychiatry*, **148**, 292–305.

Matsuda, H., Gyobu, T., Masayasu, Z. D. & Hisada, K. (1988). Increased accumulation of IMP in the left auditory area in a schizophrenic patient with auditory hallucinations. *Clinical Nuclear Medicine*, **13**, 53–5.

Matsuda, H., Jibiki, I. & Kinuya, K. (1991). HMPAO SPECT analysis of neuroleptic effects on regional brain function. *Clinical Nuclear Medicine*, **16**, 660–4.

McGuire, P. K., Shah, G. M. S. & Murray, R. M. (1993). Increased blood flow in Broca's area during auditory hallucinations in schizophrenia. *Lancet*, **342**, 703–6.

McGuire, P. K., Silbersweig, D. A., Wright, I., et al. (1995). Abnormal monitoring of inner speech: a physiological basis for auditory hallucinations. *Lancet*, **346**, 596–600.

McGuire, P. K., Quested, D. J., Spence, S. A., et al. (1998). Pathophysiology of 'positive' thought disorder in schizophrenia. *British Journal of Psychiatry*, **173**, 231–5.

Menon, R. R., Barta, P. E., Aylward, E. H., et al. (1995). Posterior superior temporal gyrus in schizophrenia: grey matter changes and clinical correlates. *Schizophrenia Research*, **16**, 127–35.

Miller, D. D., Rezai, K., Alliger, R. & Andreasen, N. C. (1997). The effect of antipsychotic medication on relative cerebral blood perfusion in schizophrenia: assessment with HMPAO-SPECT. *Biological Psychiatry*, **41**, 550–9.

Morretti, J. L., Caglar, M. & Weinmann, P. (1995). Cerebral perfusion imaging tracers for SPECT: which one to chose? *Journal of Nuclear Medicine*, **36**, 359–63.

Mozley, L. H., Gur, R. C., Gur, R. E., Mozley, D. & Alavi, A. (1996). Relationships between verbal memory performance and the cerebral distribution of fluorodeoxyglucose in patients with schizophrenia. *Biological Psychiatry*, **40**, 443–51.

Musalek, M., Podreka, I., Walter, H., et al. (1989). Regional brain function in hallucinations: a study of regional cerebral blood flow with 99m-Tc-HMPAO-SPECT in patients with auditory hallucinations, tactile hallucinations and normal controls. *Comprehensive Psychiatry*, **30**, 99–108.

Nakashima, Y., Momose, T., Sano, I., et al. (1994). Cortical control of saccade in normal and schizophrenic subjects: a PET study using a task-evoked rCBF paradigm. *Schizophrenia Research*, **12**, 259–64.

Nasrallah, H. A., Olsen, S. C., McCalley-Whitters, M., et al. (1986). Cerebral ventricular enlargement in schizophrenia: a preliminary follow-up study. *Archives of General Psychiatry*, **43**, 157–9.

Nelson, M. D., Saykin, A. J., Flashman, L. A. & Riordan, H. J. (1998). Hippocampal volume reduction in schizophrenics as assessed by MRI. *Archives of General Psychiatry*, **55**, 433–40.

Nestor, P. G., Shenton, M. E., McCarley, R. W., et al. (1993). Neuropsychological correlates of MRI temporal lobe abnormalities in schizophrenia. *American Journal of Psychiatry*, **150**, 1849–55.

Nimgaonkar, V. L., Wessely, S., Lune, L. E. & Murray, R. M. (1988). Response to drugs in schizophrenia: the influence of family history, obstetric complications and ventricular enlargement. *Psychological Medicine*, **18**, 583–92.

Noga, J. T., Aylward, E., Barta, P. E. & Pearlson, G. D. (1995). Cingulate gyrus in schizophrenic patients and normal volunteers. *Psychiatry Research: Neuroimaging*, **61**, 201–8.

Noga, J. T., Bartley, A. J., Jones, D. W., Torrey, E. F. & Weinberger, D. R. (1996). Cortical gyral anatomy and gross brain dimensions in monozygotic twins discordant for schizophrenia. *Schizophrenia Research*, **22**, 27–40.

Nopoulos, P., Torres, I., Flaum, M., et al. (1995). Brain morphology in first-episode schizophrenia. *American Journal of Psychiatry*, **152**, 1721–3.

Nordstrom, A-L., Farde, L., Eriksson, L. & Halldin, C. (1995). No elevated D2 dopamine receptors in neuroleptic-naive schizophrenic patients revealed by PET and [11C]N-methylspiperone. *Psychiatry Research: Neuroimaging*, **61**, 67–83.

O'Callaghan, E., Buckley, P., Redmond, O., et al. (1992). Abnormalities of cerebral structure in schizophrenia on magnetic resonance imaging: interpretation in relation to the neurodevelopmental hypothesis. *Journal of the Royal Society of Medicine*, **85**, 227–31.

Ohnuma, T., Kimura, M., Takahashi, T., Iwamoto, N. & Arai, H. (1997). A magnetic resonance imaging study in first-episode disorganized-type patients with schizophrenia. *Psychiatry & Clinical Neurosciences*, **51**, 9–15.

Owens, D. G. C., Johnstone, E. C., Crow, T. J., et al. (1985). Lateral ventricular size in schizophrenia: relationship to the disease process and its clinical manifestations. *Psychological Medicine*, **14**, 27–41.

Pakkenberg, B. (1987). Post-mortem study of chronic schizophrenic brains. *British Journal of Psychiatry*, **151**, 744–52.

Paulman, R. G., Devous, M. D., Gregory, R. R., et al. (1990). Hypofrontality and cognitive impairment in schizophrenia: dynamic SPET neuropsychological assessment of schizophrenic brain function. *Biological Psychiatry*, **27**, 377–99.

Pearlson, G. D., Kim, W. S., Kubos, K. L., et al. (1989). Ventricle–brain ratio, computed tomography density and brain area in 50 schizophrenics. *Archives of General Psychiatry*, **41**, 690–7.

Pearlson, G. D., Wong, D. F., Tune, L. E., et al. (1995). In vivo D$_2$ dopamine receptor density in psychotic and non-psychotic patients with bipolar disorder. *Archives of General Psychiatry*, **52**, 471–7.

Pearlson, G. D., Barta, P. E., Powers, R. E., et al. (1997). Medial and superior temporal gyral volumes and cerebral asymmetry in schizophrenia versus bipolar disorder. *Biological Psychiatry*, **41**, 1–14.

Petty, R. G., Barta, P. E., Pearlson, G. D., et al. (1995). Reversal of asymmetry of the planum temporale in schizophrenia. *American Journal of Psychiatry*, **152**,

715–21.

Pickar, D., Su, T-P., Weinberger, D. R., et al. (1996). Individual variation in D2 receptor occupancy in clozapine-treated patients. *American Journal of Psychiatry*, **153**, 1571–8.

Pilowsky, L. S., Costa, D. C., Ell, P. J., Murray, R. M., Verhoeff, N. L. P. G. & Kerwin, R. W. (1992). Clozapine, SPET, and the dopamine receptor blockade hypothesis of schizophrenia. *Lancet*, **340**, 199–202.

Pilowsky, L. S., Costa, D. C., Ell, P. J., Murray, R. M., Verhoeff, N. L. P. G. & Kerwin, R. W. (1993). Antipsychotic medication, D2 receptor blockade and clinical response: a IBZM- SPET study. *Psychological Medicine*, **23**, 791–7.

Plante, E. & Turkstra, L. (1991). Sources of error in the quantitative analysis of MRI scans. *Magnetic Resonance Imaging*, **9**, 589–95.

Raichle, M. E., Grubb, R. L., Gado, M. H., et al. (1976). Correlation between regional cerebral blood flow and oxidative metabolism. *Archives of Neurology*, **33**, 523–6.

Rauch, S. L., Savage, C. R., Alpert, N. M., et al. (1995). A PET study of simple phobic symptom provocation. *Archives of General Psychiatry*, **52**, 20–8.

Rauch, S. L., Van der Kolk, B. A., Fisler, R. E., et al. (1996). A symptom provocation study in post traumatic stress disorder using PET and script driven-imagery. *Archives of General Psychiatry*, **53**, 380–7.

Raz, S. & Raz, N. (1990). Structural brain abnormalities in the major psychoses: a quantitative review of the evidence from CT. *Psychological Bulletin*, **108**, 93–108.

Reiman, E. M., Raichle, M. E., Butler, F. K., Herscovitch, P. & Robins, E. (1984). A focal brain abnormality in panic disorder, a severe form of anxiety. *Nature*, **310**, 683–5.

Reith, J., Benkelfat, C., Sherwin, A., et al. (1994). Elevated dopa decarboxylase activity in living brain of patients with psychosis. *Proceedings of the National Academy of Sciences*, **91**, 11651–4.

Renshaw, P. F., Yurgelun-Todd, D. A., Tohen, M., et al. (1995). Temporal lobe MRS of patients with first-episode psychosis. *American Journal of Psychiatry*, **152**, 444–6.

Resnick, S. M., Gur, R. E., Alavi, A., et al. (1988). PET and subcortical glucose metabolism in schizophrenia. *Psychiatry Research*, **24**, 1–11.

Reveley, A. M., Reveley, M. A., Clifford, C. A. & Murray, R. M. (1982). Cerebral ventricular size in twins discordant for schizophrenia. *Lancet*, **i**, 540–1.

Roland, P. E. (1993). *Brain Activation*. Chichester: John Wiley.

Rodriguez, V. M., Andree, R. M., Castejon, M. J. P., Garcia, E. C., Delgado, J. L. C. & Vila, F. J. R. (1996). SPECT study of regional cerebral perfusion in neuroleptic-resistant schizophrenic patients who responded or did not to clozapine. *American Journal of Psychiatry*, **153**, 1343–6.

Rossi, A., Stratta, P., Mancini, F., et al. (1994). Magnetic resonance imaging findings of amygdala-hippocampus shrinkage in male patients with schizophrenia. *Psychiatry Research*, **52**, 43–53.

Roy, M-A., Flaum, M. A., Arndt, S. V., Crowe, R. R. & Andreasen, N. C. (1994). MRI in familial versus sporadic cases of schizophrenia. *Psychiatry Research*, **54**, 25–36.

Rubin, P., Holm, S., Friberg, L., et al. (1991). Altered modulation of prefrontal and subcortical brain activity in newly diagnosed schizophrenia and schizophreniform disorder: a rCBF study. *Archives of General Psychiatry*, **48**, 987–95.

Rubin, T., Holm, S. & Madsen, P. L. (1994). Regional cerebral blood flow distributed in newly diagnosed schizophrenia and schizophreniform disorder. *Psychiatry Research*, **53**, 57–75.

Sabri, O., Erkwoh, R., Schreckenberger, M., Owega, A., Sass, H. & Buell, U. (1997). Correlation of positive symptoms exclusively to hyperperfusion or hypoperfusion of cerebral cortex in never-treated schizophrenics. *Lancet*, **349**, 1735–9.

Sagawa, K., Kawakutsu, S., Shibuya, I., et al. (1990). Correlation of regional cerebral blood flow with performance on neuropsychological tests in schizophrenic patients. *Schizophrenia Research*, **3**, 241–6.

Schild, H. H. (1990). *MRI Made Easy*, Berlin: Heenemann.

Schlaepfer, T. E., Harris, G. J., Tien, A. Y., et al. (1994). Decreased regional gray matter volume in schizophrenia. *American Journal of Psychiatry*, **151**, 842–8.

Schroder, J., Buchsbaum, M. S., Siegel, B. V., et al. (1994). Patterns of cortical activity in schizophrenia. *Psychological Medicine*, **24**, 947–55.

Schroder, J., Bubeck, B., Sauer, H., Demisch, S. (1995a). Benzodiazepine receptors in schizophrenia: a study with Iomazenil-SPET. *Schizophrenia Research*, **15**, 97–8.

Schroder, J., Wenz, F., Schad, L. R., Baudendistel, K. & Knopp, M. (1995b). Sensorimotor cortex and supplementary motor area changes in schizophrenia: a study with functional magnetic resonance imaging. *British Journal of Psychiatry*, **167**, 197–201.

Schroder, J., Buchsbaum, M. S., Siegel, B. V., et al. (1996). Cerebral metabolic activity correlates of subsyndromes in chronic schizophrenia. *Schizophrenia Research*, **19**, 41–53.

Schwartz, J. M., Stoessel, P. W., Baxter, L. R., Martin, K. M. & Phelps, M. E. (1996). Systematic changes in cerebral glucose metabolic rate after successful behaviour modification treatment of obsessive–compulsive disorder. *Archives of General Psychiatry*, **53**, 109–13.

Schwartzkopf, S. B., Nasrallah, H. A., Olson, S. C., et al. (1991). Family history and brain morphology in schizophrenia: an MRI study. *Psychiatry Research*: *Neuroimaging*, **40**, 49–60.

Scottish Schizophrenia Research Group. (1998). Regional cerebral blood flow in first epsiode schizophrenia patients before and after antipsychotic drug treatment. *Acta Psychiatrica Scandinavica*, **97**, 440–9.

Sedvall, G., Farde, L., Persson, A. & Wiesel, F-A. (1986). Imaging of neurotransmitter receptors in the living human brain. *Archives of General Psychiatry*, **43**, 995–1005.

Seeman, P., Niznik, H. B., Guan, H-C., et al. (1990). Elevation of dopamine D_2 receptors in schizophrenia is underestimated by radioactive raclopride. *Archives of General Psychiatry*, **47**, 1170–2.

Seeman, P., Guan, H-C., Van Tol, H. M. (1993). Dopamine D4 receptors elevated in schizophrenia. *Nature*, **365**, 441–5.

Selemon, L. D., Rajkowska, G. & Goldman-Rakic, P. S. (1995). Abnormally high neuronal density in the schizophrenic cortex. *Archives of General Psychiatry*, **52**, 805–18.

Shapiro, R. M. (1993). Regional neuropathology in schizophrenia: Where are we? Where are we going? *Schizophrenia Research*, **10**, 187–239.

Sharma, T., Lewis, S., Barta, P., et al. (1996). Loss of cerebral asymmetry in familial schizophrenia – a volumetric MRI study using unbiased stereology. *Schizophrenia Research*, **18**, 184 (abstract).

Shenton, M. E., Kikinis, R., McCarley, R. W., et al. (1991). Application of automated MRI volumetric measurement techniques to the ventricular system in schizophrenics and normal controls. *Schizophrenia Research*, **5**, 103–13.

Shenton, M. E., Kikinis, R., Jolesz, F. A., et al. (1992). Abnormalities of the left temporal lobe and thought disorder in schizophrenia: a quantitative magnetic resonance imaging study. *New England Journal of Medicine*, **327**, 604–12.

Sheppard, G., Gruzelier, J., Manchanda, R., et al. (1983). ^{15}O-PET scanning in predominantly never-treated acute schizophrenic patients. *Lancet*, **ii**, 1148–52.

Sherer, J., Tatsch, K., Schwartz, J., et al. (1994). D_2-dopamine receptor occupancy differs between patients with and without extrapyramidal side effects. *Acta Psychiatrica Scandinavica*, **90**, 266–8.

Siegel, B. V., Buchsbaum, M. S., Bunney, W. E., et al. (1993). Cortical-striatal-thalamic circuits and brain glucose metabolic activity in 70 unmedicated male schizophrenic patients. *American Journal of Psychiatry*, **150**, 1325–6.

Silbersweig, D. & Stern, E. (1996). Functional neuroimaging of hallucinations in schizophrenia: toward an integration of bottom-up and top-down approaches. *Molecular Psychiatry*, **1**, 367–75.

Silbersweig, D. A., Stern, E., Frith, C., et al. (1996). A functional neuroanatomy of auditory hallucinations. *Nature*, **378**, 176–9.

Spence, S. A., Brooks, D. J., Hirsch, S. R., et al. (1997). A PET study of voluntary movement in schizophrenic patients experiencing passivity phenomena (delusions of control). *Brain*, **120**, 1997–2011.

Spence, S. A., Hirsch, S. R., Brooks, D. J. & Grasby, P. M. (1998). Prefrontal cortex activity in people with schizophrenia and control subjects. *British Journal of Psychiatry*, **172**, 316–23.

Stanley, J. A., Williamson, P. C., Drost, D. J., et al. (1995). An in vivo study of the prefrontal cortex of schizophrenic patients at different stages of illness via MRS. *Archives of General Psychiatry*, **52**, 399–406.

Steinberg, J. L., Devous, M. D. Sr. & Paulman, R. G. (1996). WCST activated rCBF in first break and chronic schizophrenic patients and normal controls. *Schizophrenia Research*, **19**, 177–87.

Stevens, J. R. (1982). Neuropathology of schizophrenia. *Archives of General Psychiatry*, **39**, 1131–9.

Suddath, R. L., Casanova, M. F., Goldberg, T. E., Daniel, D. G., Kelsoe, J. R. & Weinberger, D. R. (1989). Temporal lobe pathology in schizophrenia: a quantitative MRI study. *American Journal of Psychiatry*, **146**, 464–72.

Suddath, R. L., Christison, G. W., Torrey, E. F., et al. (1990). Anatomical abnormalities in the brains of monozygotic twins discordant for schizophrenia. *New England Journal of Medicine*, **322**, 789–94.

Suga, H., Hayashi, T. & Mitsugi, O. (1994). SPECT findings using N-Isopropyl-p-[^{123}I]iodoamphetamine (^{123}I-IMP) in schizophrenia, and atypical psychosis. *Japanese Journal of Psychiatry*, **48**, 833–48.

Suzuki, M., Yuasa, S., Minabe, Y., Murata, Y. & Kurachi, M. (1993). Left superior temporal blood flow increases in schizophrenic and schizophreniform patients with auditory hallucinations: a longitudinal case study using IMP SPECT. *European Archives of Psychiatry and Clinical Neuroscience*, **242**, 257–61.

Swayze, V. W., Andreasen, N. C., Alliger, R. J., et al. (1992). Subcortical and temporal structures in affective disorder and schizophrenia: A magnetic resonance imaging study. *Biological Psychiatry*, **32**, 221–40.

Szechtman, H., Nahmias, C., Garnett, S., et al. (1988). Effect of neuroleptics on altered cerebral glucose metabolism in schizophrenia. *Archives of General Psychiatry*, **45**, 523–32.

Tamminga, C. A., Thaker, G. K., Buchanan, R., et al. (1992). Limbic system abnormalities identified in schizophrenia using positron emission tomography with fluorodeoxyglucose and neocortical alterations with deficit syndrome. *Archives of General Psychiatry*, **49**, 522–30.

Tune, L. E., Wong, D. F., Pearlson, G., et al. (1993). Dopamine D2 receptor density estimates in schizophrenia: a PET study with ^{11}C-N-Methylspiperone. *Psychiatry Research*, **49**, 219–37.

Turetsky, B., Cowell, P. E., Gur, R. C., et al. (1995). Frontal and temporal lobe brain volumes in schizophrenia. *Archives of General Psychiatry*, **52**, 1061–70.

Turner, S. W., Toone, B. K. & Breet-Jones, J. R. (1986). CT scan changes in early chronic schizophrenia – their relationship to perinatal trauma, family history and alcohol intake: preliminary findings. *Psychological Medicine*, **14**, 219–25.

Van Heertum, R. L. & Tikofsky, R. F. (1995). *Cerebral SPECT Imaging*, 2nd edn. New York: Raven Press.

Van Horn, J. D. & McManus, I. C. (1992). Ventricular enlargement in schizophrenia: a meta-analysis of studies of the VBR. *British Journal of Psychiatry*, **160**, 687–97.

Vita, A., Sacchetti, E., Calzeroni, A. & Cazzullo, C. L. (1988). Cortical atrophy in schizophrenia: prevalence and associated features. *Schizophrenia Research*, **1**, 329–37.

Vita, A., Dieci, M., Giobbio, G. M., et al. (1994). A reconsideration of the relationship between cerebral structural abnormalities and family history of schizophrenia. *Psychiatry Research*, **53**, 41–55.

Vita, A., Dieci, M., Giobbio, G. M., et al. (1995a). Language and thought disorder in schizophrenia: brain morphological correlates. *Schizophrenia Research*, **15**, 243–51.

Vita, A., Bressi, S., Perani, D., et al. (1995b). High-resolution SPECT study of regional cerebral blood flow in drug-free and drug-naive schizophrenic patients. *American Journal of Psychiatry*, **152**, 876–82.

Volkow, N. D., Brodie, J. D., Wolf, A. P., Angrist, B., Russell, J. & Cancro, R. (1986). Brain metabolism in patients with schizophrenia before and after acute neuroleptic administration. *Journal Neurology, Neurosurgery and Psychiatry*, **49**, 1199–202.

Volkow, N. D., Wolf, A. P., Van Gelder, P., et al. (1987). Phenomenological correlates of metabolic activity in patients with chronic schizophrenia. *American Journal of Psychiatry*, **144**, 151–8.

Waddington, J. L., O'Callaghan, E., Larkin, C., Redmond, O., Stack, J. & Ennis, J. T. (1990). Magnetic resonance imaging and spectroscopy in schizophrenia. *British Journal of Psychiatry*, **57 (supplement 9)**, 56–65.

Walker, E. F., Lewine, R. R. J. & Neumann, C. (1996). Childhood behavioural characteristics and adult brain morphology in schizophrenia. *Schizophrenia Research*, **22**, 93–101.

Warkentin, S., Nilsson, A., Risberg, J., et al. (1990). Regional cerebral blood flow in schizophrenia: repeated studies during a psychotic episode. *Psychiatry Research: Neuroimaging*, **35**, 27–38.

Ward, K. E., Friedman, L., Wise, A. & Schulz, S. C. (1996). Meta-analysis of brain and cranial size in schizophrenia. *Schizophrenia Research*, **22**, 197–213.

Weinberger, D. R., Torrey, E. F., Neophytides, A. N. & Wyatt, R. J. (1979). Structural abnormalities of cerebral cortex in chronic schizophrenia. *Archives of General Psychiatry*, **36**, 935–9.

Weinberger, D. R., DeLisi, L. E., Perman, G. P., et al. (1982). CT scans in schizophreniform disorder and other acute psychiatric patients. *Archives of General Psychiatry*, **39**, 778–83.

Weinberger, D. R., Berman, K. F. & Zec, R. F. (1986). Physiologic dysfunction of dorsolateral pre-frontal cortex in schizophrenia, I: regional cerebral blood flow evidence. *Archives of General Psychiatry*, **43**, 114–24.

Weinberger, D. R., Berman, K. F. & Illowsky, B. P. (1988). Physiologic dysfunction of dorsolateral pre-frontal cortex in schizophrenia, III: a new cohort and evidence for a monoaminergic mechanism. *Archives of General Psychiatry*, **45**, 609–15.

Weinberger, D. R., Berman, K. F., Suddath, R. & Torrey, E. F. (1992). Evidence of dysfunction of a prefrontal-limbic network in schizophrenia: a MRI and rCBF study of discordant monozygotic twins. *American Journal of Psychiatry*, **149**, 890–7.

Wible, C. G., Shenton, M. E., Hokama, H., et al. (1995). Prefrontal cortex and schizophrenia. *Archives of General Psychiatry*, **52**, 279–88.

Wiesel, F. A., Wik, G., Sjogren, I., et al. (1987a). Regional brain glucose metabolism in drug free schizophrenic patients and clinical correlates. *Acta Psychiatrica Scandinavica*, **76**, 628–41.

Wiesel, F. A., Wik, G., Sjogren, I., et al. (1987b). Altered relationships between metabolic rates of glucose in brain regions in schizophrenic patients. *Acta Psychiatrica Scandinavica*, **76**, 642–7.

Wolkin, A., Jaeger, J., Brodie, J. D., et al. (1985). Persistence of cerebral metabolic abnormalities in chronic schizophrenia determined by PET. *American Journal of Psychiatry*, **142**, 564–71.

Wolkin, A., Angrist, B., Wolf, A., et al. (1988). Low frontal glucose utilisation in chronic schizophrenia: a replication study. *American Journal of Psychiatry*, **145**, 251–3.

Wolkin, A., Barouche, F., Wolf, A. P., et al. (1989). Dopamine blockade and clinical response: evidence for two biological sub-groups of schizophrenia. *American Journal of Psychiatry*, **146**, 905–8.

Wolkin, A., Sanfilipo, M., Wolf, A. P., et al. (1992). Negative symptoms and hypofrontality in chronic schizophrenia. *Archives of General Psychiatry*, **49**, 959–65.

Wolkin, A., Sanfilipo, M., Angrist, B., et al. (1994). Acute d-amphetamine challenge in schizophrenia: effects on cerebral glucose utilisation and clinical symptomatology. *Biological Psychiatry*, **36**, 317–25.

Wolkin, A., Sanfilipo, M., Duncan, E., et al. (1996). Blunted change in cerebral glucose utilisation after haloperidol treatment in schizophrenic patients with prominent negative symptoms. *American Journal of Psychiatry*, **153**, 346–54.

Wong, D. F., Wagner, H. N., Tune, L. E., et al. (1986). PET reveals elevated D2 receptors in drug-naive schizophrenics. *Science*, **234**, 1558–63.

Wood, F. B. & Flowers, D. L. (1990). Hypofrontal vs. hypo-Sylvian blood flow in schizophrenia. *Schizophrenia Bulletin*, **16**, 413–24.

Woodruff, P. W. R., McManus, I. C. & David, A. S. (1995). Meta-analysis of corpus callosum size in schizophrenia. *Journal Neurology, Neurosurgery and*

Psychiatry, **58**, 457–61.

Woods, B. T., Yurgelun-Todd, D., Benes, F. M., et al. (1990). Progressive ventricular enlargement in schizophrenia: comparison to bipolar affective disorder and correlation with clinical course. *Biological Psychiatry*, **27**, 341–52.

Woods, B. T., Douglass, A. & Gescuk, B. (1991). Is the VBR still a useful measure of changes in the cerebral ventricles. *Psychiatry Research: Neuroimaging*, **40**, 1–10.

Woods, B. T., Yurgelun-Todd, D., Goldstein, J. M., Seidman, L. J. & Tsuang, M. T. (1996). MRI brain abnormalities in chronic schizophrenia: one process or more? *Biological Psychiatry*, **40**, 585–96.

Wright, I. C., McGuire, P. K., Poline, J. B., et al. (1995). A voxel-based method for the statistical analysis of gray and white matter density applied to schizophrenia. *Neuroimage*, **2**, 244–52.

Yuasa, S., Kurachi, M., Suzuki, M., et al. (1995). Clinical symptoms and regional cerebral blood flow in schizophrenia. *European Archives of Psychiatry and Clinical Neuroscience*, **246**, 7–12.

Yurgelun-Todd, D. A., Waternaux, C. M., Cohen, B. M., Gruber, S. A., English, C. D. & Renshaw, P. F. (1996). Functional magnetic resonance imaging of schizophrenic patients and comparison of subjects during word production. *American Journal of Psychiatry*, **153**, 200–5.

Zaidel, D. W., Esiri, M. M. & Harrison, P. J. (1997). Size, shape and orientation of neurons in the left and right hippocampus: investigation of normal asymmetries and alterations in schizophrenia. *American Journal of Psychiatry*, **154**, 812–18.

Zakzanis, K. K. & Hansen, K. T. (1998). Dopamine D_2 densities and the schizophrenic brain. *Schizophrenia Research*, **32**, 201–6.

Zipursky, R. B., Lim, K. O. & Pfefferbaum, A. (1991). Volumetric assessment of cerebral asymmetry from CT scans. *Psychiatry Research: Neuroimaging*, **35**, 71–89.

Zipursky, R. B., Lim, K. O., Sullivan, E. V., Brown, B. W. & Pfefferbaum, A. (1992). Widespread cerebral gray matter volume deficits in schizophrenia. *Archives of General Psychiatry*, **49**, 195–205.

Zipursky, R. B., Marsh, L., Lim, K. O., et al. (1994). Volumetric MRI assessment of temporal lobe structures in schizophrenia. *Biological Psychiatry*, **35**, 501–16.

Zohar, J., Insel, T. R., Berman, K. F., Foa, E. B., Hill, J. L. & Weinberger, D. R. (1989). Anxiety and cerebral blood flow during behavioural challenge. *Archives of General Psychiatry*, **46**, 505–10.

6

The neuropsychology of schizophrenia

Introduction

As mentioned in the introduction to the previous chapter, neuropsychological study of schizophrenia has undergone something of a renais-
sance in recent years. Kraepelin and Bleuler did not think that cognitive
function was noticeably impaired in their patients, and thought that any
'feeble-mindedness' was non-progressive and could recover. This view held
sway for the first half of this century, such that clearly impaired performance on various tests of intelligence were interpreted as due to a non-
specific failure of cooperation or motivation. (see Brody, 1941). Studies
from the 1960s onwards, however, as reviewed by Heaton et al. (1978),
consistently showed that patients with schizophrenia – whether acute or
chronic – exhibited an 'organic' pattern of deficits. Subsequent studies have
not only shown that schizophrenics have pronounced global intellectual
deficits, but have demonstrated difficulties in other areas of cognition –
particularly attention/executive function and memory – and have tried to
identify associations between these and clinical phenomena.

It should be appreciated that neuropsychology was originally a method
of detecting and localizing specific brain lesions. Thus, general tests of
intelligence led on to the development of comprehensive neuropsychological test batteries which included sub-tests of what was described as frontal,
temporal or parietal lobe function. It is only recently that such 'location-
ism' has been recognized as over-simplistic for most tasks and most neuropsychiatric patients, and researchers have taken to referring to particular
abilities or 'modules'. In addition, some have devised 'everyday' tests of
these domains that might more accurately reflect the daily living problems
of neuropsychiatric patients than do tests devised to identify sites of gross
brain damage. Another recent development, quite distinct from the empirical and essentially atheoretical approach of classical neuropsychology, has

become known as 'cognitive neuropsychology' – where attempts are made to explain symptoms or the disease as a whole in terms of abnormal cognitive processes, often as measured with inventive novel tests for each particular experiment.

This chapter will therefore summarize the main findings and current issues in the classical neuropsychology of schizophrenia – under the headings of general intelligence, attention/executive function, memory and others (including language, perception, spatial and motor abilities) – before describing some of the more successful cognitive approaches to explaining symptoms.

Global intelligence

It is now well recognized that patients with schizophrenia, as a group, have global intellectual impairments and that these pre-date the onset of psychotic symptoms by many years (see reviews by Dunkley & Rogers, 1994; Barber et al., 1996). The main issues of current interest are to what extent, if any, these deficits progress and how they are best measured so that any more specific deficits in other cognitive domains can be reliably assessed.

Several researchers have suggested that there is some general intellectual decline in schizophrenia, but the effects are mild and generally thought to occur in the first five years of the illness rather than progressively over time (Nelson et al., 1990; Frith et al., 1991). Indeed, some have found that cognitive function may improve with time and clinical stabilization (Sweeney et al., 1991; Hoff et al., 1991; Nopoulos et al., 1994). This does not of course disprove a progressive element, if only in some patients, just as other cross-sectional or short follow up studies that report deterioration do not prove it (Goldstein & Zubin, 1990; Goldstein et al., 1991; Bilder et al., 1992; Harvey et al., 1994; Hyde et al., 1994). Of the few long term (five years or more) prospective follow up studies in the literature, two have reported some decline (Schwartzmann & Douglas, 1962; Waddington & Yousef, 1996), but only in chronic institutionalized patients, whereas four others do not (Smith, 1964; Klonoff et al., 1970; Waddington et al., 1990; Russell et al., 1997). The small minority of patients who approach dementia levels, with for example 'age disorientation' (Liddle & Crow, 1984), also tend to be chronically institutionalized and this phenomenon has also been described in those with psychotic affective disorders (Lombardi et al., 1995).

Nonetheless, current IQ and any decline from pre-morbid levels is an important research issue when other more specific deficits are being examined. A full Wechsler Adult Intelligence Scale (WAIS) to quantify these factors will tire patients and reduce their compliance with the subsequent tests of prime interest. Quicker assessments are available – the most commonly used being the National (or New) Adult Reading Test (NART). This simple test assesses pre-morbid intelligence by irregular word pronunciation – a task that was presumed to be resistant to most neuropsychiatric disorders. Its ease of use has led to a veritable 'NART industry', but this has unfortunately found evidence that NART performance may be impaired in at least some patients with chronic schizophrenia (and other disorders), possibly due to a lack of educational attainment (Crawford et al., 1992). Its cautious use can however be justified, particularly in community patients, but it is best used in conjunction with other baseline measures such as years in education or paternal social class (O'Carroll et al., 1992).

Attention and executive functioning

The study of various aspects of attention in schizophrenia can be traced back to Broadbent's theory (1958) about defective filtering or inhibition of irrelevant sensory information. Although there has been little empirical support for this assertion, many other aspects of attention have been studied and found to be abnormal in schizophrenia.

The most studied aspect of attention has been vigilance or so-called 'sustained attention' as measured with a Continuous Performance Test (CPT), which requires subjects to respond to certain stimuli but not to others. Early CPT studies found performance to be abnormal in both acute and remitted cases (Wohlberg et al., 1973) and several researchers have since shown deficits in those who are at risk for psychosis but not affected (Wolf & Cornblatt, 1996). CPT abnormalities have been found in both unmedicated and medicated patients, and to correlate with positive symptoms (Pandurangi et al., 1994; Servan-Schreiber et al., 1996), although they have also been reported to be greater in deficit than non-deficit patients (Buchanan et al., 1997).

Focused or selective attention (the ability to avoid distraction) has also been widely studied and found to be abnormal, usually with the Stroop test (e.g. Hepp et al., 1996). During the Stroop test, subjects have to read a list of words describing colours which are printed in different colours, e.g. the word blue would be printed in red. Recently, Buchanan et al. (1994a) have found that deficit patients perform more poorly than non-deficit patients on the Stroop test, while Brebion et al. (1996) have suggested that Stroop deficits may be correlated with 'reality monitoring' performance (see below).

Other tests of attention have been used that tap into more complex aspects of 'frontal lobe function', i.e. the ability to form concepts, think abstractly and plan actions. The most used test is the Wisconsin Card Sort Test (WCST) which requires subjects to sort cards by colour, shape or number according to shifting rules – a test of the ability to change attentional set. There can be no doubt that schizophrenics perform badly (perseverate) on the WCST, as seen in numerous activation scanning studies described in the previous chapter, but this impairment could be explained by general attention problems. Nonetheless, similar results have been reported from groups using other traditional and more novel everyday set-shifting tests (Elliott et al., 1995; Morice & Delahunty, 1996; Evans et al., 1997). WCST performance has also been linked to dopaminergic mechanisms and a study in monkeys has shown that the administration of phencyclidine causes perseverative responses to novel situations that can be ameliorated by clozapine (Jentsch et al., 1997).

Impairments on the seemingly simple task of word production, or verbal fluency, could also be attributable to various difficulties in for example, the word store or processing speed. However, the number of words produced is consistently lower in patients with schizophrenia (Gruzelier et al., 1988; Allen et al., 1993; Crawford et al., 1993), and recent work suggests that the underlying problem is in access to the word store (Allen et al., 1993) as cueing improves performance (Joyce et al., 1996).

These consistently described deficits suggest impairments in attending to several tasks that may reflect a more generalized deficit in executive function, i.e., the allocation of attention to discrete modules for particular tasks. General deficits in executive functioning have indeed been described by several workers and these have often been reported to be greater than deficits in other domains (Shallice et al., 1991; Morrison-Stewart et al., 1992; Morice & Delahunty, 1996). Some have attributed this to a failure of a 'supervisory attentional system' (Shallice et al., 1991), which bears some similarities to Broadbent's original formulation. On the other hand, there are also a large number of reports suggesting specific problems in memory – although these too could be attributed to an overall executive deficit.

Memory

Memory deficits have been observed in schizophrenia for some time, such as impaired paired associates and digit span (Johnstone et al., 1978), but they have only been studied specifically in the past few years. The classification of memory functions is complex, being sub-divided into short and long term, declarative and non-declarative, and according to the particular cognitive operations in for example, encoding or retrieving memories. Suffice it to say that although deficits in virtually all aspects of memory have been reported in schizophrenia, current interest is mainly focused on short term/working and long term, declarative (episodic and semantic) problems, particularly on verbal memory tests.

This may be largely attributable to influential studies from America that showed disproportionate verbal memory impairment in discordant monozygotic twins (Goldberg et al., 1990, 1993a) and in both medicated and unmedicated patients (Saykin et al., 1991, 1994). It is only very recently that a working memory deficit in schizophrenia, as measured by the digit span task, has been shown to be independent of attentional/executive factors (Goldberg et al., 1998), McKenna et al. (1990) reported a substantial deficit on a test designed to test everyday long term episodic (personal) memory functioning – the Rivermead Behavioural Memory Test (RBMT, Wilson et al., 1985). The deficit was so great as to be comparable to an amnesic syndrome (Tamlyn et al., 1992), and has since been replicated (Duffy & O'Carroll, 1994). However, semantic memory (of general knowledge or external facts) may be affected to an even greater extent (Duffy & O'Carroll, 1994; Chen et al., 1994). More recently, some researchers have found that schizophrenics are not impaired on 'implicit' or pre-conscious personal memory tasks, but are only impaired on explicit or concious recollection (Huron et al., 1995; Bazin & Perruchet, 1996).

These findings have particular appeal because they may be linked to temporal lobe volume deficits and a number of investigators have reported potentially important clinical associations. We have found that treatment resistant patients selectively exhibit greater deficits on the RBMT of episodic memory than responsive patients, whereas other tests of global, executive and memory function did not differentiate the groups after controlling for the number of years in education (Lawrie et al., 1995). Others have found that semantic memory disturbance predicts outcome at one year (Goldman et al., 1993) and both have been associated with chronicity (Tamlyn et al., 1992; Duffy & O'Carroll, 1994). Episodic or personal memory problems could result in, for example, a failure of insight and/or poor compliance with medication or other care arrangements, while general or semantic memory deficits could be related to unusual interpretations of external events (see below). However, deficits in attention (Smith et al., 1992) and global cognitive impairment have also been related to a poor outcome or treatment response (e.g. Johnstone et al., 1978; Nelson et al., 1990; Frith et al., 1991). Reviewing this literature, Green (1996) concluded that both memory and vigilance appeared crucial for adequate functional outcome in schizophrenia.

Language, perception, spatial and motor abilities

These 'modules' are included more for completeness than because they are selectively impaired in schizophrenia. Despite the clinical observation that various aspects of language are frequently abnormal in schizophrenia, and the similarities between dysphasia and formal thought disorder, there are no consistently replicated experimental findings (see Cutting, 1985 for review). Similarly, although perceptual abnormalities characterize schizophrenia, these are generally thought to reflect abnormal interpretations of essentially normal perceptions (e.g. Schneider's 'delusional perception'). There are some suggestions that the perception of form, of faces and ambiguous stimuli, may be disturbed but these have not been shown to be disproportionate to overall intellectual impairment (Cutting, 1985). There is little clinical support for visuo-spatial dysfunction in schizophrenia nor much in the way of research evidence either. The inconsistent results of studies looking at these abilities independently are in keeping with the results from studies using comprehensive neuropsychological testing batteries which report no greater impairments on language, perception and spatial skills than that expected from general difficulties (Goldberg et al., 1990; Saykin et al., 1991). However, such abnormalities have been shown to be, probably in a non-specific way, more common in children who go on to develop schizophrenia than those who do not, as have some motor anomalies. These 'soft' neurological signs – of reduced motor co-ordination and speed – have been commonly reported in schizophrenia, their unaffected relatives and children at high risk. They have also been shown to be associated with obstetric complications, structural imaging abnormalities and other neuropsychological deficits, and are very much in keeping with the neurodevelopmental model of schizophrenia (Walker, 1994).

Other issues

Continuing examination of putative laterality effects on neuropsychological functioning in schizophrenia can be traced to the association between temporal lobe epilepsy with left-sided foci and schizophreniform psychosis, and to suggestions from the imaging literature of greater abnormalities on the left side and anomalies of cerebral asymmetry. Divided visual field and dichotic listening tests have been commonly used to examine possible abnormalities of asymmetrical information processing and inter-hemispheric transfer, particularly as regards the domains of attention, learning and memory. However, both the left and right hemispheres and connections in both directions have been implicated, and whether these deficits are any greater than global problems remains to be established. Few conclusions can be made, save that information processing and integrated brain function is somehow disturbed in schizophrenia (see review by Gruzelier, 1996). The inconsistencies in this literature may however be attributable to the difficulties in controlling for handedness, sexual dimorphism in neuropsychological functioning and possible differences in symptomatology between patients' groups (Gruzelier, 1996). There is no simple excess of left or right handedness in schizophrenia, but there are suggestions that ambiguous handedness may be over-represented (Gruzelier, 1996).

Another test of information processing, that of 'backward masking', has however provided more consistent evidence of abnormalities in schizophrenia (and their unaffected relatives). Briefly, a stimulus (usually visual) is presented to subjects and the perception of this is 'masked' by presenting another stimulus after a variable length of time (0–300 ms). In schizophrenia, the minimum time between stimuli allowing the perception of both without interference is longer than for healthy controls. Although similar abnormalities have been reported in other actively psychotic patients, antipsychotic medication if anything normalizes performance (see Green & Neuchterlein, 1994 for review). These issues, of disease specificity and the effects of medication, will now be considered as they relate to neuropsychological testing in schizophrenia in general.

Disease specificity

Ideally, of course, such neuropsychological abnormalities will be demonstrably different from patients with other psychoses, whether 'organic' or 'functional', and those with neuroses. There is some evidence that schizophrenia appears to have a relatively distinct cognitive profile as compared with other neuropsychiatric disorders. Early studies could not reliably distinguish schizophrenia and organic disorders (Heaton et al., 1978), and latter studies have shown that the pattern of memory dysfunction may be similar in schizophrenia and the dementias. However, Alzheimers patients demonstrate more rapid forgetting (Heaton et al., 1994) and patients with sub-cortical dementias have more slowed thinking and motor abnormalities (Hanes et al., 1996). Moreover, there are recent suggestions that patients with schizophrenia have more severe neuropsychological impairments than those with either bipolar or unipolar affective disorders – although it remains to be established whether these differences are most marked on executive (Goldberg et al., 1993b) or memory tasks (Jeste et al., 1996).

More exciting yet, as alluded to above, certain cognitive deficits apparent in schizophrenia are also evident in children at high risk of developing the disorder and in unaffected genetic relatives and those with schizotypal personality disorder. This is particularly true of abnormalities of attention, executive function and verbal memory (Wolf & Cornblatt, 1996; Byrne et al., 1998). Not only do these findings suggest a link between genotype and phenotype, they also suggest that these abnormalities could serve as trait markers for early intervention or even preventative programmes.

Medication effects

Medication effects are of course potentially very important confounders of apparent problems with cognition. Sedation from many drugs could non-specifically affect any neuropsychological testing, while benzodiazepines and anticholinergics have been shown to have particular adverse effects on memory. However, most studies at least control for such exposure (e.g. Lawrie et al., 1995) and several of the above anomalies have been reported in unmedicated patients (e.g. Saykin et al., 1994). Even more convincing, antipsychotics generally tend to normalize attention and general cognitive functioning as the illness itself improves (see reviews by King, 1990 and Goldberg & Weinberger, 1996), as has been shown in some functional imaging studies, although the mechanisms of such improvement are unknown. It is unlikely therefore that medication effects can account for the more consistent findings in the neuropsychology of schizophrenia, but some of these abnormalities could reflect the abuse of alcohol and illicit drugs that is so common in schizophrenia and which has such well known adverse effects on neuropsychological functioning.

A current area of considerable research interest is whether atypical neuroleptics, with their different modes of action to the typical antipsychotics, have different effects on neuropsychological test performance. Most published reports have considered clozapine as compared with typical antipsychotics, but other new drugs are now receiving intensive study. Goldberg et al. (1993c) found that clinical improvements on clozapine were not associated with changes in cognitive function, as did Classen & Laux (1988). Other groups have reported improvements or deteriorations in various cognitive domains with clozapine treatment. Improvements on various aspects of attention and verbal fluency have been replicated in both chronic (Buchanan et al., 1994b; Zahn et al., 1994; Hoff et al., 1996) and treatment resistant patients (Hagger et al., 1993; Lee et al., 1994). Clozapine also seems to have consistently adverse effects on some motor and memory tasks (Zahn et al., 1994; Hoff et al., 1996; Vrtunski et al., 1996). The effects of risperidone have been reported by three groups. Improvements have been described on selective attention and general alertness (Stip & Lussier, 1996), and in attention, memory and executive function (Rossi et al., 1997), but these studies were uncontrolled and practice effects are a possible explanation of the findings. However, Green et al. (1997) have described an improvement in verbal memory performance in treatment resistant patients on risperidone as compared with similar patients treated with 15 mg of haloperidol daily.

Cognitive neuropsychology

As described above there are a few examples of significant correlations between particular, usually negative, symptoms and cognitive deficits. However, relatively specific findings of associations between, for example, verbal fluency and alogia (Joyce et al., 1996) are about equal in number to reports of general relationships between, for example, executive function and negative symptoms (Allen et al., 1993; Stolar et al., 1994). More specific models of symptoms or sub-syndromes and cognitive deficits are clearly required and three main proposals described below have appeared since Broadbent (1958). 1) Hemsley (1987) saw the fundamental problem as an abnormal experience of actions rather than perceptions. Specifically, he proposed that 'past regularities of experience exerted less influence on current perceptions' so that information is less prioritized. He linked this to all the symptoms of schizophrenia in various ways, but the model has most obvious relevance to the relationship between semantic memory processes and delusions. 2) Frith, on the other hand, has proposed differing underlying mechanisms for particular symptoms. Initially, negative symptoms were attributed to a failure to initiate spontaneous action and positive symptoms to a defect in internal monitoring of action (Frith & Done, 1988). However, with the subsequent demonstration of three syndromes of schizophrenia by factor analysis (Liddle & Barnes, 1990), each tied to a particular functional imaging abnormality (Liddle et al., 1992), disorganization came to be separately regarded as a failure to suppress inappropriate responses (Frith, 1992 & 1995). 3) Finally, Gray et al. (1991) incorporated elements of both of these models and much animal experimental work into a conceptualization of schizophrenia as a disorder of motor programming and monitoring, localized to limbic and striatal networks.

Although there is as yet little empirical evidence for these theories, it has to be said that Frith's model has achieved the most widespread and consistent support. In general, negative symptoms have been linked to reduced word production (Frith et al., 1991; Allen et al., 1993) and omission errors in vigilance tasks (Frith et al., 1991); while disorganization has been associated with inappropriate responses or commissions on the same tests. More specifically, schizophrenics with first rank symptoms have been shown to be more impaired on tests assessing self-monitoring of actions, or error detection, than those without such symptoms (Frith & Done, 1989; Mlakar et al., 1994), although one group has reported poor internal error detection in all patients with schizophrenia (Leudar et al., 1994). Several groups have also found evidence supporting the view that auditory hallucinations are related to an external mis-attribution of internal thoughts (see Nayani & David, 1996).

Hemsley (1987) and Gray et al. (1991) used animal findings in latent inhibition tests and the Kamin blocking effect to support their models. Briefly, these experimental paradigms examine the effects of a pre-exposure to a stimulus in impairing subsequent learning – the extrapolation to schizophrenia being that patients with acute symptoms would show less such inhibition or blocking and actually perform relatively better on subsequent tests. The authors produced some evidence in support of their models by demonstrating differential patterns of association learning in acute and chronic patients with schizophrenia (Jones et al., 1991). However, others have not found such patterns of performance on similar tasks (O'Carroll et al., 1993; O'Carroll, 1995), or have attributed them to medication effects (Williams et al., 1998).

Frith (1992) has also recently invoked a concept borrowed from autism – 'theory of mind' or awareness that others have minds – to explain some general deficits and specific symptoms in schizophrenia. For example, this can be linked to asociality and social withdrawal, as well as to the development of delusions through misperceiving the intentions of others. Doody et al. (1998) have recently shown that theory of mind deficits are found in schizophrenia but not in affective disorder. Such a disturbance of 'metacognition' appears to be compatible with findings of disturbed social cognition (e.g. Corrigan & Green, 1993; Penn et al., 1996 & 1997) but awaits specific testing.

Conclusions

Patients with schizophrenia show deficits in global intelligence, various aspects of attention and memory, and in executive functions. The presence of essentially non-progressive impairments in many cognitive domains supports theories of a developmental cause of schizophrenia. A fundamental underlying problem in 'executive functioning' is possible but difficult to tie in with particular symptoms or disabilities. Although classical lesion-oriented neuropsychological tests reveal abnormalities in schizophrenia, there is an increasing move towards a cognitive neuropsychology that also attempts to integrate mental experiences or symptoms into the model. Too much has been made in the past of falsely localized frontal or temporal 'lobe' deficits when it is clear that both are impaired and connected (e.g. Nathaniel-James et al., 1996; Gold et al., 1997). At the same time, clinicians and researchers have been slow to realize the potential of neuropsychological testing for individualized rehabilitation (see Keefe, 1995 and Chapter 8). The resurgence of interest in neuropsychology and the rise of cognitive neuropsychology has however brought about some progress in linking the brain imaging literature in schizophrenia with the subjective experiences of patients. Further advances in this area, and possibly in non-pharmacological treatments, can be expected.

References

Allen, H. A., Liddle, P. F. & Frith, C. D. (1993). Negative features, retrieval processes and verbal fluency in schizophrenia. *British Journal of Psychiatry*, **163**, 769–75.

Barber, F., Pantelis, C., Bodger, S. & Nelson, H. E. (1996). Intellectual functioning in schizophrenia: natural history. In *Schizophrenia: A Neuropsychological Perspective*, ed. C. Pantelis, H. E. Nelson & T. R. E. Barnes, pp. 49–70. Chichester, England: John Wiley.

Bazin, N. & Perruchet, P. (1996). Implicit and explicit associative memory in patients with schizophrenia. *Schizophrenia Research*, **22**, 241–8.

Bilder, R. M., Lipschutz-Broch, L., Reiter, G., et al. (1992). Intellectual deficits in first-episode schizophrenia: evidence for progressive deterioration. *Schizophrenia Bulletin*, **18**, 437–49.

Brebion, G., Smith, M. J., Gorman, J. M. & Amador, X. (1996). Reality monitoring failure in schizophrenia – the role of selective attention. *Schizophrenia Research*, **22**, 173–80.

Broadbent, D. E. (1958). *Perception and Communication*. London: Pergamon.

Brody, M. B. (1941). A survey of the results of intelligence tests in psychosis. *British Journal of Medical Psychology*, **19**, 215–61.

Buchanan, R. W., Strauss, M. E., Kirkpatrick, B., et al. (1994a). Neuropsychological impairments in deficit vs non-deficit forms of schizophrenia. *Archives of General Psychiatry*, **51**, 804–11.

Buchanan, R. W., Holstein, C. & Breier, A. (1994b). The comparative efficacy and long-term effect of clozapine treatment on neuropsychological test performance. *Biological Psychiatry*, **36**, 717–25.

Buchanan, R. W., Strauss, M. E., Breier, A., et al. (1997). Attentional impairments in deficit and non-deficit forms of schizophrenia. *American Journal of Psychiatry*, **154**, 363–70.

Byrne, M., Hodges, A., Grant, E. & Johnstone, E. C. (1998). Evidence for executive dysfunction in young people at high risk for schizophrenia. Results of the Hayling sentence completion test *Schizophrenia Research*, **29**, 43(A).

Chen, E. Y. H., Wilkins, A. J. & McKenna, P. J. (1994). Semantic memory is both impaired and anomalous in schizophrenia. *Psychological Medicine*, **24**, 193–202.

Classen, W. & Laux, G. (1988). Sensorimotor and cognitive performance of schizophrenic inpatients treated with haloperidol, flupenthixol or clozapine. *Pharmacopsychiatry*, **21**, 295–7.

Corrigan, P. W. & Green, M. F. (1993). Schizophrenic patients' sensitivity to social cues: the role of abstraction. *American Journal of Psychiatry*, **150**, 589–94.

Crawford, J. R., Besson, J. A. O., Bremner, M., et al. (1992). Estimation of premorbid intelligence in schizophrenia. *British Journal of Psychiatry*, **161**, 69–74.

Crawford, J. R., Obonsawin, M. C. & Bremner, M. (1993). Frontal lobe impairment in schizophrenia: relationship to intellectual functioning. *Psychological Medicine*, **23**, 787–90.

Cutting, J. (1985). *The Psychology of Schizophrenia*. Edinburgh: Churchill Livingstone.

Doody, G. A., Gotz, M., Johnstone, E. C., Frith, C. D. & Owens, D. G. C. (1998). Theory of mind & psychoses. *Psychological Medicine*, **28**, 397–405.

Duffy, L. & O'Carroll, R. E. (1994). Memory impairment in schizophrenia – a comparison with that observed in the Alcoholic Korsakoff Syndrome. *Psychological Medicine*, **24**, 155–65.

Dunkley, G. & Rogers, D. (1994). The cognitive impairment of severe psychiatric illness: a clinical study. In *The Neuropsychology of Schizophrenia*, ed. A. S. David & J. C. Cutting, pp. 181–960. Hove: Lawrence Erlbaum.

Elliott, R., McKenna, P. J., Robbins, T. W. & Sahakian, B. J. (1995). Neuropsychological evidence for frontostriatal dysfunction in schizophrenia. *Psychological Medicine*, **25**, 619–30.

Evans, J. J., Chua, S. E., McKenna, P. J. & Wilson, B. A. (1997). Assessment of the dysexecutive syndrome in schizophrenia. *Psychological Medicine*, **27**, 635–46.

Frith, C. D. (1992). *The Cognitive Neuropsychology of Schizophrenia*. Hove, UK: LEA.

Frith, C. D. (1995). Schizophrenia: functional imaging and cognitive abnormalities. *Lancet*, **346**, 615–20.

Frith, C. D. & Done, D. J. (1988). Towards a neuropsychology of schizophrenia. *British Journal of Psychiatry*, **153**, 437–43.

Frith, C. D. & Done, D. J. (1989). Experiences of alien control in schizophrenia reflect a disorder in the central monitoring of action. *Psychological Medicine*, **19**, 359–63.

Frith, C. D., Leary, J., Cahill, C. & Johnstone, E. C. (1991). Disabilities and circumstances of schizophrenic patients. IV. Performance on psychological tests. *British Journal of Psychiatry*, **159 (supplement 13)**, 26–9.

Gold, J. M., Carpenter, C., Randolph, C., Goldberg, T. E. & Weinberger, D. R. (1997). Auditory working memory and Wisconsin Card Sorting Test performance in schizophrenia. *Archives of General Psychiatry*, **54**, 159–65.

Goldberg, T. E. & Weinberger, D. R. (1996). Effects of neuroleptic medications on the cognition of patients with schizophrenia: a review of recent studies. *Journal of Clinical Psychiatry*, **57 Suppl 9**, 62–5.

Goldberg, T. E., Ragland, J. D., Torrey, E. F., et al. (1990). Neuropsychological assessment of monozygotic twins discordant for schizophrenia. *Archives of General Psychiatry*, **47**, 1066–72.

Goldberg, T. E., Torrey, E. F., Gold, J. M., et al. (1993a). Learning and memory in monozygotic twins discordant for schizophrenia. *Psychological Medicine*, **23**, 71–85.

Goldberg, T. E., Gold, J. M., Greenberg, R., et al. (1993b). Contrasts between patients with affective disorders and patients with schizophrenia on a neuropsychological test battery. *American Journal of Psychiatry*, **150**, 1355–62.

Goldberg, T. E., Greenberg, R. D., Griffin, S. J., et al. (1993c). The effect of clozapine on cognition and psychiatric symptoms in patients with schizophrenia. *British Journal of Psychiatry*, **162**, 43–8.

Goldberg, T. E., Patterson, K. J., Taqqu, Y. & Wilder, K. (1998). Capacity limitations in short-term memory in schizophrenia: tests of competing hypotheses. *Psychological Medicine*, **28**, 665–73.

Goldman, R. S., Axelrod, B. N., Tandon, R., et al. (1993). Neuropsychological prediction of treatment efficacy and one-year outcome in schizophrenia. *Psychopathology*, **26**, 122–6.

Goldstein, G. & Zubin, J. (1990). Neuropsychological differences between young and old schizophrenics with and without associated neurological dysfunction. *Schizophrenia Research*, **3**, 117–26.

Goldstein, G., Zubin, J. & Pogue-Geile, M. F. (1991). Hospitalisation and the cognitive deficits of schizophrenia: the influences of age and education. *Journal of Nervous and Mental Disease*, **179**, 202–6.

Gray, J. A., Feldman, J., Rawling, J. N. P., et al. (1991). The neuropsychology of schizophrenia. *Behavioural and Brain Sciences*, **14**, 1–20.

Green, M. F. (1996). What are the functional consequences of neurocognitive deficits in schizophrenia? *American Journal of Psychiatry*, **153**, 321–30.

Green, M. F. & Neuchterlein, K. H. (1994). Mechanisms of backward masking in schizophrenia. In *The Neuropsychology of Schizophrenia*, ed. A. S. David & J. C. Cutting, pp. 79–95. Hove, UK: Lawrence Erlbaum Associates.

Green, M. F., Marshall, B. D. Jr., Wirshing, W. C., et al. (1997). Does risperidone improve verbal working memory in treatment-resistant schizophrenia? *American Journal of Psychiatry*, **154**, 799–804.

Gruzelier, J. (1996). Lateralised dysfunction is necessary but not sufficient to account for neuropsychological deficits in schizophrenia. In *Schizophrenia: A Neuropsychological Perspective*, ed. C. Pantelis, H. E. Nelson & T. R. E. Barnes, pp. 125–60. Chichester, England: John Wiley.

Gruzelier, J., Seymour, K., Wilson, L., et al. (1988). Impairments on neuropsychologic tests of temperophippocampal and frontohippocampal functions and word fluency in remitting schizophrenia and affective disorders. *Archives of General Psychiatry*, **45**, 623–9.

Hagger, C., Buckley, P., Kenny, J. T., et al. (1993). Improvement in cognitive functions and psychiatric symptoms in treatment-refractory schizophrenic patients receiving clozapine. *Biological Psychiatry*, **34**, 702–12.

Hanes, K. R., Andrewes, D. G., Pantelis, C. & Chiu, E. (1996). Subcortical dysfunction in schizophrenia: a comparison with Parkinson's disease and Huntington's disease. *Schizophrenia Research*, **19**, 121–8.

Harvey, P. D., White, L., Parrella, M., et al. (1994). The longitudinal stability of cognitive impairment in schizophrenia. *British Journal of Psychiatry*, **166**, 630–3.

Heaton, R. K., Baade, L. E. & Johnson, K. L. (1978). Neuropsychological test results associated with psychiatric disorders in adults. *Psychological Bulletin*, **85**, 141–62.

Heaton, R., Paulson, J. S., McAdams, L. A., et al. (1994). Neuropsychological deficits in schizophrenics. *Archives of General Psychiatry*, **51**, 469–76.

Hemsley, D. R. (1987). An experimental psychological model for schizophrenia. In *Search for the Causes of Schizophrenia*, ed. H. Hafner, W. F. Gattaz & W. Janzarik, pp. 179–88. Heidelberg: Springer.

Hepp, H. H., Maier, S., Hermle, L. & Spitzer, M. (1996). The Stroop effect in schizophrenic patients. *Schizophrenia Research*, 22, 187–95.

Hoff, A. L., Riordan, H., O'Donnell, D. W. & DeLisi, L. E. (1991). Cross-sectional and longitudinal test findings in first episode schizophrenic patients. *Schizophrenia Research*, 5, 197–8.

Hoff, A. L., Faustman, W. O., Wieneke, M., et al. (1996). The effects of clozapine on symptom reduction, neurocognitive function, and clinical management in treatment-refractory state hospital schizophrenic inpatients. *Neuropsychopharmacology*, 15, 361–9.

Huron, C., Danion, J.-M., Giacomoni, F., et al. (1995). Impairment of recognition memory with, but not without, conscious recollection in schizophrenia. *American Journal of Psychiatry*, 152, 1737–42.

Hyde, T. M., Nawroz, S., Goldberg, T. E., et al. (1994). Is there cognitive decline in schizophrenia? A cross-sectional study. *British Journal of Psychiatry*, 164, 494–500.

Jentsch, J. D., Redmond, D. E. Jr., Elsworth, J. D., et al. (1997). Enduring cognitive deficits and cortical dopamine dysfunction in monkeys after long-term administration of phencyclidene. *Science*, 277, 953–5.

Jeste, D. V., Heaton, S. C., Paulson, J. S., et al. (1996). Clinical and neuropsychological comparison of psychotic depression with nonpsychotic depression and schizophrenia. *American Journal of Psychiatry*, 153, 490–6.

Johnstone, E. C., Crow, T. J., Frith, C. D., et al. (1978). The dementia of dementia praecox. *Acta Psychiatrica Scandinavica*, 57, 305–24.

Jones, S. H., Hemsley, D. R. & Gray, J. A. (1991). Contextual effects on choice reaction time and accuracy in acute and chronic schizophrenia. *British Journal of Psychiatry*, 159, 415–21.

Joyce, E. M., Collinson, S. L. & Crichton, P. (1996). Verbal fluency in schizophrenia: relationship with executive function, semantic memory and clinical alogia. *Psychological Medicine*, 26, 39–49.

Keefe, R. S. E. (1995). The contribution of neuropsychology to psychiatry. *American Journal of Psychiatry*, 152, 6–15.

King, D. J. (1990). The effect of neuroleptics on cognitive and motor function. *British Journal of Psychiatry*, 157, 799–811.

Klonoff, H., Fibiger, C. H. & Hutton, G. H. (1970). Neuropsychological patterns in chronic schizophrenia. *Journal of Nervous and Mental Disease*, 150, 291–300.

Lawrie, S. M., Ingle, G., Santosh, C., et al. (1995). MRI and SPET in treatment responsive and treatment resistant schizophrenia. *British Journal of Psychiatry*, 167, 202–10.

Lee, M. A., Thompson, P. A. & Meltzer, H. Y. (1994). Effects of clozapine on cognitive function in schizophrenia. *Journal of Clinical Psychiatry*, 55 **Suppl. B**, 82–7.

Leudar, I., Thomas, P. & Johnston, M. (1994). Self-monitoring in speech production: effects of verbal hallucinations and negative symptoms. *Psychological Medicine*, 24, 749–61.

Liddle, P. F. & Barnes, T. R. E. (1990). Syndromes of chronic schizophrenia. *British Journal of Psychiatry*, 157, 558–61.

Liddle, P. F. & Crow, T. J. (1984). Age disorientation in chronic schizophrenia is associated with global intellectual impairment. *British Journal of Psychiatry*, 144, 193–9.

Liddle, P. F., Friston, K. J., Frith, C. D., et al. (1992). Patterns of cerebral blood flow in schizophrenia. *British Journal of Psychiatry*, **160**, 179–86.

Lombardi, J., Harvey, P. D., White, L., et al. (1996). Age disorientation in chronically hospitalised patients with mood disorders. *Psychiatry Research*, **60**, 87–90.

McKenna, P. J., Tamlyn, D., Lund, C. E., et al. (1990). Amnesic syndrome in schizophrenia. *Psychological Medicine*, **20**, 967–72.

Mlakar, J., Jensterle, J. & Frith, C. D. (1994). Central monitoring deficiency and schizophrenic symptoms. *Psychological Medicine*, **24**, 557–64.

Morice, R. & Delahunty, A. (1996). Frontal/executive impairments in schizophrenia. *Schizophrenia Bulletin*, **22**, 125–37.

Morrison-Stewart, S. L., Williamson, P. C., Corning, W. C., et al. (1992). Frontal and non-frontal neuropsychological tests performance and clinical symptomatology in chronic schizophrenia. *Psychological Medicine*, **22**, 353–9.

Nathaniel-James, D. A., Brown, R. & Ron, M. A. (1996). Memory impairment in schizophrenia: its' relationship to executive function. *Schizophrenia Research*, **21(2)**, 85–96.

Nayani, T. & David, A. (1996). The neuropsychology and neurophenomenology of auditory hallucinations. In *Schizophrenia: A Neuropsychological Perspective*, ed. C. Pantelis, H. E. Nelson & T. R. E. Barnes, pp. 345–72. Chichester, England: John Wiley.

Nelson, H. E., Pantelis, C., Carruthers, K., et al. (1990). Cognitive functioning and symptomatology in chronic schizophrenia. *Psychological Medicine*, **20**, 357–65.

Nopoulos, P., Flashman, L., Flaum, M., Arndt, S. & Andreasen, N. (1994). Stability of cognitive functioning early in the course of schizophrenia. *Schizophrenia Research*, **14**, 29–37.

O'Carroll, R. E. (1995). Associative learning in acutely ill and recovered schizophrenic patients. *Schizophrenia Research*, **15**, 299–301.

O'Carroll, R. E., Walker, M., Dunan, J., et al. (1992). Selecting controls for schizophrenia research studies: the use of the NART as a measure of pre-morbid ability. *Schizophrenia Research*, **8**, 137–41.

O'Carroll, R. E., Murray, C., Austin, M. P., Ebmeier, K. P., Goodwin, G. M. & Dunan, J. (1993). Proactive interference and the neuropsychology of schizophrenia. *British Journal of Psychiatry*, **32**, 353–6.

Pandurangi, A. K., Sax, K. W., Pelonero, A. L. & Goldberg, S. C. (1994). Sustained attention and positive formal thought disorder in schizophrenia. *Schizophrenia Research*, **13**, 109–16.

Penn, D. L., Spaulding, W., Reed, D. & Sullivan, M. (1996). The relationship of social cognition to ward behaviour in chronic schizophrenia. *Schizophrenia Research*, **20**, 327–35.

Penn, D. L., Corrigan, P. W., Bentall, R. P., Racenstein, J. M. & Newman, L. (1997). Social cognition in schizophrenia. *Psychological Bulletin*, **121**, 114–32.

Rossi, A., Mancini, F., Stratta, P., et al. (1997). Risperidone, negative symptoms and cognitive deficit in schizophrenia: an open study. *Acta Psychiatrica Scandinavica*, **95**, 40–3.

Russell, A. J., Munro, J. C., Jones, P. B., Hemsley, D. R. & Murray, R. M. (1997). Schizophrenia and the myth of intellectual decline. *American Journal of Psychiatry*, **154**, 635–9.

Saykin, A. J., Gur, R. C., Gur, R. E., et al. (1991). Neuropsychological function in schizophrenia: selective impairment in memory and learning. *Archives of General Psychiatry*, **48**, 618–24.

Saykin, A. J., Shtasel, D. L., Gur, R. E., et al. (1994). Neuropsychological deficits in neuroleptic naive patients with first-episode schizophrenia. *Archives of General Psychiatry*, **51**, 124–31.

Schwartzman, A. E. & Douglas, V. I. (1962). Intellectual loss in schizophrenia – part II. *Canadian Journal of Psychology*, **16**, 161–8.

Servan-Schreiber, D., Cohen, J. D. & Steingard, S. (1996). Schizophrenic deficits in the processing of context. *Archives of General Psychiatry*, **53**, 1105–12.

Shallice, T., Burgess, P. W. & Frith, C. D. (1991). Can the neuropsychological case-study approach be applied to schizophrenia? *Psychological Medicine*, **21**, 661–73.

Smith, A. (1964). Mental deterioration in chronic schizophrenia. *Journal of Nervous and Mental Disease*, **139**, 479–87.

Smith, R. C., Largen, J., Vroulis, G. & Ravichandran, G. K. (1992). Neuropsychological test scores and clinical response to neuroleptics in schizophrenic patients. *Comprehensive Psychiatry*, **33**, 139–45.

Stip, E. & Lussier, I. (1996). The effect of risperidone on cognition in patients with schizophrenia. *Canadian Journal of Psychiatry*, **41 (Suppl 2)**, S35–40.

Stolar, N., Berenbaum, H., Banich, M. T. & Barch, D. (1994). Neuropsychological correlates of alogia and affective flattening in schizophrenia. *Biological Psychiatry*, **35**, 164–72.

Sweeney, J. A., Haas, G. L., Keilp, J. G. & Long, M. (1991). Evaluation of the stability of neuropsychological functioning after acute episodes of schizophrenia: one-year follow-up study. *Psychiatry Research*, **38**, 63–76.

Tamlyn, D., McKenna, P. J., Mortimer, A. M., et al. (1992). Memory impairment in schizophrenia: its extent, affiliations and neuropsychological character. *Psychological Medicine*, **22**, 101–15.

Vrtunski, P. B., Konicki, P. E., Kwon, K. Y., Jaskiw, G. J. & Jaskiw, G. E. (1996). Effect of clozapine on motor function in schizophrenic patients. *Schizophrenia Research*, **20**, 187–98.

Waddington, J. L. & Youssef, H. A. (1996). Cognitive dysfunction in chronic schizophrenia followed perspectively over ten years and its longitudinal relationship to the emergence of tardive dyskinesia. *Psychological Medicine*, **26**, 681–8.

Waddington, J. L., Youssef, H. A. & Kinsella, A. (1990). Cognitive dysfunction in schizophrenia over five years, and its longitudinal relationship to the emergence of tardive dyskinesia. *Psychological Medicine*, **20**, 835–42.

Walker, E. F. (1994). Neurodevelopmental precursors of schizophrenia. In *The Neuropsychology of Schizophrenia*, ed. A. S. David & J. C. Cutting, pp. 119–29. Hove, UK: Lawrence Erlbaum Associates.

Williams, J. H., Wellman, N. A., Geaney, D. P., et al. (1998). Reduced latent inhibition in people with schizophrenia: an effect of psychosis or of its treatment. *British Journal of Psychiatry*, **172**, 243–9.

Wilson, B., Cockburn, J. & Baddeley, A. (1985). *The Rivermead Behavioural Memory Test*. Reading: Thames Valley Test Company.

Wohlberg, G. W. & Kornetsky, C. (1973). Sustained attention in remitted schizophrenics. *Archives of General Psychiatry*, **28**, 533–7.

Wolf, L. E. & Cornblatt, B. A. (1996). Neuropsychological functioning in children at high risk of schizophrenia. In *Schizophrenia: a Neuropsychological Perspective*, ed. C. Pantelis, H. E. Nelson & T. R. E. Barnes, pp. 161–82. Chichester, England: John Wiley.

Zahn, T. P., Pickar, D. & Haier, R. J. (1994). Effects of clozapine, fluphenazine, and placebo on reaction time measures of attention and sensory dominance in schizophrenia. *Schizophrenia Research*, **13**, 133–44.

7

Epidemiology and genetics

More than one hundred years after Emil Kraepelin (1896) defined, as dementia praecox, the disease concept which came to be known as schizophrenia, the cause or causes of the disorder remain unknown. This very important question has been addressed from numerous angles by many individuals. It does not seem likely that all of the points of view will ever be able to be fully reconciled. A major division of opinion lies between those who believe schizophrenia to be a biological brain disease and those for whom the disorder can only be understood in psychological terms, as a manifestation of the individual's inner conflicts or of his/her dysfunctional relationships. As McKenna (1994) points out, one or other of these camps has held the upper hand for decades at a time, the other being forced very much to the sidelines. Presently the biologists are in the ascendant. Current views are clearly expressed by Weinberger (1995):

Our understanding of the pathogenesis of schizophrenia has changed dramatically in recent years. Decades of scientifically unfounded psychological and social theories that blamed families and society have given way to increasingly compelling scientific evidence that schizophrenia is a brain disorder.

The evidence certainly can be described as compelling, but the picture is not yet entirely clear and much requires to be confirmed and clarified. While it is worth remembering that the race is not yet over and many a favourite has fallen at the last fence, if we take the view that adequate objective evidence implicating the brain in schizophrenia has now been gathered, and that there is underlying brain pathology in a large proportion of patients (Weinberger, 1995), we must still concede that we do not know what causes that pathology. Genetic factors are known to be relevant and will be described in detail below, but it seems very unlikely indeed that no additional factor is involved. Eighty nine per cent of patients have parents who are not schizophrenic – 81% have no affected first degree relatives, and 63% will show no family history of the disease whatsoever (Gottesman, 1991). Estimates of concordance in monozygotic twins vary, but average about 50% (Gottesman, 1991), certainly very far short of the 100% that would be expected from genetically identical individuals if no other factors were involved.

It has of course long been known that illnesses phenomenologically typical of schizophrenia may occur in association with, and perhaps because of, organic disease of various kinds (Davison & Bagley, 1969; Davison, 1983). Such disorders have aroused much interest, largely because of the possibility that study of the mechanism underlying them may shed light upon the pathogenesis of the generality of schizophrenia. They are not common. In the Northwick Park First Episodes Study, 6% of cases were found to have an organic condition of definite or possible aetiological significance for their psychosis (Johnstone et al., 1987). This frequency is in keeping with the generality of the literature in the area (Lewis, 1995) and it is clear that underlying organic disease of this type which can be demonstrated and diagnosed by currently available techniques cannot account for the proportion of schizophrenic illness which cannot be plausibly attributed to genetic causes. Epidemiological methods can be of great value in demonstrating patterns of disease which suggest possible aetiologies and which allow better focused clinical and laboratory research to take place. Such methods have greatly illuminated understanding of disorders as diverse as rubella, encephalopathy, pellagra and kuru. Wide-ranging epidemiological studies of schizophrenia have been conducted over a long period and have not yet provided the great gains in understanding that have occurred in some other disorders, although they have provided replicable findings, the full meaning of which is probably yet to be understood.

Schizophrenia has some particular difficulties for epidemiologists. A central difficulty is the uncertain nature of the disease concept. The diagnosis continues essentially to be made upon the basis of the patient's account of his inner experiences. Although recent findings have been encouraging, there is still no structural or functional abnormality of the brain which is reliably found in cases of schizophrenia and not in other people. There is no objective diagnostic test which can provide a validating criterion for the clinical diagnostic concept.

In interpreting epidemiological findings in schizophrenia, the variation in concepts and the wide range of methods used require to be acknowledged and emphasis requires to be given to findings which are replicable in spite of these problems. The difficulties resulting from variation in the concept of schizophrenia are illustrated by the findings of the US–UK diagnostic project (Cooper et al., 1972) described in Chapter 1, in which substantial discrepancies between American and British psychiatric practice in the differentiation of schizophrenia from affective illness were highlighted. It is clear that at that time the concept of schizophrenia in New York was wider than that in London, and that the breadth of this concept was occurring at the expense of the affective disorder. These and similar findings have encouraged the use of operational rules for defining psychiatric disorders, including schizophrenia.

Measuring the prevalence, incidence and morbid risk of schizophrenia to provide a framework for research into risk factors and possible causes requires a diagnostic assessment which will (by using operational rules) select cases which conform to accepted clinical concepts of the disorder and the capacity for identifying in a given population at least the great majority of affected individuals (case finding). Most case finding exercises involve the detection of cases among populations in clinical contact with either general practice, psychiatric services or hospitals. Other methods involving samples of the population who have not necessarily been in contact with the services, e.g. door to door surveys or follow-up studies of birth cohorts, may also be used but are much less common. The WHO International Pilot Study of Schizophrenia (WHO, 1973, 1979) demonstrates that it is possible by the use of standardized methods of diagnostic classification (PSE/Catego, Wing et al., 1974) to achieve a similar concept of schizophrenia, in diverse cultures. Morbidity can be measured by prevalence (number of cases per 1000 persons at risk in a population over a given time period), incidence (annual number of new cases in a defined population per 1000 individuals at risk), or morbid risk (the probability that an individual born into a particular population or group will develop the disease if he/she survives throughout the entire period of risk for that disease). Most studies, apart from those concerning small isolated populations, e.g. in North Sweden, which may consist of genetic isolates (Böök et al., 1978), have estimated morbid risk at 0.50–1.60%, which provides a basis for the crude estimate of 1% which is often used (Jablensky, 1995). Whether or not significant differences exist in the rate of occurrence of schizophrenia is a matter of debate. Taking into account the inherent difficulties of the method and the size of the populations surveyed, some statistically significant differences are bound to occur. As Jablensky (1995) points out, 'whether such differences are epidemiologically salient is another matter'. Accepting that there are pockets of unusual frequency, Jablensky is of the view that these are exceptions to the general rule and that the weight of the current evidence does not suggest the existence of major population differences in the incidence and disease expectancy of schizophrenia such as are known to occur in common multifactorial diseases such as diabetes or heart disease.

Reporting on the initial evaluation phase of the WHO Collaborative Study on Determinants of Outcome of Severe Mental Disorders, Sartorius et al. (1986) concluded that the results provide strong support for the notion that schizophrenic illnesses occur with comparable frequency in different populations. On the other hand, Torrey (1987) expressed the view that the almost two-fold (but non-significant) difference in rates between centres using a narrow definition of schizophrenia and the three-fold (and significant) difference using a broad definition of schizophrenia found in the study described by Sartorius et al. (1986) could perhaps be interpreted differently, and that the issue of variable frequency requires further study, possibly with emphasis upon populations showing unusual rates, e.g. Northern Swedes (Böök et al., 1978), and Western Irish (Torrey et al., 1984). He does, however, point out that other major diseases in which both genetic and non-genetic factors are thought to be important have significant prevalence differences – six-fold for heart disease (Thom et al., 1985), 10-fold for rheumatoid arthritis (Utsinger et al., 1985), while diabetes (Type 1) and multiple sclerosis are said to show 30-fold (Marble et al., 1975) and 50-fold differences respectively. Against this background the frequency of schizophrenia does seem remarkably uniform throughout the world.

Certain important replicable facts have however emerged from epidemiological studies, and they may well represent clues to the aetiology of schizophrenia. Gender has been consistently shown to be significantly related to major aspects of schizophrenia. The finding of an earlier mean age of onset in men than in women has been repeatedly demonstrated (Lewine, 1981; Hafner et al., 1993). Recent studies of a large series of first admissions in Germany, together with a comparison of German and Danish case register data (Hafner, 1993) and analysis of data from two WHO multinational studies (Hambrecht et al., 1992a,b) indicate that this finding is robust and does not depend upon the diagnostic system used, that it occurs across cultures and that it is specific to schizophrenia. It appears that men and women show different age incidence curves in relation to the development of schizophrenia (Hafner, 1993), such that onsets in men peak at ages 20–24, thereafter remaining constant at a rather lower level, whereas in women there is a less prominent peak in the early twenties, followed by another increase in incidence in age groups older than 35. The question as to whether the total lifetime risks for men and women are the same or different is presently unresolved and findings are much affected by the operational definition for schizophrenia used. Clearly the use of definitions such as DSM III, which have an upper age limit of 45 for the diagnosis, will mean that women of older age onsets are not included and may suggest that the disorder is commoner in men, and it is possible that if samples are followed up until very late ages, findings will be quite different (Jablensky, 1995). Male–female differences have also been reported in relation to the course of the illness – women having better premorbid functioning and in general a less disabling course (WHO, 1979; Childers & Harding, 1990). Such findings have been widely replicated, but they could obviously, at least to some extent, be explained by the later onset and the generally more protected role that women occupy in society in most cultures. It is difficult to see how such factors could affect the robust differences in age of onset between the sexes, and this may well be a clue to the 'underlying morbid condition' of schizophrenia. A neuromodulating effect of oestrogens on D_2 receptors (Hafner, 1993), a protective effect of the earlier CNS maturation in females (Saugstad, 1989) and a genetic effect (De Lisi, 1992) have all been suggested as possibilities.

The excessive mortality of schizophrenic patients has long been known, and in recent years has remained at about twice that of the general population (Herrman et al., 1983; Allebeck & Wistedt, 1986). The high mortality rates among schizophrenic patients from infectious diseases, particularly tuberculosis, reported for periods from the 1920s to the 1940s were considered at one time to perhaps represent an unusual susceptibility to such disorders. This high mortality was, however, shown not to be specific for schizophrenia but to be characteristic of the mental hospital population as a whole (Alstrom, 1942). The current high mortality largely but not entirely relates to an excess of suicides and avoidable deaths (Herrman et al., 1983; Anderson et al., 1991).

The lower fertility of both men and women diagnosed as schizophrenic is well established (Essen-Möller, 1935; Larson & Nyman, 1973; Odegaard, 1980). Although there have been claims that rates of schizophrenia are declining (Munk-Jorgensen, 1986; Eagles et al., 1988; Harrison et al., 1991) it is far from clear that these findings cannot be explained by changes in diagnostic and administrative practices, changes in treatment modalities and settings, etc. (Jablensky, 1995) and it is probably appropriate still to say that the disorder seems stable over time as well as over place. This is difficult to reconcile with a disorder in which genetic effects have an aetiological role and where fertility is clearly reduced, unless either some biological advantage for relatives can be shown, or a high rate of mutation in the general population can be demonstrated. With regard to the former, the fertility of siblings of schizophrenic probands has therefore been examined by several research groups (Lindelius, 1970; Buck et al., 1975; Erlenmeyer-Kimling, 1978) but no differences have been found which are indicative of any reproductive advantage for the non-psychotic biological first degree relatives of schizophrenic individuals and which would offset the low fertility and high mortality of the condition.

Epidemiological findings relating to season of birth, ethnicity, the occurrence of epidemics of influenza and perinatal events have all been interpreted as offering support for the idea that insults of various kinds very early in life may result in the later development of schizophrenia. The season of birth effect in schizophrenia has long been known (Tramer, 1929) and an excess of schizophrenic births in the winter has been found in both northern and southern hemispheres (Bradbury & Miller, 1985; Boyd et al., 1986). This is a robust finding which is generally interpreted as indicating that some noxious agent which is seasonally related and may concern, for example, variables related to infection, nutrition or temperature, affects individuals during fetal life or around the time of birth in such a way as to cause them to develop schizophrenia later. Such views are to some extent undermined by the argument that this finding could be due to the fact that as, at ages of maximal frequency, the risk of schizophrenia increases with age, individuals born early in a year will have a higher rate than individuals born later in the same year. Furthermore, seasonality occurs in depression, neurotic illness, personality disorders and learning disability as well as in schizophrenia (Hafner, 1987).

In 1932 Odegaard demonstrated that Norwegians who had emigrated to the United States had higher rates of schizophrenia than those who had remained in Norway, and the phenomenon of relatively high rates of schizophrenia in immigrants has since been shown in numerous studies, including that of Cochrane (1977) in which most immigrant groups to England and Wales, including Asians, West Indians and Poles, were shown to have higher hospital admission rates for schizophrenia than English or Scottish people. Such findings were generally interpreted as being due to phenomena such as selective migration of unsettled (and therefore prepsychotic) people, the stresses of living in a foreign land and mistaken diagnosis as a result of cultural and language barriers. Interest in the relationship between immigration and schizophrenia was, however, much enhanced by the demonstration of substantially increased rates of disorder in second generation (i.e. U.K. born) Afro Caribbean immigrants to the

United Kingdom (Harrison et al., 1988; Wessely et al., 1991; Bhugra et al., 1997). These findings are difficult to interpret because of a lack of reliable figures on the size and age structure of the Afro Caribbean population in the U.K., and there may well be a denominator error. If the findings can be consistently substantiated, however, there are a number of possible explanations for this intriguing result, one of which is that the mothers of the affected individuals, on arriving in this country as young women, were unusually susceptible to some noxious agent which affected them during pregnancy and resulted in the much later development of schizophrenia in their children. An example of such a mechanism is provided by the work of Fahy et al. (1992) which demonstrated an excess of births in March 1958 of Afro Caribbeans who went on to develop schizophrenia. The authors suggest that this may be due to the effects upon their mothers of the influenza epidemic of 1957. The relationship of maternal infection with influenza to the later development of schizophrenia in the adult offspring has been much more widely explored.

In 1988 Mednick et al. reported that there was a significantly increased rate of schizophrenia in individuals who had been in the second trimester of fetal life during the 1957 influenzia epidemic. This finding has been further investigated using data sets from Denmark (Barr et al., 1990), Scotland (Kendall & Kemp, 1989; Kendell & Adams, 1991) and England and Wales (Sham et al., 1992). The data are suggestive of there being a link between epidemics of influenza and the later development of schizophrenia in those who were in utero during the epidemic. Such data can only provide a very indirect link between influenzal infection and schizophrenia. The work of Done et al., 1991, studying individuals who were subjects of the National Child Development Study in 1958 and who went on later to develop schizophrenia, had the possibility of studying this issue more directly because the subjects of the National Child Development study were born between the 3rd and the 9th March 1958 and were thus in the second trimester of fetal life during the influenza epidemic in October 1957. Detailed accounts of each mother's health during the pregnancy had been obtained by a midwife as a part of the 1958 study, and it was possible to compare the rates for the later development of schizophrenia in the offspring of those mothers who gave a history of having been affected by the influenza epidemic, with the rates in the offspring of mothers who gave no such history. The children of the mothers who had been affected by influenza did not show a significantly increased rate of development of schizophrenia (Crow & Done, 1992). The timing of the National Child Development Study in relation to the influenza epidemic was entirely fortuitous, and although these data provide a more direct means of addressing the issue of the relationship between fetal infection with the influenza virus and the later development of schizophrenia than might ordinarily be expected to be available, these negative findings cannot be regarded as conclusive, because of course the diagnosis of influenza was based upon the mother's account at the time. It is perfectly possible that subclinical infections took place and that not all infections were recollected and reported some months later.

The relationship between exposure to a noxious agent during fetal life and the later development of schizophrenia has also been explored in relation to maternal starvation. Famines, sadly, are not infrequent but usually such circumstances tend to be associated with a breakdown of organized record-keeping in relation to registration of births, etc. In Holland at the end of the Second World War, during what came to be known as the Dutch Hunger Winter of 1944–45, the population was severely deprived of food. This deprivation was relatively circumscribed in time and affected pregnant women as well as the rest of the population. The organization of society was maintained and record keeping continued. An increased rate of schizophrenia was found in the female offspring of women who suffered severe food deprivation during the first trimester of pregnancy (Susser & Lin, 1992).

The effects of both influenza and food deprivation are suggested as affecting the brain during a critical period of brain development, and thus are held to support the neurodevelopment hypothesis of schizophrenia. More generalized complications of pregnancy and birth have also been studied in relation to schizophrenia. This is a difficult field, as much work has relied upon the maternal recollection of the births of known cases of schizophrenia and prospective studies have been relatively few.

The field is well reviewed by McNeil (1991) and overall most work does support an association between pregnancy and birth complications and the later development of schizophrenia, although there have certainly been negative studies (Done et al., 1991; McCreadie et al., 1992). The type of obstetric difficulty which is most relevant to the later development of schizophrenia is not at all clear. It has been suggested that as there is an association between abnormal fetal development and abnormal delivery, the relationship between pregnancy and birth complications and the later development of schizophrenia may be interpreted in neurodevelopmental terms (Weinberger, 1995).

The familial occurrence of schizophrenia has been studied over many years. After defining dementia praecox, Kraepelin (1907) expressed the idea that 'defective heredity is a very prominent factor'. A study of the familiality of the disorder was undertaken in Kraepelin's department (Rudin, 1916) and the issue has received continued investigation since that time (Falconer, 1965; Slater & Cowie, 1971; Kendler et al., 1985). Demonstrating familiality does not necessarily imply that an inherited genetic factor is causing the disorder, since families often share a common environment as well as common genes, but the matter was clarified by an elegant series of studies (Rosenthal et al., 1971; Kety et al., 1975). These investigations of children adopted away from their biological parents at birth showed that they were at significantly greater risk of the later development of schizophrenia if there was schizophrenia among their biological relatives, but not if it was present among their adoptive relatives. It was thus clear that the enhanced tendency to develop schizophrenia was not due to a shared environment but to shared genetic material, unless it is argued that shared environment before adoption (during pregnancy and the neonatal period) is critical. It is evident from this work and from the twin studies that have been conducted comparing concordance for the disease between members of monozygotic twin pairs and members of dizygotic twin pairs (Fischer, 1971; Tienari, 1975; Gottesman & Shields, 1972; Kringlen, 1976) that genetic factors play a major, but not absolute, role in developing schizophrenia, but the mode of transmission remains uncertain. Studies of the pattern of inheritance in families with schizophrenia and examination of the risks to various classes of relatives are unable to demonstrate a simple Mendelian mode of transmission in the great majority of cases. The pattern of inheritance is complex or irregular, and it is not clear whether the familial clustering in schizophrenia is due to a single gene, to a few genes or to many genes, or, as is perhaps more likely, to all three different mechanisms operating in different sub-populations of the condition. The technique of genetic modelling involves assessing the probability of the observed family data under alternative models to see what kind of genetic and environmental factors are most compatible with the data. The numerous studies that have attempted to discriminate a single gene from a polygenic inheritance for schizophrenia have produced conflicting results (Baron, 1986). It has been suggested (Meehl, 1973) that in schizophrenia the expression of a single major gene is modified by interaction with a number of other genes, each of only small effect. This 'mixed model' has been the subject of several studies (Carter & Chung, 1980; Risch & Baron, 1984; Vogler et al., 1990). This work provides some evidence in favour of multifactorial as opposed to single major gene models of inheritance, but has not been able to provide conclusive results (Asherson et al., 1995). Indeed, given that genetic heterogeneity is probable, the solution of this problem may be very difficult without prior knowledge of definite acting genetic loci. Pedigrees multiply affected with individuals who have schizophrenia are uncommon, but can provide considerable power to detect sites on chromosomes that may contain genes for the condition (McGuffin & Owen, 1991). Linkage analysis, which tests for the co-segregation of the condition with polymorphic marker probes, has been used to define loci for genes involved in a wide range of inherited medical illnesses, and it is the first step in gene isolation by the method now generally termed positional cloning. Although it does not rely on an understanding of the disease pathophysiology, the method is sensitive to assumptions about the mode of inheritance, the penetrance, the definition of caseness, and its power is markedly diminished by heterogeneity in the study sample. The method has, however, been successful with major psychiatric disorders such as the identification of the Chromosome 14 locus linked to the majority of familial Alzheimer's disease, pedigrees which paved the way for the detection of the presenilin I gene and its relevant mutations (Sherrington et al., 1995). Studies of families multiply affected with schizophrenia initially produced positive results in relation to Chromosome 5 (Sherrington et al., 1988) but these findings have not been replicated in numerous subsequent studies, e.g. St. Clair et al. (1989). Studies relating to Chromosome 6 (Schwab et al., 1995; Mowry et al., 1995) and Chromosome 22 (Pulver et al., 1994; Vallada et al., 1995) have similarly produced conflicting findings and at present no reliably replicable findings in this area have been made (Sham, 1996; Delisi, 1997). Heterogeneity may be a major stumbling block to such studies, and the examination of single very large pedigrees able to generate significant linkage results by themselves may be a more useful approach. Candidate gene approaches may be used in the investigation of disorders with simple Mendelian inheritance where there are genes which are known or suspected to have a role in the pathophysiology of the disease (candidate genes). An alternative to cloning genes through a known chromosomal position is by the so-called functional cloning strategy. Candidate genes are defined through their assumed importance in the pathophysiology of the disease and can be screened directly for mutations. This approach has been successful in identifying the disease gene of Marfan's syndrome and autosomal dominant retinitis pigmentosa (Strachan, 1992).

Other analytical methods can be applied to complex disorders, such as schizophrenia, without a simple, single, defined mode of inheritance. Association studies of marker polymorphisms in case and control populations can point to genetic loci for genes of minor as well as major effect.

Successful examples include cleft lip and palate (Holder et al., 1992) and insulin dependent diabetes mellitus (Chiu et al., 1993; Bell et al., 1984). As yet such studies have produced conflicting results in schizophrenia (Asherson et al., 1995). Sib-pair analysis, based on the degree of allele sharing between affected pairs of siblings, can also be used in complex disorders, although large sample sizes are predicted to be required (Craddock & Owen, 1996).

The situation at present therefore is that there is compelling evidence from family, twin and adoption studies that genetic factors are important in the transmission of schizophrenia, although they do not account for all of the variance in liability to the disorder, so that some environmental factors must be relevant. The nature of the genetic transmission remains unknown, in spite of intensive investigation. It may very well be that the nature of the genetic substrate is not the same in all families, and indeed examination of the pattern of inheritance in different families suggests that this is likely. If genetic heterogeneity exists, it is entirely possible that there are single genes of major effect in the multiply affected pedigrees where the condition looks as though it could be dominant (McGuffin & Owen, 1991). If this is the case, linkage strategies have the potential of localizing these genes in the foreseeable future. There is of course no firm evidence that single major genes are involved and the demonstration of modes of transmission by a few genes of moderate effect or many genes of small effect will be more difficult. The molecular basis of other common complex disorders has, however, been demonstrated by molecular genetic approaches, which in spite of recent disappointments remain one of the most promising techniques in the investigation of the biological basis of schizophrenia.

References

Allebeck, P. & Wistedt, B. (1986). Mortality in schizophrenia. *Archives of General Psychiatry*, **43**, 650–3.

Alstrom, C. H. (1942). Mortality in mental hospitals with especial regard to tuberculosis. *Acta Psychiatrica et Neurologica Scandinavica*, **(Suppl 24)**.

Anderson, A., Connelly, J., Johnstone, E. C. & Owens, D. G. C. (1991). Cause of death. *British Journal of Psychiatry*, **Suppl 13**, 30–3.

Asherson, P., Mont, R. & McGuffin, P. (1995). Genetics and schizophrenia. In *Schizophrenia*, ed. S. R. Hirsch & D. R. Weinberger, pp. 253–74. Oxford: Blackwell Science Ltd.

Baron, M. (1986). Genetics of schizophrenia. I. Familial patterns and mode of inheritance. *Biological Psychiatry*, **21**, 1051–66.

Barr, C. E., Medrick, S. A. & Munk–Jorgensen, P. (1990). Exposure to influenza epidemics during gestation and adult schizophrenia: a 40 year study. *Archives of General Psychiatry*, **47**, 869–74.

Bell, G. I., Hortas, S. & Karam, J. H. (1984). A polymorphic locus near the human insulin gene is associated with insulin dependent diabetes mellitus. *Diabetes*, **33**, 176–83.

Bhugra, D., Leff, J. Mallett, R., et al. (1997). Incidence and outcome of schizophrenia in Whites, African Caribbeans and Asians in London. *Psychological Medicine*, **27**, 791–8.

Böök, J. A., Wettenberg, L. & Modrzewska, K. (1978). Schizophrenia in a North Swedish geographical isolate, 1900–1977: epidemiology, genetics and biochemistry. *Clinical Genetics*, **14**, 373–94.

Boyd, J. H., Pulver, A. E. & Stewart, W. (1986). Season of birth: schizophrenia and bipolar disorder. *Schizophrenia Bulletin*, **12**, 173–85.

Bradbury, T. N. & Miller, G. A. (1985). Season of birth in schizophrenia: a review of the evidence, methodology and aetiology. *Psychological Bulletin*, **98**, 569–94.

Buck, C., Hobbs, G. E., Simpson, H. & Winokur, J. M. (1975). Fertility of the sibs of schizophrenic patients. *British Journal of Psychiatry*, **127**, 235–9.

Carter, C. L. & Chung, C. S. (1980). Segregation analysis of schizophrenia under a mixed model. *Human Heredity*, **30**, 350–6.

Childers, S. E. & Harding, C. M. (1990). Gender, premorbid social functioning and long term outcome in DSM III schizophrenia. *Schizophrenia Bulletin*, **16**, 309–18.

Chiu, K. C., Tanizawa, Y. & Permott, M. A. (1993). Glucokinase gene variants in the common form of NIDDM. *Diabetes*, **42**, 579–82.

Cochrane, R. (1977). Mental illness in immigrants to England & Wales: an analysis of mental hospital admissions, 1971. *Social Psychiatry*, **12**, 25–35.

Cooper, J. E., Kendell, R. E., Gurland, B. J., et al. (1972). Psychiatric diagnosis in New York and London. *Maudsley Monograph 20*, Oxford: Oxford University Press.

Craddock, N. & Owen, M. J. (1996). Modern molecular genetic approaches to psychiatric disease. In *Biological Psychiatry. British Medical Bulletin*, **52 (3)**, 434–52.

Crow, T. J. & Done, D. J. (1992). Prenatal exposure to influenza does not cause schizophrenia. *British Journal of Psychiatry*, **161**, 390–3.

Davison, K. (1983). Schizophrenia-like psychoses associated with organic cerebral disorders: a review. *Psychiatric Developments*, **i**, 1–34.

Davison, K. & Bagley, C. R. (1969). Schizophrenia-like psychoses associated with organic disorders of the nervous system: a review of the literature. In *Current Problems in Neuropsychiatry*, ed. R. N. Herrington, pp. 173–84. Ashford, Kent: Headley Bros.

De Lisi, L. E. (1992). The significance of age of onset for schizophrenia. *Schizophrenia Bulletin*, **18**, 209–15.

De Lisi, L. E. (1997). The genetics of schizophrenia: past present and future concepts. *Schizophrenia Research*, **28**, 163–75.

Done, J. D., Johnstone, E. C., Frith, C. D., et al. (1991). Complications of pregnancy and delivery in relation to psychosis in adult life: data from the British Perinatal Mortality Survey Sample. *British Medical Journal*, **302**, 1576–86.

Eagles, J. M., Hunter, D. & McCance, C. (1988). Decline in the diagnosis of schizophrenia among first contacts with psychiatric services in North East Scotland, 1969–1984. *British Journal of Psychiatry*, **152**, 793–8.

Erlenmeyer-Kimling, L. (1978). Fertility of psychotics: demography. In *Annual*

Review of the Schizophrenia Syndrome, Vol. 5, ed. R. Canero, pp. 298–333. New York: Brunner/Mazel.

Essen-Möller, E. (1935). Untersuchungen über die Fruchtbankeit gewisser Gruppen von Geisteskranken. *Acta Psychiatrica et Neurologica Scandinavica*, **Suppl. 8.**

Fahy, T. A., Jones, P. B. & Sham, P. C. (1992). Schizophrenia in Afro-Caribbeans in the U.K. following prenatal exposure to the 1957 A_2 influenza epidemic. *Schizophrenia Research*, **6**, 98–9.

Falconer, D. S. (1965). The inheritance of liability to certain diseases, estimated from the incidence among relatives. *Annals of Human Genetics*, **29**, 51–76.

Fischer, M. (1971). Psychoses in the offspring of schizophrenic monozygotic twins and their normal co-twins. *British Journal of Psychiatry*, **118**, 43–52.

Gottesman, I. I. (1991). *Schizophrenia Genesis: The Origins of Madness*. New York: Freeman.

Gottesman, I. I. & Shields, J. (1972). *Schizophrenia and Genetics: A Twin Vantage Point*. New York: Academic Press.

Hafner, H. (1987). Epidemiology of Schizophrenia. In *Search for the Causes of Schizophrenia*, ed. H. Hafner, W. Gattaz & W. Janzarik, pp. 47–74. Berlin & Heidelberg: Springer Verlag.

Hafner, H. (1993). What is schizophrenia? *Neurology, Psychiatry & Brain Research*, **2**, 36–52.

Hafner, H., Maurer, K., Löffler, W. & Riecher-Rassler, A. (1993). The influence of age and sex on the onset and early course of schizophrenia. *British Journal of Psychiatry*, **162**, 80–6.

Hambrecht, M., Maurer, K., Sartorius, N. & Hafner, H. (1992a). Transnational stability of gender differences in schizophrenia? An analysis based on the WHO study in determinants of outcome of severe mental disorders. *European Archives of Psychiatry & Clinical Neurosciences*, **242**, 6–12.

Hambrecht, M., Maurer, K. & Hafner, H. (1992b). Gender differences in schizophrenia in three cultures. Results of the WHO collaborative study on psychiatric disability. *Social Psychiatry & Psychiatric Epidemiology*, **27**, 117–21.

Harrison, G., Owens, D., Holton, A., Neilson, D. & Boot, D. (1988). A prospective study of severe mental disorder in Afro-Caribbean patients. *Psychological Medicine*, **18**, 643–57.

Harrison, G., Cooper, J. E. & Gancarczyk, R. (1991). Changes in the administrative incidence of schizophrenia. *British Journal of Psychiatry*, **159**, 811–16.

Herrman, H. E., Baldwin, J. A. & Christie, D. (1983). A record linkage study of mortality and general hospital discharge in patients diagnosed as schizophrenic. *Psychological Medicine*, **13**, 581–93.

Holder, S. E., Vintiner, G. M. & Farren, B. (1992). Confirmation of an association between RFLPs at the transforming growth factor-alpha locus and non-syndromic cleft lip and palate. *Journal of Medical Genetics*, **29**, 390–2.

Jablensky, A. (1995). Schizophrenia: the epidemiological horizon. In *Schizophrenia*, ed. S. R. Hirsch & D. R. Weinberger, pp. 206–52. Oxford: Blackwell Scientific Press.

Johnstone, E. C., Macmillan, J. F. & Crow, T. J. (1987). The occurrence of organic disease of possible or probable aetiological significance in a population of 268 cases of first episode schizophrenia. *Psychological Medicine*, **17**, 371–9.

Kendell, R. E. & Adams, W. (1991). Unexplained fluctuations in the risk for schizophrenia by month and year of birth. *British Journal of Psychiatry*, **158**, 758–63.

Kendell, R. E. & Kemp, I. W. (1989). Maternal influenza in the aetiology of schizophrenia. *Archives of General Psychiatry*, **46**, 878–82.

Kendler, K. S., Gruenberg, A. M. & Tsuang, M. T. (1985). Psychiatric illness in first degree relatives of schizophrenics and surgical control patients. *Archives of General Psychiatry*, **42**, 770–9.

Kety, S. S., Rosenthal, D., Wender, P. I. L. et al. (1975). Mental illness in the biologic and adoptive families of adopted individuals who become schizophrenic. In *Genetic Research in Schizophrenia*, ed. R. R. Fieve, D. Rosenthal & H. Brill., pp. 147–65. Baltimore: Johns Hopkins University Press.

Kraepelin, E. (1896). *Lehrbuch der Psychiatrie*, 5th edn. Leipzig: Barth.

Kraepelin, E. (1907). *Lehrbuch der Psychiatrie* (translated A. R. Diefendorf). New York: Macmillan.

Kringlen, E. (1976). Twins – still our best method. *Schizophrenia Bulletin*, **2**, 429–33.

Larson, C. A. & Nyman, G. E. (1973). Differential fertility in schizophrenia. *Acta Psychiatrica Scandinavica*, **49**, 272–80.

Lewine, R. J. (1981). Sex differences in schizophrenia: timing or subtypes. *Psychological Bulletin*, **90**, 432–44.

Lewis, S. W. (1995). The secondary schizophrenics. In *Schizophrenia*, ed. S. R. Hirsch & D. R. Weinberger, pp. 324–40. Oxford: Blackwell.

Lindelius, R. (1970). A study of schizophrenia: a clinical, prognostic and family investigation. *Acta Psychiatrica Scandinavica*, **Suppl. 216**.

McCreadie, R. G., Hall, D. J., Berry, I. J., et al. (1992). The Nithsdale schizophrenia surveys. X: Obstetric complications, family history and abnormal movements. *British Journal of Psychiatry*, **161**, 799–805.

McGuffin, P. & Owen, M. (1991). The molecular genetics of schizophrenia: an overview and forward view. *European Archives of Clinical Neuroscience*, **240**, 169–73.

McKenna, P. J. (1994). *Schizophrenia and Related Syndromes*, p. 98. Oxford: Oxford University Press.

McNeil, T. F. (1991). Obstetric complications in schizophrenic patients. *Schizophrenia Research*, **5**, 89–101.

Marble, A., Krall, L. P., Bradley, R., et al. (1975). *Joslin's Diabetes Mellitus*. Philadelphia: Lea & Febiger.

Mednick, S. A., Machon, R. A., Huttunen, M. O. & Bonett, D. (1988). Adult schizophrenia following prenatal exposure to an influenza epidemic. *Archives of General Psychiatry*, **45**, 189–92.

Meehl, P. E. (1973). *Psychodiagnosis: Selected Papers*. Minneapolis: University of Minnesota Press.

Mowry, B. J., Nancarrow, D. J., Lennon, D. P., et al. (1995). Schizophrenia susceptibility and chromosome 6p 24–22. *Nature Genetics*, **11**, 233–4.

Munk-Jorgensen, P. (1986). Decreasing first-admission rates of schizophrenia among males in Denmark from 1970–1984. *Acta Psychiatrica Scandinavica*, **13**, 645–50.

Odegaard, O. (1932). Emigration and insanity: a study of mental disease among Norwegian-born population of Minnesota. *Acta Psychiatrica et Neurologica Scandinavica*, **Suppl 4**.

Odegaard, O. (1980). Fertility of psychiatric first admissions in Norway,

1936–1975. *Acta Psychiatrica Scandinavica*, **62**, 212–20.

Pulver, A. E., Karayiongou, M., Laseker, V. K. et al. (1994). Follow up of a report of a potential linkage for schizophrenia on chromosome 22q 12–13.1. Part 2. *American Journal of Medical Genetics*, **54**, 44–50.

Risch, N. & Baron, M. (1984). Segregation analysis of schizophrenia and related disorders. *American Journal of Human Genetics*, **36**, 1039–59.

Rosenthal, D., Wender, P. H., Kety, S. S., Welner, J. & Schulsinger, F. (1971). The adopted away offspring of schizophrenics. *American Journal of Psychiatry*, **128**, 397–411.

Rudin, E. (1916). *Zur Vererbung und Neuentstehung der Dementia Praecox*. Berlin: Springer-Verlag.

Sartorius, N., Jablensky, A., Korten, A., et al. (1986). Early manifestations and first contact incidence of schizophrenia in different cultures. *Psychological Medicine*, **16**, 909–28.

Saugstad, L. F. (1989). Age at puberty and mental illness. Towards a neurodevelopmental aetiology of Kraepelin's endogenous psychoses. *British Journal of Psychiatry*, **155**, 536–44.

Schwab, S. C., Albus, M., Hallmyer, J., et al. (1995). Evaluation of a susceptibility gene for schizophrenia on chromosome 6p by multipoint affected sub-pair linkage analysis. *Nature Genetics*, **11**, 325–7.

Sham, P. (1996). Genetic epidemiology. *British Medical Bulletin*, **52(3)**, 408–33.

Sham, P. C., O'Callaghan, E., Takei, N., et al. (1992). Schizophrenia following prenatal exposure to influenza epidemics between 1939 and 1960. *British Journal of Psychiatry*, **160**, 461–6.

Sherrington, R., Brynjolffsen, J., Peterson, H., et al. (1988). Localisation of a susceptibility locus for schizophrenia on chromosome 5. *Nature*, **336**, 164–7.

Sherrington, R., Rogaev, E. I., Liang, Y., et al. (1995). Cloning of a gene bearing missense mutations in early onset familial Alzheimer's disease. *Nature*, **375**, 754–60.

Slater, E. & Cowie, V. (1971). *The Genetics of Mental Disorder*. Oxford: Oxford University Press.

St. Clair, D., Blackwood, D., Muir, W., et al. (1989). No linkage of 5q11–q13 markers to schizophrenia in Scottish families. *Nature*, **339**, 305–9.

Strachan, T. (1992). *The Human Genome*. Oxford: Bios Scientific Publishers.

Susser, E. S. & Lin, S. P. (1992). Schizophrenia after prenatal exposure to the Dutch Hunger Winter of 1944–1945. *Archives of General Psychiatry*, **49**, 983–8.

Thom, T. J., Epstein, F. H., Feldman, J. J. & Leaventon, P. E. (1985). Trends in total mortality and mortality from heart disease in 26 countries from 1950–1978. *International Journal of Epidemiology*, **4**, 510–20.

Tienari, P. (1975). Scizophrenia in Finnish male twins. *Acta Psychiatrica Scandinavica*, **39**, (5.171), 1–195.

Torrey, E. F. (1987). Prevalence studies of schizophrenia. *British Journal of Psychiatry*, **150**, 598–608.

Torrey, E. F., McGuire, M., O'Hare, A., Walsh, D. & Spellman, M. P. (1984). Endemic psychosis in Western Ireland. *American Journal of Psychiatry*, **141**, 966–9.

Tramer, M. (1929). Uber die biologische Bedeutung des Geburtsmonats insbesondere für die Psychosenerkrankung Schweizer. *Archiv für Neurologie, Neurochirurgie und Psychiatrie*, **24**, 17–24.

Utsinger, P. D., Zvaifler, N. J. & Ehrlich, G. E. (eds) (1985). *Rheumatoid Arthritis*.

Philadelphia: J. B. Lippincott.

Vallada, H. P., Collier, D., Sham, P. C., et al. (1995). Linkage studies on chromosome 22 in familial schizophrenia. *American Journal of Medical Genetics*, **60**, 139–46.

Vogler, G. P., Gottesman, I. I., McGue, M. K. & Rao, D. C. (1990). Mixed model analysis of schizophrenia in the Lindelius Swedish pedigrees. *Behavioural Genetics*, **20**, 461–72.

Weinberger, D. R. (1995). From neuropathology to neurodevelopment. *Lancet*, **346**, 552–7.

Wessely, S., Castle, D., Der, G. & Murray, R. (1991). Schizophrenia in Afro-Caribbeans: a case-control study. *British Journal of Psychiatry*, **139**, 795–801.

World Health Organization (1973). *Report of the International Pilot Study of Schizophrenia.* **Vol. I**. Geneva: WHO.

World Health Organization (1979). *Schizophrenia. An International Follow-up Study.* Chichester: Wiley.

Wing, J. K., Cooper, J. E. & Sartorius, N. (1974). *The Description and Classification of Psychiatric Symptoms.* An instruction manual for the PSE and Catego systems. Cambridge: Cambridge University Press.

8

Service provision: the clinical perspective

Introduction

The provision of services for those suffering from schizophrenia is problematic. In part, this reflects our limited understanding of the disorder. While we have learned much about the central nervous system in schizophrenia and advances have been made in the social and pharmacological approaches to patient management, the pathogenesis of the illness remains unknown and the factors which determine treatment response are unclear. For any one individual, prediction of the course of the illness is uncertain. It is not easy to estimate the degree of impairment in functioning which a given patient will experience or when an end-state will be reached. (Johnstone & Lang, 1994).

Not all people with schizophrenia demonstrate the progressive deterioration which Kraepelin (1896) originally considered was intrinsic to the condition but many have persistent and severe psychosocial and vocational disabilities. This is illustrated by a large number of follow up studies carried out in the UK.

In a study of over 500 discharged schizophrenic patients Johnstone found that in the previous month 14% had not been in a shop, even to buy a newspaper or cigarettes, 44% had not been in any place of entertainment or social interaction, and that in an area where unemployment rates for the general population did not reach 5%, only 28% were in paid employment (Johnstone, 1991). These findings were mirrored in the results of a more recent study of 193 schizophrenic patients in Edinburgh, where 13% had not been on public transport in the past month, 25% had not had anyone visit them and only 6% were in paid work (Lang et al., 1997a).

Disturbing as these statistics may be, in themselves they cannot convey the distress of the sufferers. The young patient who fails to graduate and who must watch from the sidelines as their peers establish themselves in a career, marry and have children is a scenario all too familiar to those working with schizophrenic patients. The disappointment and indeed despair of the patients is often shared by their families. Both must try to come to terms with what the diagnosis and the limitations of current treatments will mean for the patient. In addition the family, as carers, may have to face considerable changes in their day to day lifestyles, and accept the loss of their own plans for the future. They are also faced with unending concern about the long term welfare of the sufferer.

From a clinical perspective, the problems which face those charged with responsibility for service planning and the provision of care do not appear to have changed much in the last 20 years and indeed are probably little different from the problems faced throughout this century. Now, as in the past, the variable, complex and changing nature of patients' needs poses many challenges for patient care.

Over the last 20–30 years in the UK the USA and indeed much of the Western World there has been a move away from the idea that patients with serious mental illnesses should be cared for in institutions. Care in the community has become the favoured policy and the move towards this pattern of care has intensified over the past 10 years. The move away from inpatient management has increased the challenges of delivery of care and currently, there are many uncertainties concerning appropriate planning and provision of services. The nature of suitable provision for patients (especially the young and those with co-morbid drug and alcohol dependency) who are reluctant to engage with community services is unclear and it may not be realistically possible to provide long term care in the community for the most severely affected patients.

Against this background major reforms in the delivery of health care have taken place in many countries, over the last 10 years. As far as mental health services are concerned it is relatively easy to describe these in the context of the United Kingdom where essentially there is a monopoly service provided by the National Health Service. Although of course, private care does exist in the UK it is used very little for serious mental disorders such as schizophrenia and there is very little statutory variation in services throughout the country. This is very different from the situation in the United States where provision of care and legislation vary from state to state.

In recent years there has been a dramatic increase in the amount of health service based research which has been undertaken, but the incorporation of research evidence into day to day clinical practice is another matter. In our own recent study in Scotland we found that the care which similarly affected patients were receiving differed greatly; many patients were still being cared for predominately in hospital, others had very little contact with services of any kind and only a minority had access to a comprehensive and co-ordinated range of services which were community based (Lang et al., 1997a).

This diversity in patients' care arrangements may to some extent at least reflect differing levels of needs and be associated with satisfactory outcomes for patients, but this is by no means certain as treatment plans had been made without objective evaluation of patients' needs or outcomes of care.

Although a number of different approaches to service provision has been advocated over the past 300 years, the history of service delivery is one of circular change. A policy of community care was first adopted in the seventeenth century, then rejected as institutional based care came to be viewed as the optimal way of addressing patients' needs and now once again, some 300 years later, community based care has found favour; the majority of the old asylums have been closed and the number of inpatient beds is steadily declining. There are therefore very few, if any, ideas on the care of the mentally ill which have not been round at least once before (Allderidge, 1979).

Unfortunately, however, as each approach has fallen into disrepute there has been a tendency to assume that any change will be for the better (Bennett & Freeman, 1991) and little interest has been shown in clarifying the reasons why difficulties have arisen. Lessons have therefore not been learned from the mistakes of the past and although each 'new' approach has been greeted with much enthusiasm and expressions of certainty that it will offer the definitive solution to patient care, in most instances such optimism has quickly been shown to have been misplaced.

Regardless of the particular approach which has been adopted at any one time, it is possible to identify certain constant factors which have had a major influence on service provision, and which continue to contribute to the difficulties that are presently experienced in effectively caring for those who suffer from schizophrenia.

Arguably, the most important of these has been the segregation of the care of the mentally ill from the rest of the medical services and from those providing for social care. The voluntary hospitals of the early nineteenth century, if they were prepared to accept the mentally ill at all, housed them in a separated ward or annexe (Mayou, 1989) and with the building of the asylums this geographical separation from mainstream medicine was further extended. Today, despite the increasing emphasis on the integration of services, the majority of hospital beds for those with severe mental illness are still not to be found in the general hospital setting and mental health continues to be afforded a lesser status than the acute specialties and to attract a smaller percentage of any available resources (Bosanquet, 1986). As attempts have been made to expand the provision of care in the community the separate nature of the health and social services has become increasingly apparent and the major differences that currently exist in the administrative, planning and financial frameworks within which each service operates have served to hinder joint planning and financing initiatives.

The important role played by public opinion in determining service provision is not always acknowledged and yet since the time of Bedlam the public have been interested in the mentally ill, and their views and values have been of major importance in shaping the delivery of care. It was public concern about the neglect and mistreatment of the mentally ill which led to the establishment of the asylums in the early nineteenth century and it was the same concerns 150 years later which initiated the policy that was to lead to their closure.

Today's public, while no less 'alarm minded and action oriented' than previous generations is (Jones, 1972), however, better informed, thanks to a media who report almost daily on some aspect of mental illness (Barnes & Earnshaw, 1993; Scott, 1994). Scott, in her review of the articles on psychiatry reported in six national daily papers and their associated UK Sunday papers over a period of three consecutive months, found that the median prevalence of articles per newspaper per month was nineteen. The articles emphasized forensic issues and frequently promoted the view that dangerousness is synonymous with mental illness. The tone and attitude of the articles describing psychiatrists and individuals with mental health problems were predominately negative. This applied to both the tabloid and broadsheet press. Articles concerning patients with schizophrenia tended to focus on violent acts. These articles and their sensational headlines portraying those with schizophrenia as a 'possessed patient...' (*The Sun*, 7 March, 1996) a 'disturbed killer...' (*Independent*, 2 February, 1996) have understandably caused considerable distress to patients and carers alike. They have also served to heighten public concern that the Government's community care policies are 'failing' the mentally ill and placing the public at risk. As a result, service provision for patients with schizophrenia continues to be the subject of much public debate and in some areas of the UK, such has been the intensity of the media interest in the crimes of violence committed by those suffering from schizophrenia, that it has been likened to a 'campaign of fear' (*Daily Telegraph*, 2 June, 1997) which has been shown to have hindered the development of local community based services.

In seeking to evaluate developments in service provision, it is thus important to acknowledge that 'no system of care can be understood except in relation to the underlying social and political structures of the society it serves' (Wing, 1979). In retrospect, however, it is often difficult to determine the extent to which such factors may have influenced service reforms. Nonetheless, the changes which have taken place in service provision, as the pendulum of professional, public and political opinion has swung to and fro between community and institutional care cannot be shown to have been based on any clear rationale. It would appear that changes in the approaches to service provision have developed more in response to concerns that what was provided would be morally and ethically acceptable to the society of the day, than to whether it would work in practice or offer any real advantage in clinical terms, over what had gone before.

With the increasing emphasis on the practice of evidence based medicine, this position becomes ever more difficult to defend and it is important that we are able to demonstrate the efficacy and cost-effectiveness of any given approach to patient management. It is to be hoped that with the continuing expansion in health service research, we will be able to identify ways in which improvements can be afforded in the care that is available for those suffering from schizophrenia. Many patients continue to experience severe levels of disability in a number of aspects of their daily lives and their relatives bear considerable burdens in supporting them (Johnstone, 1991; Lang et al., 1997a).

The history of service provision

The present community based approach to service provision, enshrined in the legislative framework of the 1990 NHS and Community Care Act (House of Commons, 1990), is not of course a new solution to the old problems. A policy of community care was first advocated in the seventeenth century, when the Poor Law of 1601 charged each parish with responsibility for maintaining those in the local community who were unable to look after themselves. During the eighteenth century, it became apparent that the 'care' thus provided was often harsh and inadequate and as is the case today, these early 'failures' of community care aroused much

Table 8.1. *The size of mental hospital (county asylums) 1827–1930*

1 Jan. Year	No. of county borough and city asylums	Total patients in public asylums	Average number of patients per asylum
1827	9	1046	116
1850	24	7140	297
1860	41	15 845	386
1870	50	27 109	542
1880	61	40 088	657
1890	66	52 937	802
1900	77	74 004	961
1910	91	97 580	1072
1920	94	93 648 (104 298)	996 (1109)
1930	98	119 659	1221

Note: Source: Annual Reports of the Lunacy Commissioners before 1913, Board of Control after 1913.

public concern. Thus the view developed that the provision of institutional care would afford an improvement in the treatment of the mentally ill and with the growth of the humanitarian movement came the establishment of hospitals for the insane and support for the Moral Treatment pioneered by William Tuke (Digby, 1985). The era of the public asylums began with the passing of the Asylum Act in 1808. However, it was soon realized that the scale of provision required had been seriously under-estimated. The size of the population was increasing and the majority of those admitted to the asylums were severely unwell and their condition apparently incurable. As a result, overcrowding became commonplace, the asylums thus took on a largely custodial function and the problems associated with institutionalization added to the significant degree of impairment already experienced by many patients. Although the deficiencies in institutional care were acknowledged in public expressions of concern as early as 1813 (Jones, 1972), the asylums continued to expand in number throughout the nineteenth century (see Table 8.1). It was not until the end of the First World War that significant developments took place in the provision of outpatient based services and there was renewed interest in the treatment of psychiatric disorders outside the mental hospital setting.

During the 1930s, there was a steady expansion in such services and in the provision of psychiatric treatment within general hospitals, developments which in part reflected the more liberal and enlightened approach to patient management made possible by the legislative changes embodied in the Mental Treatment Act of 1930 (Unsworth, 1987).

Despite such developments, the majority of patients with schizophrenia continued to be cared for in an institutional setting and the results of a national survey, conducted at the time of the outbreak of the Second World War, clearly highlighted the fact that deficiencies still existed in mental health service provision (Blacker, 1946). Most mental hospitals continued to have more than a thousand inpatients and only one in four hospitals had a psychiatric social worker. When the National Health Service came into operation, however, service provision remained below the optimum level which the Blacker Report had outlined (Blacker, 1946) and little progress was made towards actively tackling the deficiencies in the care provided within the asylums until the early 1950s, when the so called three 'revolutions': pharmacological (see Chapter 1), administrative and legislative, (Jones, 1972) paved the way for fundamental changes in service provision and the development of community based alternatives to the care provided in these 'really hopeless buildings' (Robinson, 1954).

The introduction of chlorpromazine into routine clinical practice, therefore, while it cannot be said to have been solely responsible for the decline in the number of inpatients (which was first noted in the 1950s) can at least be credited with having facilitated the changes, which were already taking place in clinicians' and society's attitudes, to service provision, as admissions became shorter in duration, and there was a renewed interest in treating patients at home, without recourse to admission to hospital. The administrative changes which took place reflected the growing awareness of the value of a medicosocial approach to patient care, as outlined in the 1953 report of The World Health Organisation (WHO, 1953). New forms of service provision, day hospitals, industrial therapy, and hostels, began to be developed and attempts were made to explore more flexible ways of delivering care, in which inpatient treatment no longer had a dominant role to play. These developments in service provision were facilitated by the legislative changes outlined in the Mental Health Act of 1959 which removed the remaining legal barriers to the implementation of a more community orientated approach to patient care.

Thus it was, that throughout the 1960s, continued attempts were made to increase the provision of community based facilities. It was recognized that there was a need to integrate such developments with the existing hospital provision. Nonetheless there was still considerable public and professional uncertainty as to what benefits, if any, patients were deriving from the care provided in the mental hospitals. This was fuelled by a growing awareness of the negative effects of institutional life (Goffman, 1962; Barton, 1959) and reports of mistreatment in the asylums (DHSS, 1969).

From a political perspective, however, the future direction for the mental health services appeared to be quite clear cut and the two thousand delegates who gathered at the Annual Conference of the National Association for Mental Health in Britain in 1961 to hear the inaugural speech of the then Minister of Health, the Right Honourable Enoch Powell, were left in no doubt as to Government policy; there was to be '... nothing less than the total elimination of by far the greater part of this country's mental hospitals'. No longer were patients to receive hospital treatment in the '... great isolated insitutions...' which stood '... isolated, majestic, imperious...' '... brooded over by the gigantic water tower and chimney combined...' but in wards or wings of general hospitals (Powell, 1961).

There were, however, considerable concerns about the statistical projections upon which the British Government's predictions of the future requirements for hospital beds had been calculated (Tooth & Brooke, 1961) and that the policy to move away from institutional care had been '... based on assumptions none of which were empirically tested' (Jones, 1981). The crisis in institutional care and the establishment of the welfare state had led to a belief that for most if not all patients, care could be provided in the community and that such care would represent an improvement on that currently provided. No clear understanding, however, had emerged as to what should take the place of the asylums and the Hospital Plan (Ministry of Health, 1962) did not give details of the costs which would be incurred in implementing the changes in service provision nor did it outline how such developments were to be funded and organized (Freeman, 1983). There was also little evidence to support the widely expressed view at the time, that the public now had a more enlightened attitude towards the mentally ill (Ministry of Health, 1958; Scull, 1984) and such a change in public opinion would be necessary if the new services were to be successfully implemented.

The move away from institutional based care, however, had begun but it was not until 1971 that community care was embodied in national policy (DHSS, 1971) and that the essential elements of a comprehensive and integrated hospital and community service were formally outlined. Unfortunately, it quickly became apparent that what was being proposed failed to acknowledge the clinical reality that the majority of patients suffering from severe mental illnesses such as schizophrenia would require support in the longer term and by the time that *Better Services for the Mentally Ill* (DHSS, 1975) was published, only four years later, it was very evident that policy makers had adopted 'a blithely over optimistic attitude' (House of Commons, 1985) in planning on the basis of there being a dramatic reduction in the need for long term care.

In the years that have followed, however, although the flawed assumptions which underpinned these initial policy statements have become ever more apparent, mental hospitals have continued to close in Britain, the United States and Europe, as Governments, regardless of their political persuasion, have wholeheartedly embraced the concept of community based care for the mentally ill. Many have argued that this is largely the result of economic pressures.

In Britain, the developments in community services have taken place against a background of seemingly continuous change in the organization and management of the National Health Service and the Social Services. In practice, if the intention was that a comprehensive and coordinated community based approach to patient care should be developed, such changes have only added to the complexity of the problems to be overcome. The organizational changes have largely failed to address the fundamental issues which have led to the present deficiencies in service provision.

Reorganization of the social services has led to the dissolution of mental health teams (Jones, 1979) and thus the changes have had a detrimental effect on patient care. Not surprisingly, perhaps, it has been those individuals suffering from chronic illnesses such as schizophrenia, where the need for a joint social work and medical approach to their care is greatest, who have been most disadvantaged.

It was partly in an attempt to address such difficulties in coordinating care and to focus the service on the severely mentally ill that the NHS and Community Care Act was introduced in 1990 (House of Common, 1990). This Act gave a statutory basis to the measures which had previously been outlined in two white papers; *Working for Patients* (Dept. of Health 1989a) and *Caring for People* (Dept. of Health 1989b).

The first of these white papers, *Working for Patients*, outlined the legislative framework for the establishment of hospital Trusts and for fundholding in general practice. In so doing, it paved the way for what has been the most fundamental reorganization of the National Health Service since its inception in 1948. In the second white paper, *Caring for People*, guidelines were laid down for the restructuring of community based services in the 1990s; local social services and health authorities were now required to agree community care plans jointly and to ensure that, at a local level, needs based care plans were being developed for those patients with severe and enduring mental illness.

While it was envisaged that the changes which were being proposed would afford an improvement in patient care, it was financial considerations which had been of paramount importance in influencing the drafting of this legislation. The growing demand for services and the escalation in the costs of care had led to an increase in public expenditure and it had become imperative, in a climate of economic constraint, that changes were made which would allow the service to operate more efficiently.

The chosen solution was the creation of an internal market, based on the principles of managed competition. This was made possible by separating the role of purchaser of care from that of provider, and these arrangements have indeed served to focus the service on cost containment. The community care section of the Act (which was not implemented until 1993) has however not led to developments in joint approaches to patient care.

In part, the failure of the new legislation to deliver improvements in care reflects the lack of adequate preparation given to planning and investment before the changes in practice were implemented. Dialogue between purchasers and providers has been limited. Insufficient bridging funds have been made available to allow the appropriate community facilities to be developed before hospital based services have been run down and the resources that have been provided have not been ringfenced (Audit Commission, 1986). At present, therefore, while the development of community based services remains the central tenet of government policy, community care programmes still lack coherence and clear objectives and there continue to be deficiencies in service provision. Some of the difficulties which have arisen in providing adequate care for patients with schizophrenia have attracted media attention and have caused both the public and profession alike to question whether it is feasible or even desirable to care for the severely mentally ill in the community. Doubts have been expressed as to whether it will be possible to implement properly community developments within the present circumstances and foreseeable socio-economic constraints.

Developing a community based service

Attempts to develop services in the community for patients with schizophrenia, must take into account the fact that the illness may have a very variable course and that for many patients the outcome will be disappointing. Eighty per cent of patients can expect to have periods of relapse and remission. Over 50% will demonstrate an increasing degree of impairment with each successive episode and will thus not return to their premorbid level of social functioning (Shepherd et al., 1989). Most patients, therefore, will have complex and varied health and social care needs and while these may change over time, many patients will experience considerable difficulty in maintaining an independent lifestyle.

Essential features of successful community care include: availability of appropriate medical and nursing care, both at times of crisis and on a consistent long-term basis. In addition, care must be able to provide suitable accommodation, day time and recreational activities, and assistance in undertaking everyday tasks of daily living. However, this spectrum of care is not easy to provide.

Much research has been undertaken in an attempt to clarify how best such a spectrum of care can be developed. There have been many innovations in service provision which have sought to provide an alternative to hospital based treatment. Acutely unwell patients have been managed in a day hospital setting, the duration of hospital admission has been shortened, and care has been provided to patients, at home, at times of crisis and relapse. The features of schizophrenia in themselves may impair the ability of the patient to seek appropriate support and therefore care which is provided solely on the basis of demand will not necessarily guarantee that patients are adequately and appropriately managed. In order to address such issues, community teams have been established whereby an 'assertive' approach to patient management can be provided.

The most widely studied model of such an approach to community treatment and one which has consistently been shown to be of benefit to patients and relatives is the comprehensive programme of community care which was pioneered in the United States by Stein and Test (Stein & Test, 1980) and which has since been successfully replicated in many other countries including Canada, Australia and the United Kingdom. (Fenton et al., 1979; Hoult & Reynolds, 1993; Marks et al., 1994). This model of care is based on a multidisciplinary team which operates 24 hours per day, seven days per week, has close links with primary care and other community services, has direct control over hospital admission and discharge and actively seeks to involve both the patient and their informal carers in treatment. In managing patients, staff adopt an 'assertive' approach and a case management model is used whereby the individual members of the team have total responsibility for providing patients with basic health care, social support and assistance with everyday tasks of daily living.

This style of management aims to provide patients with a flexible, yet cohesive package of care designed for their individual needs. The intention is that crises will be pre-empted, hospital admissions reduced and continuity of care will be provided to ensure that patients are not lost to follow-up.

Several studies have now shown that such community based alternatives to hospital care can afford as good and in some cases a better outcome for patients (Braun et al., 1981; Cambridge & Knapp, 1988; Burns & Santos,

1995), and may reduce their need for inpatient treatment (Stein & Test, 1980; Muijen et al., 1992; Burns et al., 1993; Marks et al., 1994). Patients and their relatives prefer the care that is provided outside of a hospital environment (Johnstone, 1991; Marks, 1992; Anderson et al., 1993). It is important to acknowledge, however, the limitations of existing research. Studies of new approaches to treatment are not usually conducted on unselected clinical populations. Some patients, usually those who would be considered to be the more difficult to manage, rarely take part in research studies. The resources that are provided to fund innovative projects often far exceed those that are available in routine clinical practice and the staff who take part in such projects are specially chosen and thus highly motivated.

The limited efficacy of available treatments means that the majority of patients will remain significantly disabled by their illness. Their level of functioning is likely to deteriorate if care is not provided over an extended period of time (Test, 1990; Audini et al., 1994; Marks, 1995). For the successful outcome of community based alternatives to inpatient care to be maintained it would be necessary for the staff to have a considerable amount of direct patient contact over a sustained period of time. Such continuous support can only be provided if there is a high staff to patient ratio and if staff are committed to working with patients. The excitement of a research project is very different from ongoing routine care and in practice sustained care of this kind has not been easy to provide (Dedman, 1993; Connolly et al., 1996; Prosser et al., (1996).

The services required to ensure that the many and varied needs of this patient group can be met have not been easy to develop. To date, community developments have failed to keep pace with hospital closures (Audit Commission, 1986). At present, as has been evident from the inquiry reports which have been published on the 26 homicides and other serious untoward incidents involving people with serious mental illness which have taken place between 1988 and 1996, for the majority of patients the provision of a comprehensive service and seamless approach to the delivery of care is an ideal as yet to be realized (Coid, 1994a,b; Ritchie, 1994). There are a number of major and seemingly intractable problems facing the mental health services and the majority of patients are not in receipt of a programme of care which is based on their individual needs, delivered in a continuous and organized manner. The present deficiencies in service provision have been most keenly felt in the inner city areas, where it has proved especially difficult to develop adequate community services, and where a significant percentage of patients are either out of contact with the specialist teams or make little use of the services which are available

(Johnson et al., 1997; McCreadie et al., 1997). In their study of patients in London, McCreadie et al. found that only 13–39% were attending a day hospital and that a minority, 19–35%, were receiving support from a community psychiatric nurse. In a similar study of service provision for patients, only 24% of patients reported having seen a social worker in the previous six months (Lang et al., 1997a).

Current UK policy is that social workers have a central role in the organization and coordination of services for patients with schizophrenia and thus this lack of social work involvement in patient care is a cause for concern. It would seem that following the reorganization of the social services, social work with the mentally ill does not have a high priority. Consequently, there has been a deterioration in the service which social workers are able to provide for patients with mental illness and especially for those patients who are the most seriously unwell.

In part, the expansion which has taken place in the community psychiatric nursing service was an attempt to counteract this 'vacuum created by the genericism of the social worker' (House of Commons, 1985). There are still, however, relatively few nurses working in the community, in London there is only an estimated 0.02 per 1000 of the population (McCreadie et al., 1997). Just over half of the patients on an average Community Psychiatric Nurse's caseload have a diagnosis of schizophrenia (Wooff et al., 1988) and the contact which nursing staff have with these patients is usually brief, 10 minutes or less, and is mainly focused on the administration of depot medication (Wooff et al., 1988).

These findings may reflect Community Psychiatric Nurses' preference for working with other patient groups. Primary care physicians are able to refer directly to these nurses and the majority of their patients present with minor psychiatric morbidity (White, 1991). Greater emphasis is now being placed in the UK on the purchasing of services by general practitioners and they have increasing influence in shaping service contracts (NHS Executive, 1994). If we are to be able to provide an adequate service for patients with schizophrenia, it will be necessary for us to address the issues of the boundaries of the Community Psychiatric Nurse's role and the relationship of their contribution to patient care to that of the other professionals involved in service provision (Tyrer et al., 1990).

Barriers to the development of community services

The body of research evidence supporting the view that it is possible to care effectively for patients in the community allows the argument that the present deficiencies in service provision reflect our failure to apply what we already know, rather than a lack of understanding of the elements of an appropriate community service. The planning and implementation of community services, have been hindered by a number of factors: the change from hospital care to a community based service has not been evidence based but has been politically driven, the time scales for implementing the changes in service provision have been very short and the resources provided have been limited.

It has been difficult to generate commitment from staff, in both the health and social services, to a shared approach to patient care. As yet, however, at both a national and local level scant attention has been paid to barriers and tensions which presently exist between the health and social services and between staff working in primary and secondary care settings. The different aims and objectives of the staff, the competing demands on their time and on the resources available within each service have not been formally assessed nor have attempts been made to constructively address such issues. Little real progress has thus been made towards the establishment of joint working practices and as yet no clear understanding has emerged as to how the present divide between the primary care and specialist services and between health and social care can best be bridged (Warden, 1997).

There are substantial problems in persuading some patients, especially the young, to accept the services offered (Johnson et al., 1997). Such patients may be acutely disturbed, lack motivation and insight into their condition and in spite of a very assertive approach to their care may be retained in contact with services only with great difficulty.

Attention must also therefore be paid to the nature of the care that is available and to the accessibility of the services; if patients do not view the care that is available as acceptable and relevant to their needs and if they cannot easily access services then they are unlikely to have confidence in the care that is being offered and may thus have little motivation to engage in treatment. Such problems have perhaps been most clearly demonstrated in the studies concerning services provided for patients from the ethnic minorities, where research has clearly shown that at present the services which are available do not adequately address the concerns of these communities, are often not acceptable to them and that consequently considerable difficulties have been encountered in engaging members of these groups in treatment and in ensuring that they receive adequate care (Johnson et al., 1997).

While the aim of a community based service is to provide care as close as possible to a patient's own home, there will continue to be a percentage of patients who will require to be admitted to hospital, albeit in some cases for a shorter period of time than without the intensive support that community services may offer (Tantum, 1985). At present patients with schizophrenia are continuing to make significant use of inpatient facilities (Lang et al., 1997a). The provision of such care remains a priority in service planning but it has not been easy to establish the number of beds that will ultimately be required, nor is it entirely clear why some patients have proved so difficult to manage in the community (Hirsch, 1988; Watson, 1994; Thornicroft & Strathdee, 1994). Given the current 'bed crisis' (Lelliot et al., 1995) in acute psychiatric units, the importance of clarification of these issues is obvious.

Hospital or community – a false dichotomy

In our enthusiasm to develop community services, therefore, it is important that we do not lose sight of the fact that hospital care must remain an integral part of any service, complementary to the care that is available in the community and not an alternative to it (Lawrence et al., 1991; Bennett & Freeman, 1991). The provision of inpatient care in the UK, however, has been afforded low priority in recent service planning. Relatively little interest has been shown in clarifying the factors which determine bed use and although several studies have demonstrated that it is possible to effectively provide continuous nursing care outside of a ward setting (Wykes, 1982; Goldberg et al., 1985; Hyde et al., 1987; Trieman & Leff, 1996) there have been few attempts to develop such services.

The national UK survey of acute bed usage which has recently been conducted is thus a welcome addition to the literature (Shepherd et al., 1997). This work confirms the findings of previous studies (Mann & Cree, 1976; Bewley et al., 1981; McCreadie et al., 1983), to the effect that acute units have accumulated a number of long stay patients. The results of Shepherd et al. (1997) indicate, however, that no one subgroup of patients is responsible for the current lack of acute beds and that correspondingly there is no single solution to the problem. Some patients do indeed need care in the longer term, but in only a minority of cases do they need to receive such care in a hospital setting. Many patients could be managed in the community if appropriate accommodation were available and if they had access to additional sources of support. Thus despite the calls that there have been for more acute beds (Watson, 1994; Hollander & Slater, 1994) and an end to bed closures (National Schizophrenia Fellowship,

1994), it appears that providing more inpatient beds will not solve the present problems in service provision. Additional services will be required in the community and there is a particular need to develop more specialist accommodation for the most severely disabled patients which is not short term.

The role of the general practitioner (primary care physician)

Although patients with schizophrenia represent less than 5% of all those who attend with psychiatric symptoms in general practice (Goldberg, 1979), it has long been recognized that they place considerable demands on the primary care team (Parkes et al., 1962). Over the past 30 years, as the number of hospital beds has steadily declined, the number of patients who now live in the community and are in regular contact with their general practitioner has increased (Lang et al., 1997b) and the nature of these demands has thus changed considerably (Kendrick et al., 1991).

The developments in community care policies have therefore had important implications for primary care physicians (Kendell, 1989), many of whom have limited experience of caring for the mentally ill, feel ill prepared to treat such patients and may be reluctant to become more actively involved in their management. Currently there is considerable debate amongst clinicians working in both the primary and secondary care services as to what role, if any, primary care physician should have in managing patients with severe and enduring mental illness. Although the majority of doctors consider that joint working with the psychiatric services is the most desirable way of caring for such patients (Kendrick et al., 1991) there is still no consensus as to the form which such collaboration should take (Mitchell, 1985).

Resolution of this issue will require adequate information on the reasons why schizophrenic patients contact their local surgery, what benefit they think they are deriving from such contact and how the care provided in primary care relates to that provided by the specialist services. In practice it has proved very difficult to obtain such data. Few general practices have adopted a standardized method for assessing patients or for documenting their contacts with primary care (Lang et al., 1997b). Research findings have therefore largely been based on discussions with physicians and patients. It is not easy to determine the validity or reliability of such information.

Consequently, we still know relatively little of the way in which schizophrenia is managed in primary care (Nazereth et al., 1993) and individual roles and responsibilities remain unclear. It is thus not surprising that despite the widening interface between the primary and secondary care services, it has proved difficult to develop collaborative approaches to patient management. It is still the exception, rather than the rule, that in caring for patients with schizophrenia, psychiatrists and primary care physicians are working together in a structured and coordinated way and that the services provided are appropriately integrated.

Patients therefore continue to experience considerable difficulties in moving from one service and care setting to another, as their needs dictate. Some patients are still lost to follow up. Where such cases have come to media attention there has been much criticism of community care policies and considerable public concern that the move away from institutional based care has created a situation of community neglect.

In the absence of clear and agreed policies for the development of shared models of care, any attempts that have been made to facilitate joint working practices have progressed in a rather ad hoc fashion. A number of different approaches has been advocated. Those based on a liaison– attachment model of service provision (Williams & Clare, 1981), whereby a psychiatrist regularly visits the practice to see patients, discuss issues of mutual interest and provide an educational input to practice meetings, have proved to be the most viable (Creed & Marks, 1989; Tyrer et al., 1990). In recent years, this model has gained increasing acceptance (Pullen & Yellowlees, 1988; Kendrick et al., 1991, Strathdee & Williams, 1984) and over 20% of psychiatrists in the UK now have such direct links with general practice (Strathdee & Williams, 1984).

Many general practitioners welcome this opportunity for closer liaison with their specialist colleagues. It has been shown that for some patients this model of service provision has led to a reduction in the amount of time they are required to spend in hospital (Williams & Balestrieri, 1989; Tyrer et al., 1984). In the case of patients with schizophrenia, provision of an outpatient service within the local surgery setting provides a basis for collaborative working and may directly benefit patients if it enables them to more readily access specialist help. By this means it may increase the likelihood that patients will remain in contact with the services in the longer term.

It was hoped that the recent legislative changes regarding patient discharge and the introduction of the Care Programme Approach (Dept. of Health, 1990) would facilitate joint working between the primary and secondary services and might thus address the criticisms that have been levied against the present community care policies. As has been the case with previous government directives regarding the care of those with severe mental illness, general practitioners are seen as having a central role to play in the successful implementation of these reforms and it has been assumed that they will be willing to share the responsibility which the specialist services now have to target services at the severely mentally ill.

In day to day practice, however, there is very little evidence to suggest that this is the case and it is becoming increasingly apparent that the majority of doctors have a very different perspective on resource allocation from that of their psychiatric colleagues. They have had limited involvement in the planning of the recent reforms (Grace et al., 1996), they know relatively little about them and many consider that they are remote and theoretical (Robinson, 1993). It is also the case, however, that many general practitioners are aware of the assumptions which underpin the proposed changes in patient management but are reluctant to take on additional responsibility for patients with severe mental illness. They do not wish to devote resources, which they consider could be more efficiently and cost-effectively deployed elsewhere, to providing services for such a small group of individuals who previously and many consider more appropriately were cared for by the specialist services.

With the continuing emphasis on the establishment of a primary care led National Health Service, such financial considerations are likely to become of increasing importance in decisions on resource allocation. Implementation of the changes in service provision, necessary to allow for the expansion of community based facilities, will not be helped by the fact that the current incentives mitigate against this. Unless ways are found to reconcile these differing perspectives services will become more fragmented (Lelliott & Audini, 1996) and there may be greater inequalities in access to health care, (Coulter, 1995). Patients with schizophrenia are often the least able to make their voice heard.

Services for relatives

Since the mid 1950s it has been recognized that caring for a relative who is mentally unwell has a significant impact on a family (Clausen & Yarrow, 1955). As attempts have been made to develop alternatives to hospital based care there has been an increased awareness of the role which families now play in supporting their ill relative, especially at times of crisis and relapse. There has therefore been much interest in determining how such changes in service provision have affected relatives and the ways in which family relationships may influence a patient's symptoms and level of functioning.

Many studies have demonstrated that psychosocial interventions can enable a family to cope better with the patient's symptoms (Liberman et al., 1981; Falloon et al., 1982; Leff et al., 1982; Barraclough & Tarrier, 1984), but the burdens which relatives experience in caring for a family member with schizophrenia are often not fully appreciated nor do we understand the degree to which relatives feel able or indeed wish to take on such reponsibility and how services can best be arranged to support them. In part, this reflects the difficulties that have been encountered in conceptualizing and measuring burden (Platt, 1985) and in translating such measurements into an assessment of need which then can be used as a basis for service planning.

Grad & Sainsbury (1963) were among the first to assess relative burden. The results of this and other early studies (Wing et al., 1964; Waters & Northover, 1965; Mandelbrote & Folkard, 1961) highlighted the considerable levels of objective and subjective burden (Hoenig & Hamilton, 1966) which relatives bore and that such burdens had increased with the move away from institutional based care.

While subsequent work has shown that it is possible to reduce the length of hospital admissions without increasing the burden on relatives (Hirsch et al., 1979) and that comprehensive programmes of community care can in fact offer a better means of supporting those caring for a patient (Stein & Test, 1980; Dean et al., 1993), many relatives continue to report considerable levels of difficulty. In particular it is the negative symptoms of the illness – the patient's apathy, lack of motivation and limited conversation which they find most disturbing. The severe restrictions which caring is placing on their own lifestyles and the detrimental effect which it is having on their relationships with other family members (National Schizophrenia Fellowship, 1974) are also distressing for them.

Regardless, however, of such difficulties and distress, few relatives wish the patient to be re-admitted to hospital (Johnstone et al., 1986). In part, this may be because they prefer to care for their relative themselves and that they feel that they should be able to cope on their own. It may also, however, reflect the fact that many relatives do not know what services are, or ideally should be, available. It may be that in the past when they have sought help they have been unsuccessful in obtaining assistance or that they have found that the help that was offered was of little benefit to them (DHSS, 1991).

Many relatives are very tolerant and accepting in their attitude (NSF, 1974), so that the relationship between an objective description of the tasks a relative performs and the relative's feelings about these responsibilities is by no means straightforward (Creer et al., 1982) and relatives may underestimate their difficulties and their need for help.

Developments in community based services mean that many relatives now have a greater degree of direct involvement in patient care. If relatives are to be adequately supported in a caring role, a range of services must be provided for them, so that they may obtain information and advice about the illness and be offered practical assistance and emotional support in managing the patient (Fadden et al., 1987).

Despite the recognition of the need for carefully organized support (Brown, 1985; Mechanic & Aitken, 1987), relatively little has been done to improve the help that is offered to relatives. Thus in terms of the services that are available to them little has changed (Sargeant, 1993). While at a local level there have been innovations in practice (Mullen et al., 1992), in general the response of the health and social services has been meagre (Kreisman & Joy, 1994). It is from the voluntary rather than the statutory agencies that relatives receive most help.

Improvements in the services presently available will only occur if the valuable contribution which relatives are making is recognized and reflected in changes in clinical practice and community care policies (Atkinson & Coia, 1991).

Conclusions

Although policies of hospital closure have been advocated for almost 40 years, providing care in the community for patients with schizophrenia remains problematic; services are still not planned on the basis of need, little progress has been made in developing joint working between the health and social services and the roles and responsibilities of staff in primary and secondary care remain unclear.

For the majority of patients, therefore, the provision of an integrated and coordinated programme of care which is delivered in a flexible but continuous manner is an ideal as yet to be realized. Patients are still making significant use of inpatient facilities and their relatives continue to experience considerable difficulties in supporting them.

While the introduction of measures such as the Care Programme Approach and Supervision Registers may go some way to addressing the present problems in service provision they are unlikely in themselves to afford any real improvement in care and have indeed been criticized as offering no more than a 'bureaucratic solution to what is essentially a problem of inadequate resources' (Holloway, 1994).

Additional funds are certainly needed, but the successful development of community services will not depend on resources and manpower alone. More detailed information is needed on local patient populations and clear policies that prioritize care for chronic mentally ill are required. Ways must be found of increasing the involvement which patients and relatives have in service planning and of reconciling the differing and conflicting perspectives that exist between purchasers and providers and between the health and social services.

Unless these fundamental issues are addressed no number of protocols, checklists or registers will ensure that patients receive a more comprehensive and coordinated approach to their care and as recent tragedies have shown (Ritchie, 1994), there may be a high price to be paid when services fail to meet the needs of patients with schizophrenia.

References

Allderidge, P. (1979). *Hospitals, Madhouses and Asylums: A History of the York Retreat*. Cambridge: Cambridge University Press.

Anderson, J., Dayson, D., Wills, W., et al. (1993). The Taps Project. 13: Clinical and social outcomes of long-stay psychiatric patients after one year in the community. *British Journal of Psychiatry*, **162, (Suppl 19)**, 45–56.

Atkinson, J. M. & Coia, D. A. (1991). Carers, the community and the White Paper. *Psychiatric Bulletin*, **15**, 763–4.

Audini, B., Marks, I. M., Lawrence, R. E., Connolly, J. & Watts, V. (1994). Home-based versus out-patients care for people with serious mental illness. Phase II of a controlled study. *British Journal of Psychiatry*, **165**, 204–10.

Audit Commission. (1986). *Making a Reality of Community Care*. London: HMSO.

Barnes, R. C. & Earnshaw, S. (1993). Mental illness in British newspapers. *Psychiatric Bulletin*, **17**, 673–4.

Barraclough, C. & Tarrier, N. (1984). 'Psychosocial' interventions with families and their effects on the course of schizophrenia: a review. *Psychological Medicine*, **14**, 629–42.

Barton, W. R. (1959). *Institutional Neurosis*. Bristol: Wright.

Bennett, D. H. & Freeman, H. L. (1991). *Community Psychiatry*. London: Churchill Livingstone.

Bewley, T. H., Bland, M., Mechen, D. & Walch, E. (1981). 'New chronic' patients. *British Medical Journal*, **283**, 1161–4.

Blacker, C. P. (1946). *Neurosis and the Mental Health Services*. Oxford: Oxford University Press.

Bosanquet, N. (1986). *Public Expenditure on the NHS: Recent Trends and Outlook*. York: Centre for Health Economics, University of York.

Braun, P., Kochansky, G., Shapiro, R., et al. (1981). Overview: deinstitutionalisation of psychiatric patients, a critical review of outcome studies. *American Journal of Psychiatry*, **136**, 736–49.

Brown, P. (1985). *The Transfer of Care: Psychiatric Deinstitutionalisation and its Aftermath*. London: Routledge and Kegan Paul.

Burns, B. J. & Santos, A. B. (1995). Assertive community treatment: an update of randomised controlled trials. *Psychiatric Services*, **46**, 669–75.

Burns, T., Raffery, J., Beadsmoore, A., McGuigan, S. & Dickson, M. (1993). A controlled trial of home-based acute psychiatric services II: Treatment patterns and costs. *British Journal of Psychiatry*, **163**, 55–61.

Cambridge, P. & Knapp, M. (1988). *Demonstrating Successful Care in the Community*. Canterbury PSSU: University of Canterbury.

Clausen, J. A. & Yarrow, M. R. (1955). The impact of mental illness on the family. *Journal of Social Issues*, **11**, 3–14.

Coid, J. W. (1994a). 'The Christopher Clunis enquiry'. *Psychiatric Bulletin*, **18**, 449–52.

Coid, J. W. (1994b). Failure in community care: psychiatrists' dilemma. *British Medical Journal*, **308**, 805–6.

Connolly, J., Marks, I., Lawrence, R., et al. (1996). Observations from community care for serious mental illness during a controlled study. *Psychiatric Bulletin*, **20**, 3–7.

Coulter, A. (1995). General Practice Fundholding: time for a cool appraisal. *British Journal of General Practice*, **45**, 119–20.

Creed, F. & Marks, B. (1989). Liaison psychiatry in general practice: a comparison of a liaison attachment scheme and the shifted outpatient model. *Journal of the Royal College of General Practitioners*, **39**, 514–17.

Creer, C., Sturt, E. & Wykes, T. (1982). *The Role of Relatives in Long-term Community Care: Experience in a London Borough*, ed. J. K. Wing. Cambridge: Cambridge University Press.

Daily Telegraph (1997). *Mentally Ill Patients Face 'Campaign of Fear'*. 2nd June, p. 8.

Dean, C., Phillips, J., Gadd, E. M., Joseph, M. & England, S. (1993). Comparison of community based service with hospital based service for people with acute, severe psychiatric illness. *British Medical Journal*, **307**, 437–76.

Dedman, P. (1993). Home treatment for acute psychiatric disorder. *British Medical Journal*, **306**, 1359–60.

Department of Health and Social Services (1969). *Report of the Committee of Inquiry into Allegations of Ill Treatment of Patients and other Irregularities at the Ely Hospital Cardiff*. Cmnd 3975. London: HMSO.

Department of Health and Social Services (1971). *Hospital Services for the Mentally Ill*. London: HMSO.

Department of Health and Social Security (1975). *Better Services for the Mentally Ill*. Cmnd 6233. London: HMSO.

Department of Health (1989a). *Working for Patients*. London: HMSO.

Department of Health (1989b). *Caring for People*. London: HMSO.

Department of Health (1990). *Caring for People. The Care Programme Approach for People with a Mental Illness Referred to the Specialist Psychiatric Services*. HC(90) 23/LASSL(90), **II**, London: HMSO.

Department of Health and Social Services (1991). *Carer Support in the Community*. London: HMSO.

Digby, A. (1985). *Madness, Morality and Medicine: A History of the York Retreat*. Cambridge: Cambridge University Press.

Fadden, G., Bebbington, P. & Kuipers, L. (1987). The burden of care: the impact of functional psychiatric illness on the patient's family. *British Journal of Psychiatry*, **150**, 285–92.

Falloon, I. R. H., Boyd, J. L., McGill, C. W., Razani, J., Moss, H. B. & Golderman, A. M. (1982). Family management in the prevention of exacerbations of schizophrenia. A controlled study. *New England Journal of Medicine*, **306**, 1437–40.

Fenton, F. R., Tessier, L. & Struening, L. L. (1979). A comparative trial of home and hospital psychiatric care. One year follow-up. *Archives of General Psychiatry*, **36**, 1073–9.

Freeman, H. L. (1983). District psychiatric services: psychiatry for defined populations. In *Mental Illness: Changes and Trends*, ed. P. Bean, pp. 351–78. Chichester: John Wiley.

Goffman, E. (1962). *Asylums: Essays on the Social Situation of Mental Patients and Other Inmates*. Doubleday: New York.

Goldberg, D. P. (1979). Detection and assessment of emotional disorders in a primary care setting. *International Journal of Mental Health*, **8**, 30–48.

Goldberg, D. B., Bridges, K., Cooper, W., Hyde, C., Sterling, C. & Wyatt, R. (1985). Douglas House: a new type of hostel ward for chronic psychotic patients. *British Journal of Psychiatry*, **147**, 383–8.

Grace, J., Steels, M. & Baruach, R. (1996). General Practitioners' knowledge of and views on the care programme approach. *Psychiatric Bulletin*, **20**, 643–4.

Grad, J. & Sainsbury, P. (1963). Mental illness and the family. *Lancet*, **1**, 544–7.

Hirsch, S. R. (1988). *Psychiatric Beds and Resources: Factors Influencing Bed Use and Service Planning*. London: Gaskell.

Hirsch, S. R., Platt, S., Knights, A. & Weyman, A. (1979). Shortening hospital stay for psychiatric care: effect on patients and their families. *British Medical Journal*, **1**, 442–6.

Hoenig, J. & Hamilton, M. W. (1966). The schizophrenic patient in the community and his effect on the household. *International Journal of Social Psychiatry*, **12**, 165–76.

Hollander, D. & Slater, M. S. (1994). 'Sorry no beds': a problem for acute psychiatric admissions. *Psychiatric Bulletin*, **18**, 532–4.

Holloway, F. (1994). Supervision registers – recent government policy and legislation. *Psychiatric Bulletin*, **18**, 593–6.

Hoult, J. & Reynolds, I. (1983). *Psychiatric Hospital Versus Community Treatment: A Controlled Study*. Department of Health: New South Wales.

House of Commons. (1985). *Second Report from the Social Services Committee: Community Care*. London: HMSO.

House of Commons. (1990). *The National Health Service and Community Care Act*. London: HMSO.

Hyde, C., Bridges, K., Goldberg, D., Lowson, K., Sterling, C. & Faragher, B. (1987). The evaluation of a hostel ward – a controlled study using modified cost–benefit analysis. *British Journal of Psychiatry*, **151**, 805–12.

Independent. (1996). *Disturbed killer 'too dangerous' for hospital*. 2nd. February.

Johnstone, E. C. (1991). Disabilities and circumstances of schizophrenic patients – a follow-up study. *British Journal of Psychiatry*, **159**, **(Suppl 13)**.

Johnstone, E. C. & Lang, F. H. (1994). The onset, course and outcome in schizophrenia. *Current Opinion in Psychiatry*, **7**, 56–60.

Johnstone, E. C., Owens, D. G. C., Gold, A., Crow, T. J. & Macmillan, J. F. (1986). Schizophrenic patients discharged from hospital: a follow-up study. *British Journal of Psychiatry*, **145**, 586–90.

Johnson, S., Ramsey, R., Thornicroft, G., et al. (1997). *London's Mental Health. The Report for the King's Fund London Commission*. London: King's Fund.

Jones, K. (1972). *A History of the Mental Health Services*. London: Routledge and Kegan Paul.

Jones, K. (1979). In *New Methods of Mental Health Care*, ed. M. Meader. Oxford: Pergamon Press.

Jones, K. (1981). 'Re-inventing The Wheel' in *MIND, The Future of the Mental Hospitals: a report of MIND's 1980 annual conference*. Brighton Marshalles Print Services.

Kendell, R. (1989). The future of Britain's mental hospitals. *British Medical Journal*, **299**, 1237–8.

Kendrick, T., Sibbald, B., Burns, T. & Freely, P. (1991). Role of General Practitioners in care of long-term mentally ill patients. *British Medical Journal*, **302**, 508–10.

Kraepelin, E. (1896). *Psychiatrie: Ein Lehrbuch fur Studievende und Artze 7. Auflage*. Leipzig: JA Barth.

Kreisman, D. E. & Joy, V. D. (1994). Family response to the mental illness of a relative: a review of the literature. *Schizophrenia Bulletin*, **10**, 34–57.

Lang, F. H., Forbes, J. F., Murray, G. D. & Johnstone, E. C. (1997a). Service provision for patients with schizophrenia 1. A clinical and economic perspective. *British Journal of Psychiatry*, **171**, 159–63.

Lang, F. H., Murray, G. D. & Johnstone, E. C. (1997b). Service provision for patients with schizophrenia. 11. The role of the general practitioner. *British Journal of Psychiatry*, **171**, 165–8.

Lawrence, R. E., Copas, J. B. & Cooper, P. W. (1991). Community care: does it reduce the need for psychiatric 'beds'. A comparison of two different styles of service in three hospitals. *British Journal of Psychiatry*, **159**, 334–40.

Leff, J. P., Kuipers, L., BerKowitz, R., Eberlein–Fries, R. & Sturgeon, D. (1982). A controlled trial of social intervention in schizophrenic families. *British Journal of Psychiatry*, **141**, 121–34.

Lelliott, P. & Audini, B. (1996). Fundholding and the care of the mentally ill. *Psychiatric Bulletin*, **20**, 641–2.

Lelliott, P., Audini, B. & Darroch, N. (1995). Resolving London's bed crisis: there might be a way, is there a will? *Psychiatric Bulletin*, **19**, 273–5.

Liberman, R. P., Wallace, C. J., Falloon, L. R. H. & Vaughin, C. E. (1981). Interpersonal problem solving for schizophrenics and their families. *Comprehensive Psychiatry*, **22**, 627–30.

Mandelbrote, B. M. & Folkard, S. (1961). Some problems and needs of schizophrenics in relation to a developing psychiatric community service. *Comprehensive Psychiatry*, **2**, 317–28.

Mann, S. & Cree, W. (1976). 'New' long-stay psychiatric patients: a national survey of fifteen mental hospitals in England and Wales 1972/3. *Psychological Medicine*, **6**, 603–16.

Marks, I. (1992). Innovations in mental health care delivery. *British Journal of Psychiatry*, **160**, 589–97.

Marks, I. M. (1995). Synopsis of the DLP for the seriously mentally ill: A controlled comparison of home vs hospital based care. In *Community Psychiatry in Action*, ed. F. Creed & P. Tyrer, pp. 29–44. Cambridge: Cambridge University Press.

Marks, I. M., Connolly, J., Muijen, M., McNamee, G., Audini, B. & Lawrence, R. E. (1994). Home-based versus hospital-based care for people with serious mental illness. *British Journal of Psychiatry*, **165**, 179–94.

Mayou, R. (1989). The history of general hospital psychiatry. *British Journal of Psychiatry*, **155**, 764–6.

Mechanic, D. & Aitken, L. (1987). Improving the care of patients with chronic mental illness. *New England Journal of Medicine*, **317**, 1634–8.

McCreadie, R. G., Wilson, D. A. & Burton, L. L. (1983). The Scottish survey of 'new chronic' inpatients. *British Journal of Psychiatry*, **143**, 564–71.

McCreadie, R. G., Leese, M., Tilak-Singh, G., Loftus, L., MacEwan, T. & Thorncroft, G. (1997). Nithsdale, Nunhead and Norwood: similarities and differences in prevalence of schizophrenia and utilisation of services in rural and urban areas. *British Journal of Psychiatry*, **170**, 31–6.

Ministry of Health. (1958). *Annual Reports*. London: HMSO.

Ministry of Health. (1962). *A Hospital Plan for England and Wales*. London: HMSO.

Mitchell, A. R. K. (1985). Psychiatrists in primary care settings. *British Journal of Psychiatry*, **147**, 371–9.

Muijen, M., Marks, I. M., Connolly, J., Audini, B. & McNamee, G. (1992). The daily living programme – preliminary comparison of community versus hospital-based treatment for the seriously mentally ill facing emergency admission. *British Journal of Psychiatry*, **160**, 379–84.

Mullen, R., Bebbington, P. & Kuipers, L. (1992). A workshop for relatives of people with chronic mental illness. *Psychiatric Bulletin*, **6**, 206–7.

National Schizophrenia Fellowship. (1974). *Living with Schizophrenia – By the Relatives*. Surbiton: NSF Publications.

National Schizophrenic Fellowship. (1994). *What's Gone Wrong?* Surbiton: NSF Publications.

Nazareth, I., King, M., Haines, A., See Tai, S. & Hall, G. (1993). Care of schizophrenia in general practice. *British Medical Journal*, **307**, 910–1.

NHS Executive. (1994). Developing NHS purchasing and GP fundholding: towards a primary care-led NHS. *EL (94) 79*, London: NHS Executive.

Parkes, C. M., Brown, G. W. & Monck, E. M. (1962). The General Practitioner and the schizophrenic patient. *British Medical Journal*, **1**, 972–6.

Platt, S. (1985). Measuring the burden of psychiatric illness on the family: an evaluation of some rating scales. *Psychological Medicine*, **15**, 388–93.

Powell, E. (1961). *Annual Conference of the National Association for Mental Health – Inaugural Speech*.

Prosser, D., Johnson, S., Kuipers, E., Szmukler, G., Bebbington, G. & Thorncroft, G. (1996). Mental health 'burnout' and job satisfaction among hospital and community-based mental health staff. *British Journal of Psychiatry*, **169**, 331–7.

Pullen, I. & Yellowlees, A. (1988). Scottish psychiatrists in primary health care settings: a silent majority. *British Journal of Psychiatry*, **153**, 663–6.

Ritchie, J. (1994). *The Report of the Inquiry in the Care and Treatment of Christopher Clunis*. London: HMSO.

Robinson, K. (1954). Parliamentary debate. *Hansard* 19th February.

Robinson, R. (1993). Moving ahead, community care in Gwent. *British Medical Journal*, **806**, 44–7.

Sargeant, R. (1993). Schizophrenia: the problems for the family. *Psychiatric Bulletin*, **17**, 14–15.

Scott, J. (1994). What the papers say. *Psychiatric Bulletin*, **18**, 489–91.

Scull, A. (1984). *Decarceration: Community Treatment and the Deviant – A Radical View*, 2nd edn. Cambridge: Polity Press.

Shepherd, G., Beadsmoore, A., Moore, C., Hardy, P. & Muijen, M. (1997). Relation between bed use, social deprivation and overall bed availability in acute adult psychiatric units, and alternative residential options: a cross sectional survey, one day census data, and staff interviews. *British Medical Journal*, **314**, 262–6.

Shepherd, M., Watt, D., Falloon, L. & Smeeton, N. (1989). The natural history of schizophrenia: a five year follow-up study of a home and prediction in a representative sample of schizophrenics. *Psychological Medicine*, (Monog. and Suppl.), **15**.

Stein, L. I. & Test, M. A. (1980). Alternative to mental hospital treatment. 1. Conceptual model, treatment program and clinical evaluation. *Archives of General Psychiatry*, **37**, 392–7.

Strathdee, G. & Williams, P. (1984). A survey of psychiatrists in primary care: the silent growth of a new service. *Journal of the Royal College of General Practitioners*, **34**, 615–18.

The Sun (1996). 'Possessed' patient killed two relatives after release. 7th March.

Tantum, D. (1985). Alternatives to psychiatric hospitalisation. *British Journal of Psychiatry*, **146**, 1–4.

Test, M. A. (1990). Theoretical and research basis of community care programmes. In *Mental Health Care Delivery: Innovations, Impediments and Implementation*, ed. I. M. Marks & R. Scott, pp. 11–16, 254–6. Cambridge: Cambridge University Press.

Trieman, N. & Leff, J. (1996). The TAPS project 36: the most difficult to place long-stay psychiatric in-patients. Outcome one year after relocation. *British Journal of Psychiatry*, **169**, 209–92.

Thornicroft, G. & Strathdee, G. (1994). How many psychiatric beds? Editorial. *British Medical Journal*, **309**, 970–1.

Tooth, G. C. & Brook, E. M. (1961). Needs and beds: trends in the mental hospital population and their effect on future planning. *Lancet*, **1**, 710–13.

Tyrer, P., Seivewright, N. & Wollerton, S. (1984). General practice psychiatric clinics – impact on psychiatric services. *British Journal of Psychiatry*, **145**, 15–19.

Tyrer, P., Hawksworth, J., Hobbs, R., et al. (1990). The place of the community psychiatric nurse in a comprehensive mental health service. *British Journal of Hospital Medicine*, **43**, 439–42.

Unsworth, C. (1987). *The Politics of Mental Health Legislation*. Oxford: Oxford University Press.

Warden, J. (1997). Changes to mental health care proposed. *British Medical Journal*, **314**, 394.

Waters, M. A. & Northover, J. (1965). Rehabilitated long-stay schizophrenics in the community. *British Journal of Psychiatry*, **11**, 258–67.

Watson, J. P. (1994). Too few beds. Editorial. *Psychiatric Bulletin*, **18**, 531–2.

White, E. (1991). *Community Psychiatric Nursing: A Research Project*. London: Hyman.

Williams, P. & Balestrieri, M. (1989). Psychiatric clinics in general practice – do they reduce admissions? *British Journal of Psychiatry*, **154**, 67–71.

Williams, P. & Clare, A. (1981). Changing patterns of psychiatric care. *British Medical Journal*, **282**, 375–7.

Wing, J. K. (1979). *New Methods of Mental Health Care*. ed. M. Meacher, p. 209. Oxford: Pergamon Press.

Wing, J. K., Monck, C. E., Brown, G. W. & Carstairs, E. M. (1964). Morbidity in the community of schizophrenic patients discharged from London mental hospitals in 1959. *British Journal of Psychiatry*, **110**, 10–21.

Wooff, K., Goldberg, D. P. & Fryers, T. (1988). The practice of community psychiatric nursing and mental health social work in Salford. Some implications for community care. *British Journal of Psychiatry*, **152**, 783–92.

World Health Organization. (1953). *Third Report of the Expert Committee on Mental Health.* WHO: Geneva.

Wykes, T. (1982). A hostel-ward for 'new' long-stay patients. In *Long Term Community Care: An Experience in a London Borough*, ed. J. K. Wing. *Psychological Medicine*, **Suppl 2**, 57–97.

9

Special problem areas

Implicit in early accounts of the development of facilities for the control and care of the insane was an acceptance that disordered and possibly dangerous behaviour might be expected at any time from those suffering under the burden of mental disease (Haslam, 1797). The term 'criminal lunatic' was itself enshrined in the British legislation of the early nineteenth century (Act for the Better Care and Maintenance of Pauper and Criminal Lunatics, 1808) and clearly implied a relationship between disorders of the mind and criminality. Furthermore this association was reinforced by subsequent emergence of the tacit understanding that the presence of various mental symptoms might substantially affect an individual's responsibility for his or her actions (West & Walk, 1977). Given the passage of time and perhaps increasing enlightenment and liberalism it might reasonably have been hoped that by the present day, ideas and attitudes about the way in which a major mental illness can affect behaviour would be better understood. Unfortunately that is far from the case and sometimes, especially when the mentally ill become involved in criminal proceedings, there is a sense in which society seems intent upon exacting a greater rather than a lesser price for the crime.

Disorganized and disturbed behaviour is often part and parcel of an acute schizophrenic illness and is acknowledged as such in modern classificatory systems for mental disorder (ICD 10, WHO, 1992; DSM IV, APA, 1994). It may take a variety of forms. Attempts to distinguish between those elements which might be within the individual's own control, and others which are not, are requently fruitless and may have little or no place in the management of the immediate clinical situation or long term treatment of the underlying disorder. To attempt to define what is often referred to as the 'behavioural' element of a course of action, as opposed to difficulties resulting directly from the patient's illness is unwise. It implies an ability to understand an individual's thinking and emotional processes, as well as physical capacities, in a way which reduces good psychiatric practice to the level of guesswork and conjecture. It changes dramatically the therapeutic relationship, alarms and confuses relatives and creates frustration and uncertainty among criminal justice workers and courts alike. Political exhortations to reduce the number of suicides or homicides by the mentally ill, and legislation which seeks primarily to impose responsibilities upon clinicians for aspects of the disorder which are as unpredictable as dangerous behaviour, or as frequent as non-accidental self-injury, may serve only to frustrate the efforts of those dealing with this gravely ill and disadvantaged group. (Gunn & Taylor, 1993; Hall et al., 1993). The public perception of the mentally ill as not only different from themselves, but also being far more likely to commit acts of violence than the mentally well (Appleby & Wessely, 1988; Levey & Howells, 1995), is fuelled by distorted and sensationalized media reporting of incidents involving mentally disordered individuals (Steadman & Cocozza, 1974; Matas et al., 1985). Such public perception is also compounded by the fact that the inaccurate portrayal of mental illness and the effects of this in the popular press and on television tends to reinforce negative stereotypes even in the face of public education (Wolff et al., 1996) and evidence to the contrary (Domino, 1983; Link & Cullen, 1986; Borinstein, 1992). Coupled with the increasing number of high profile cases and ensuing enquiries into the treatment and care of mentally disordered individuals who commit homicide (Peay, 1996), there has been a tendency in the past towards bias and discrimination and away from a rational, scientific approach to the problem of the association between mental illness and disturbed behaviour. Fortunately, more recently there has been a growing acknowledgement of the need for work in this area, paradoxically, and to some extent at least, as the result of media interest. This has given impetus to large studies of criminal behaviour and particularly violence among patients with schizophrenia worldwide.

The issues are complex and understanding is constrained by the limitations inherent in research in this difficult and underinvestigated field. Defining a specific mental illness for the purposes of investigation may be difficult enough. When in addition one is faced with the need to identify a specific form of behaviour, in particular 'violence', or address the issue of associated criminal activity, the possible pitfalls are further compounded. Coupled with sample populations limited in size (by virtue of the relatively small number of mentally disordered individuals who behave in this way), by location (frequently those in hospitals or other forms of institutional care), and by the vagaries of the admission process to health care and other settings, epidemiological data linking schizophrenia with various types of disturbed behaviour should always be interpreted with some degree of caution (Taylor, 1993). Potential difficulties with experimental methods need not prevent the conduct of research work but resources must be made available to investigate the problem thoroughly in ways which will improve service delivery and management and reduce risk.

This chapter is concerned with schizophrenia and a range of disordered behaviours, offending as a whole, violence in particular and death by suicide.

Schizophrenia and offending behaviour

Schizophrenia is a common illness (WHO, 1973) and offending is a frequent occurrence (British Crime Survey, 1996), but how often they occur together and whether one might lead to the other is still a matter of some dispute and uncertainty (Monahan & Steadman, 1983). There is evidence that in men with schizophrenia the rate of offending is much the same as that which is found among the general population. For women, however, the figure is doubled, and convictions are made as many as three times more frequently than for those with other forms of mental disorder (Wessely et al., 1994). Violent offences, although generally of a less severe type, occur four times more often in those with schizophrenia than in the general population (Lindqvist & Allebeck, 1990).

Even during the course of their first episode of illness a small but significant percentage of those with schizophrenia have had contact with the police (Macmillan & Johnson, 1987). Of that same group, as many as 16% may have committed an offence within the five year period immediately prior to their initial admission to hospital. Nearly half of these offences are closely associated with, or are directly the result of psychotic symptoms (Humphreys et al., 1994). In addition, a substantial proportion of all patients with schizophrenia, irrespective of the length of the illness, the nature of the predominant symptoms or any previous treatment, have had some involvement with the police (Mackay & Wright, 1984). More than 10% may have actually been convicted of an offence (Johnstone et al., 1991). Those who find their way to psychiatric services by virtue of contact with criminal justice agencies may not necessarily be charged with an offence, being diverted from custody at an early stage, even where the behaviour concerned has seriously threatened the safety of others (Lagos, 1977; Humphreys et al., 1992). A prosecution, if continued, may be for any sort of offence, some directly as a result of the symptoms of illness, and others not. A smaller number of patients may have been convicted of more serious offences including assault, grievous bodily harm, arson, attempted murder and murder (Johnstone et al., 1991). Others behave in a way which might very well have led to prosecution, again for a whole range of different sorts of offence from drunk and disorderly to attempted stabbing, but charges are not pressed due to the presence of obvious mental illness and in most cases immediate admission to hospital. For some individuals, criminal justice agencies, the police, courts, probation service, etc. may be their primary and sometimes only means of access to psychiatric care. This is perhaps not surprising as mentally disordered offenders are more often seen whilst committing a crime than their well counterparts (Robertson, 1988). Such offenders show a greater degree of disorganization in their actions and are likely to be arrested by a uniformed police officer immediately after committing the crime.

Increasing concern that mentally abnormal offenders were entering the criminal justice system more and more often, has led to the development of a variety of formal schemes to screen those in police custody and passing through courts etc. with a view to extricating the mentally ill as early as possible (Joseph & Potter, 1990; James & Hamilton, 1991; Wix, 1994). Curiously, despite the fact that individuals brought to the attention of psychiatrists by the police have higher rates of major mental disorder (Fahy, 1989), there is some evidence that fewer than usual are charged when compared to the mentally well (Johnstone et al., 1986; Lagos et al., 1977) and that those who are do not represent the mentally ill as a whole (Bowden, 1992), although the reasons for this are unclear. Perhaps it is because the police are able to recognize accurately mental disorder and its manifestations (Robertson et al., 1996) and identify those that need help. On the other hand it seems clear that the fate of a mentally disordered individual who becomes involved in the criminal justice system at whatever stage, depends heavily upon their location and the individuals that they meet. Other important factors include services that are available locally and the views of the individuals involved with regard to the identification of mental illness and its treatment (Humphreys et al., 1994). One of the difficulties which arises time and again in such circumstances is the difference in perception of what constitutes a mental disorder in the minds of criminal justice agency workers and court officers, and what is sometimes seen as the rather narrow, exclusive and sometimes dismissive view of assessing professionals. The intoxicated, violent, anti-social individual may create far more of a management problem in police cells or prison than the quietly disorganized, profoundly psychotic individual. The care of mentally ill patients in such circumstances can only be improved with careful inter-agency liaison founded on the will to cooperate and learn new ways and strategies for dealing with potentially difficult situations. Again adequate funds and facilities will be required.

At one time there was uncertainty about whether a schizophrenic illness renders an individual more liable to conviction for an offence (Zitrin et al., 1976). More recently the assumption, founded on earlier studies, that schizophrenia was associated with an increased rate of offending, has been questioned (Wessely & Taylor, 1991; Monahan, 1992) and systematically investigated. In their large longitudinal study of criminal behaviour in newly occurring cases of schizophrenia, Wessely et al. (1994) found an increased rate of conviction for women with schizophrenia of 3:1 when compared to those with other forms of psychiatric disorder and although they identified similar rates amongst men as an equivalent control group, there were increased rates of violence in both subject samples. In addition, there were various compounding personal and social factors which increased the risk of conviction amongst those with schizophrenia. These include unemployment, low social class and substance abuse. Despite this, the most clear association was with a prior history of offending, something which might be expected with any group of offenders, mentally ill or not.

Whatever the nature of the relationship between schizophrenia and offending behaviour, it is clear that in terms of crime as a whole, those with this diagnosis contribute relatively little to the overall picture. Nevertheless, the two occur together and the practical, clinical problems, as well as the ethical and moral dilemmas which arise as a result, have implications in terms of requirements for resources and expertise in care and management. Unfortunately, in the United Kingdom at least, the fact remains that substantial numbers of people with schizophrenia are to be found among prison populations, both those awaiting trial (Davidson et al., 1995; Brooke et al., 1996), and those convicted and serving sentences (Gunn et al., 1991). Elsewhere in the world, particularly in the United States, it is difficult to be certain that the same holds true, not least because of the size of the country and prison population concerned and also the practical and legal differences between different states. It seems likely, however, that there must be a considerable sub-set of those in most penal institutions, wherever one looks, who have immediate or long standing mental health needs and in some cases, major mental illness.

Schizophrenia and violence

Formal studies of the relationship between mental disorder and violence are very difficult to conduct. There has, perhaps understandably, been more concern about acts of violence towards others associated with mental disorder as a whole than with any other form of disturbed behaviour. Public awareness in the UK in particular has been increased by widespread press interest and the recent publication of a large number of reports arising from the mandatory requirement for an independent enquiry following homicide by any mentally disordered individual (National Health Services Executive Circular HSG(94)27). Although these have taken various forms, each has made public details of the treatment and care of individual patients who have gone on to kill, all of whom have had a diagnosis of schizophrenia or some similar form of illness, albeit in some cases complicated by other problems such as alcohol and substance abuse or personality disorder (Crichton & Sheppard 1996; Eastman, 1996). The value of such enquiries remains uncertain (Eastman, 1996) and a matter of some considerable controversy (Crichton & Sheppard, 1996). As yet they have shed little light on the relationship between the underlying disorder in each case and the behaviour leading to the victim's death. The main concerns have been process and outcome in relation to care (Zito Trust, 1995) and to some extent they may have served to fulfil perceived needs for catharsis and perhaps for apportioning blame. This overall concern with violent acts perpetrated by mentally ill people is reflected elsewhere, especially in research activity in the US (Monahan, 1992; Swanson et al., 1990).

There does seem to have been far more media and public interest in the United Kingdom nevertheless, perhaps simply, again, as a reflection of the relative size of the country and also maybe the variation in the legislative framework and legal process from state to state in the US.

In parallel with the increased publicity given to acts of violence committed by some mentally disordered people, there have been growing doubts and scepticism about inadequate policies and resources for care. The lack of these compromises professional practice, which might otherwise have facilitated earlier intervention and reduced risk of danger (Coid, 1996). The argument in favour of increased resources and more manpower to help reduce the potential for disturbed behaviour among mentally ill patients in hospital, the community or elsewhere, is a powerful and emotive one, but rests on the assumption that such changes will in fact enable those risks to be reduced. It may also lead to the assumption that with such change alone, the difficulties will be reduced to a minimum or perhaps even eradicated entirely. This clearly is not the case. The same is true of changes in legislation intended to afford more professional control. Neither increases in funds, staffing, hospital beds or statutory instruments will enable prediction or prevention of some of the episodes of the disturbed behaviour associated with a schizophrenic illness.

Despite the obvious difficulties already outlined in relation to offending, which are very similar to those that hamper investigation of how mental illness impacts on violence, lately there has been some additional impetus to research into the relationship between physical aggression and schizophrenia. Research ranges from work including schizophrenic patients and patients with other mental disorders, studying the influence on violence in the community (Swanson et al., 1990) and descriptions of mentally abnormal groups imprisoned for violent offences (Hafner & Boker, 1973; Taylor & Gunn, 1984), to the occurrences of behaviour threatening the lives of others during the course of a first schizophrenic episode (Humphreys et al., 1994). The relationship between violence and specific symptoms was reported (Wessely et al., 1994) and, more recently still, cognitive and neuropsychological deficits in schizophrenia have been associated with physical aggression (Lapierre et al., 1995; Heads, 1996).

In relation to mental illness as a whole and schizophrenia in particular, there has been a swing towards the view that the possibility of violence is greater among those with this form of disorder than the population as a whole (Lindqvist & Allebeck, 1990; Swanson et al., 1990; Link et al., 1992; Hodgins, 1992; Wessely et al., 1994). On the other hand, there is no doubt that people with a mental illness commit only a very small percentage of acts of violence. In some ways it is perhaps surprising that the two are not more frequently found together given the facts that, like offending, violence occurs often, that schizophrenia can be expected to affect nearly one per cent of the population, and that there is frequent association of psychotic illness with disorganized and disturbed behaviour. In the past, schizophrenic patients were thought to be second only in number to aggressive psychopaths among the mentally disordered as perpetrators of violence (Henderson & Gillespie, 1969). Studies of psychiatric hospital populations have always found more patients with schizophrenia involved in violent incidents than those with any other diagnosis (Fottrell, 1980). This may be perhaps because there were far more patients in hospital with this illness than any other, although there is some evidence that those with schizophrenia are disproportionately represented amongst hospitalized patients in terms of violent behaviour (Noble & Roger, 1989).

With more and more emphasis being placed upon the need to predict and thus prevent violent disturbed behaviour among those with a mental illness, the focus has tended towards attempts to identify risk factors in terms of history, and in particular signs or symptoms which may accompany or drive violent behaviour (Taylor & Monahan, 1996). In the past, claims have been made that certain personality traits, identifiable before the onset of illness, were the most important factors in aggression among patients with schizophrenia (Blackburn, 1968), but it has become increasingly clear that for some patients disturbed behaviour, not just violence, comes with the onset of the disorder (Humphreys et al., 1992) and for others this behaviour emerges with chronic deteriorating illness (Taylor & Hodgins, 1994).

Increasingly there is evidence that violence committed by people with schizophrenia is associated with symptoms of the psychosis (Taylor, 1985), not simply the positive phenomena, but also the disorganized, disruptive behaviour which can result from misinterpretation of actions and events or from having no other apparent means of self-expression. There is now general agreement that hallucinations play relatively little part in motivating violent behaviour among patients with schizophrenia (Hellerstein et al., 1987; Rogers et al., 1988), but that some types of delusion are more commonly associated with dangerous behaviour, particularly those of morbid jealousy (Mowat, 1966), delusions of being poisoned (Mawson, 1985; Varsamis et al., 1972), or a combination of these possibly associated with somatic hallucinations and sexual delusions (Humphreys et al., 1992). In addition, confirmation of the work of Link & Stueve (1994) shows an increased risk of violence among patients with a particular constellation of psychotic symptoms to do with perceived threat from others, delusions of control and being plotted against or followed, which in combination lead, for some individuals, to the inability to overcome the impulse to respond violently to the preceived persecutor (Swanson et al. 1996).

Some clinical features more frequently associated with dangerous behaviour such as previous violence, lack of support of family or friends, specific threats or alcohol and drug misuse and dependence are more easily identified. Findings which relate to symptom specific episodes are less clear even now with the examples given earlier applying to only very small numbers of patients (Buchanan, 1993). Risk assessment and management, not only in relation to the possibility of harm to others, but also vulnerability and non-accidental self-injury, have become almost an industry in their own right and an end in themselves. This may mean that what should be the ultimate aim, namely to reduce the possibility of harmful untoward events, becomes lost in preoccupation with the process itself. As well as reasonable resources, training and an effective legal framework, the pressing need is for large scale population based longitudinal studies of risk over time, carefully conducted and with painstaking attention to detail. The fact is that even though statistically patients with schizophrenia commit only a tiny proportion of the total number of violent acts that occur anywhere and at any time (Wessely, 1993), a small minority do behave in a dangerous way towards others. By virtue of their illness they have characteristics that may be changed by treatment and thus there is the potential for the course of events to be altered.

Suicide

Suicide, the act of killing oneself intentionally, has been known throughout history and is popularly associated with abnormalities of the mind to an even greater extent than outwardly directed violence affecting others. This is, in all likelihood, an accurate perception, with as many as nine out of every ten people who succeed in taking their own lives having had some sort of mental disorder in the broadest sense of the term (Barraclough et al., 1974).

Rates of suicide among the general population, in the United Kingdom at least, have remained much the same in recent years, although there has been concern that among some sections of society, especially young males (Hawton, 1992), they are on the increase. The accuracy of suicide statistics has always been a matter of some uncertainty, due not only to differences in reaching and recording verdicts, but also to social and religious considerations and stigmatization. Suicide is no longer a criminal offence but still carries with it connotations of despair, neglect, lack of care and social support. It usually comes with no warning, causes shock and distress and for the family of someone who has had a serious mental illness, and serves only to compound the suffering associated with both the acute and long term aspects of the disorder. Feelings of guilt and recrimination among professional staff who may have been involved with a patient who takes his/her own life can impair the ability of the most objective individual to understand what has happened and may have a devastating effect on working relationships within a clinical team.

As with violent behaviour, much effort has been directed towards the search for the causes of suicide and more particularly risk factors associated with it (Barraclough et al., 1974). Even until the present time there has been a tendency to assume an understanding that the presence of a psychiatric disorder increases the risk of suicide (Steering Committee of the Confidential Enquiry into Homicides and Suicides by Mentally Ill People, 1996) and a failure to emphasize the fact that, with some notable exceptions (Appleby, 1992), suicide is a recognized outcome for significant numbers of people with some forms of mental illness, in particular major affective disorder and schizophrenia. The difficulty lies in the fact that when death by suicide occurs the focus tends, perhaps understandably, to be on the individual concerned rather than the existence of the illness. We speak of cancer and other diseases 'killing' sufferers, but in the case of suicide by an individual with schizophrenia death is ascribed to the behaviour, and hence the individual, rather than the disorder. Perhaps as with disturbed behaviour of other sorts found in cases of psychotic illness, it might be more helpful to think in terms of the illness as the major mediator and hence retain a sense of being able to effect change or reduce risk by means of treatment. This can only come with experience and the support of colleagues for mental health professionals, but may prove an impossible, or indeed unhelpful, concept to bereaved relatives or friends of the patient.

However it is measured, there is an increased relative risk of death among those who have had previous contact with psychiatric services (Appleby, 1992) and although patients with schizophrenia only account for a small percentage of all of those who commit suicide, most longer term follow up studies have shown that around 10% of patients with schizophrenia die by suicide (Rennie, 1939; Miles, 1977), although Allebeck & Wistedt (1986), in a careful study of over 1000 patients found that only 3.9% died by suicide or other non-specific causes. The risk remains nevertheless and much effort has been put into attempts to quantify this, and to determine the underlying reasons why, not only among patients with schizophrenia, but also among those with other psychiatric diagnoses (King & Barraclough, 1990; Roy, 1982; Drake & Cotton, 1986). In fact it seems that schizophrenia, and more particularly, associated specific mental state characteristics, are the clearest indicators of risk of suicide irrespective of independent social variables (Appleby, 1992). The relationship, however, is not a straightforward one. Delusions and hallucinations, as far as one can see on the basis of retrospective analysis, play little if any part in driving suicidal behaviour (Roy, 1982). For a long time depression was believed to be the major contributory factor to suicide among patients with a long standing schizophrenic illness (Roy, 1982), but the risk has been more specifically defined in terms of the existence of a sense of hopelessness (Drake & Cotton, 1986) thought likely to be due to the recognition of loss and failure due to chronic illness which may never improve but is only likely to worsen with the passage of time. Of course, it should always be remembered that the exact details of the state of mind of the individual which might indicate a particular emotional set are more often than not unlikely to have been noted or recorded since, paradoxically, suicide is of course not something which could necessarily have been predicted otherwise action would have been taken to prevent it.

Even now there are some inconsistencies in the findings from the various studies which have been undertaken, most of which have been retrospective. Some point clearly to the patient's state of mind as being the most important factor (Drake & Cotton, 1986) leading to suicide in schizophrenia. Others (Allebeck & Wistedt, 1986) seem to indicate that demographic, social and historical aspects are central and suggest that there is probably not an insight related cause in most cases. All of this makes prediction of risk difficult, even in a restricted sense and in relation to just one psychiatric diagnosis. Careful interpretation of the available evidence suggests that among patients with schizophrenia, young men, with few if any social supports, who have lost status and many of their previous abilities, and are filled with a sense of despair about their future, are most at risk of suicide, particularly where there is evidence of the presence of suicidal ideas or previous attempts at self harm. Prevention has to do with successful treatment of the illness and recognition of the risk for all patients with schizophrenia from the outset.

The provision of psychiatric care for patients who exhibit disturbed behaviour, sometimes of a severe sort, is challenging but vital. It is important to keep in mind the fundamental nature of an illness like schizophrenia in doing so and the fact that treatment, despite seemingly overwhelming evidence to the contrary in any given individual case, may effect a change, not only in specific symptoms but also patterns of self injurious, assaultive, dangerous or socially disruptive actions. At present all that we can do is continue the search for indicators of vulnerability and risk, and with increasing understanding and knowledge, incorporate into our clinical examination of patients with schizophrenia questions and enquiries which allow us to gain knowledge of those areas of the individual's mental state and hence hope to identify early features which might indicate the possibility of any form of disturbed behaviour.

References

Allebeck, P. & Wistedt, B. (1986). Mortality and schizophrenia. A 10 year follow up based on the Stockholm County inpatient register. *Archives of General*

Psychiatry, **43**, 650–3.

Appleby, L. (1992). Suicide in psychiatric patients: risk and prevention. *British Journal of Psychiatry*, **161**, 749–58.

Appleby, L. & Wessely, S. (1988). Public attitudes to mental illness: the influence of the Hungerford massacre. *Medicine, Science and the Law*, **28**, 291–5.

Barraclough, B., Bunch, J., Nelson, B. & Sainsbury, P. (1974). A hundred cases of suicide: clinical aspects. *British Journal of Psychiatry*, **125**, 355–73.

Blackburn, R. (1968). Emotionality, extroversion and aggression in paranoid and non-paranoid schizophrenic offenders. *British Journal of Psychiatry*, **114**, 1301–2.

Borinstein, A. (1992). Public attitudes towards persons with mental illness. *Health Affairs*, **11**, 186–96.

Bowden, P. (1992). Mentally disordered offenders. In *Principles and Practice of Forensic Psychiatry*, ed. R. Bluglass & P. Bowden. Edinburgh: Churchill Livingstone.

British Crime Survey (1996). *Home Office Statistical Bulletin.* Issue 19/96.

Brooke, D., Taylor, C., Gunn, J. & Maden, A. (1996). Point prevalence of mental disorder in unconvicted male prisoners in England and Wales. *British Medical Journal*, **313**, 1524–7.

Buchanan, A. (1993). Acting on delusions: a review. *Psychological Medicine*, **23**, 123–34.

Coid, J. W. (1996). Dangerous patients with mental illness: increased risks warrant new policies, adequate resources, and appropriate legislation. *British Medical Journal*, **312**, 965–9.

Crichton, J. & Sheppard, D. (1996). Psychiatric enquiries: learning the lessons. In *Enquiries After Homicide*, ed. J. Peay. London: Duckworth.

Davidson, M., Humphreys, M. S., Johnstone, E. C. & Cunningham-Owens, D. G. (1995). Prevalence of psychiatric morbidity among remand prisoners in Scotland. *British Journal of Psychiatry*, **167**, 545–8.

Domino, G. (1983). Impact of the film 'One Flew Over the Cuckoo's Nest' on attitudes towards mental illness. *Psychological Reports*, **53**, 179–82.

Drake, R. E. & Cotton, P. G. (1986). Depression, hopelessness and suicide in chronic schizophrenia. *British Journal of Psychiatry*, **148**, 554–9.

Eastman, N. (1996). Enquiry into homicides by psychiatric patients: systematic audit should replace mandatory enquiries. *British Medical Journal*, **313**, 1069–71.

Fahy, T. (1989). The police as a referral agency for psychiatric emergencies – a review. *Medicine, Science and the Law*, **29**, 315–22.

Fottrell, E. (1980). A study of violent behaviour among patients in psychiatric hospitals. *British Journal of Psychiatry*, **136**, 216–21.

Gunn, J. & Taylor, P. J. (eds) (1993). *Forensic Psychiatry: Clinical, Legal and Ethical Issues.* Oxford: Butterworth Heineman.

Gunn, J., Maden, A. & Swinton, M. (1991). Treatment needs of prisoners with psychiatric disorders. *British Medical Journal*, **303**, 338–41.

Hafner, H. & Boker, W. (1973). *Crimes of Violence by Mentally Abnormal Offenders.* (Trans. H. Marshall). Cambridge: Cambridge University Press.

Hall, P., Brockington, I. F., Levings, J. & Murphy, C. (1993). A comparison of responses to the mentally ill in two communities. *British Journal of Psychiatry*, **162**, 99–108.

Haslam, J. (1797). *Observations on Insanity.* London.

Hawton, K. (1992). By their own hand. *British Medical Journal*, **304**, 1000.

Heads, T. (1996). Neuropsychological function in patients with schizophrenia and violent or offending behaviour I: clinical characteristics. *Proceedings of a Conference on Schizophrenia – Current Advances in Research and Treatment. London: Special Hospitals Service Authority.*

Hellerstein, D., Frosch, W. & Koeningsberg, H. W. (1987). The clinical significance of command hallucinations. *American Journal of Psychiatry,* **144,** 219–21.

Henderson, D. K. & Gillespie, R. D. (1969). *Textbook of Psychiatry.* Oxford: Oxford University Press.

Hodgins, S. (1992). Mental disorder, intellectual deficiency and crime. *Archives of General Psychiatry,* **144,** 219–22.

Humphreys, M. S., Johnstone, E. C., Macmillan, J. F. & Taylor, P. J. (1992). Dangerous behaviour preceding first admissions for schizophrenia. *British Journal of Psychiatry,* **161,** 501–5.

Humphreys, M. S., Johnstone, E. C. & Macmillan, J. F. (1994). Offending among first episode schizophrenics. *Journal of Forensic Psychiatry,* **5,** 51–61.

James, D. V. & Hamilton, L. W. (1991). The Clerkenwell Scheme: assessing efficacy and cost of a psychiatric liaison service to a magistrates' court. *British Medical Journal,* **303,** 282–5.

Johnstone, E. C., Crowe, T. J., Johnson, A. L. & Macmillan, J. F. (1986). The Northwick Park study of first episodes of schizophrenia. *British Journal of Psychiatry,* **148,** 115–43.

Johnstone, E. C., Leary, J., Frith, C. D. & Owens, D. G. C. (1991). Disabilities and circumstances of schizophrenic patients – a follow up study. VII: Police contact. *British Journal of Psychiatry,* **159 (Suppl. 13),** 37–9.

Joseph, P. L. & Potter, M. (1990). Mentally disordered homeless offenders: diversion from custody. *Health Trends,* **22,** 51–3.

King, E. & Barraclough, B. (1990). Violent death and mental illness. A study of a single catchment area over 8 years. *British Journal of Psychiatry,* **156,** 714–20.

Lagos, J. M., Perolmutter, K. & Saexinger, H. (1977). Fear of the mentally ill: empirical support for the common man's response. *American Journal of Psychiatry,* **134,** 1134–7.

Lapierre, D., Brawn, C. M. J., Hodgins, S., Toupin, J., Leveillee, S. & Constantineau, C. (1995). Neuropsychological correlates of violence in schizophrenia. *Schizophrenia Bulletin,* **21,** 253–362.

Levey, S. & Howells, K. (1995). Dangerousness, unpredictability and the fear of people with schizophrenia. *Journal of Forensic Psychiatry,* **6,** 19–39.

Lindqvist, P. & Allebeck, P. (1990). Schizophrenia in crime: a longitudinal follow up of 644 schizophrenics in Stockholm. *British Journal of Psychiatry,* **157,** 345–50.

Link, B. G. & Cullen, F. T. (1986). Contact with the mentally ill and perceptions of how dangerous they are. *Journal of Health and Social Behaviour,* **27,** 289–302.

Link, B. G. & Stueve, C. (1994). Psychotic symptoms and the violent/illegal behaviour of mental patients compared to community controls. In *Violence and Mental Disorder,* ed. J. Monahan & H. Steadman. Chicago: University of Chicago Press.

Link, B. J. Andrews, H. and Cullen, F. T. (1992). The violent and illegal behaviour of mental patients reconsidered. *American Sociological Review,* **57,** 275–92.

Mackay, R. & Wright, R. (1984). Schizophrenia and anti-social (criminal) behaviour – some responds from sufferers and relatives. *Medicine, Science and the Law*, **24**, 192–8.

Macmillan, J. F. & Johnson, A. L. (1987). Contact with the police in early schizophrenia: it's nature, frequency and relevance to the outcome of treatment. *Medicine, Science and the Law*, **27**, 191–200.

Matas, M., El-Guebaly, N., Peterkin, A., Green, M. & Harper, D. (1985). Mental illness and the media assessment of attitudes and communication. *Canadian Journal of Psychiatry*, **30**, 12–19.

Mawson, D. (1985). Delusions of poisoning. *Medicine, Science and the Law*, **25**, 279–87.

Miles, P. (1977). Conditions predisposing to suicide: a review. *Journal of Nervous and Mental Diseases*, **164**, 231–46.

Monahan, J. (1992). Mental disorder and violent behaviour: perceptions and evidence. *American Psychologist*, **47**, 511–21.

Monahan, J. & Steadman, H. (1983). Crime and mental illness: an epidemiological approach. In *Crime and Justice, Volume IV*, ed. M. Morris & M. Tonery, pp. 145–89. Chicago: University of Chicago Press.

Mowat, R. R. (1966). *Morbid Jealousy and Murder*. London: Tavistock Publications.

Noble, P. & Rodger, S. (1989). Violence by psychiatric inpatients. *British Journal of Psychiatry*, **155**, 384–90.

Peay, J. (ed.) (1996). *Enquiries After Homicide*. London: Duckworth.

Rennie, T. A. C. (1939). Follow up study of 500 patients with schizophrenia admitted to the hospital from 1913–1923. *Archives of Neurology and Psychiatry*, **42**, 877–91.

Robertson, G. (1988). Arrest patterns among mentally disordered offenders. *British Journal of Psychiatry*, **153**, 313–16.

Robertson, G., Pearson, R. & Gibb, R. (1996). The entry of mentally disordered people to the criminal justice system. *British Journal of Psychiatry*, **169**, 172–80.

Rogers, R., Nussbaum, D. & Gillis, R. (1988). Command hallucinations and criminality: a clinical quandary. *Bulletin of the American Academy of Psychiatry and the Law*, **16**, 251–8.

Roy, A. (1982). Suicide in chronic schizophrenia. *British Journal of Psychiatry*, **141**, 171–7.

Steadman, H. J. & Cocozza, J. (1978). Selective reporting and public's misconceptions of the criminally inance. *Public Opinion Quarterly*, **41**, 523–33.

Swanson, J. W., Borum, R., Swartz, M. S. & Monahan, J. (1996). Psychotic symptoms and disorders and the risk of violent behaviour in the community. *Criminal Behaviour and Mental Health*, **6**, 309–29.

Swanson, J. W., Holzer, C. E., Ganja, V. K. & Jono, R. T. (1990). Violence and psychiatric disorder in the community: evidence from the epidemiological catchment area surveys. *Hospital and Community Psychiatry*, **41**, 761–70.

Taylor, P. J. (1993). Schizophrenia and crime: distinctive patterns in association. In *Mental Disorder and Crime*, ed. S. Hodgins, pp. 63–85, Sage, Newbury Park.

Taylor, P. J. (1995). Schizophrenia and the risk of violence. In *Schizophrenia*, ed. S. R. Hirsch and D. R. Weinberger, pp. 163–83. Blackwell Science: Oxford.

Taylor, P. J., Gunn, J. (1984). Violence and psychosis I. Risk of violence among psychotic men. *British Medical Journal*, **228**, 1945–9.

Taylor, P. J. & Hodgins, S. (1994). Violence and psychosis critical timings.

Criminal Behaviour and Mental Health, **4**, 266–89.

Taylor, P. J. & Monahan, J. (1996). Dangerous patients or dangerous diseases. *British Medical Journal*, **312**, 967–9.

Teplin, L. A. & Pruett, N. S. (1992). Police as a street corner psychiatrist: managing the mentally ill. *International Journal of Law and Psychiatry*, **15**, 139–56.

Varsamis, J., Adamson, J. D. & Sigardson, W. F. (1972). Schizophrenics with delusions of poisoning. *British Journal of Psychiatry*, **121**, 673–5.

Wessely, S. (1993). Violence and psychosis. In *Violence: Basic and Clinical Science*, ed. C. Thompson & P. Cowen. Oxford: Butterworth Heineman.

Wessely, S. & Taylor, P. (1991). Madness and crime: criminology or psychiatry. *Criminal Behaviour and Mental Health*, **1**, 193–228.

Wessely, S. C., Castle, D., Douglas, A. J. & Taylor, P. J. (1994). Criminal careers of incident cases of schizophrenia. *Psychological Medicine*, **24**, 483–502.

West, D. J. & Walk, A. (1977). *Daniel McNaughton; his trial and the aftermath.* London: Gaskill.

Wix, S. (1994). Keeping on the straight and narrow. *Psychiatric Care*, **1**, 102–4.

Wolff, G., Patary, S., Craig, T. & Leff, J. (1996). Community knowledge of mental illness and reaction to mentally ill people. *British Journal of Psychiatry*, **168**, 191–8.

World Health Organization (1973). *Report of the International Pilot Study of Schizophrenia.* Geneva: WHO.

Zito Trust (1995). *Learning the Lessons: Mental Health Enquiry Reports Published in England and Wales Between 1969 and 1994 and their recommendations for Improving Practice.* London: The Zito Trust.

Zitrin, A., Hardesty, A. A., Burdock, E. I. & Drossman, A. K. (1976). Crime and violence among mental patients. *American of Psychiatry*, **133**, 142–9.

10

The pharmacological treatment of schizophrenia

As discussed in Chapter 2, the first antipsychotic drugs were developed in the 1950s. The first generation of these drugs (phenothiazines, butyrophenones and thioxanthenes) are referred to as typical neuroleptics. Though these drugs have had a dramatic impact on the management of schizophrenia, they have significant side-effects and they have also not proved effective in all cases. They also have little effect in alleviating the often disabling negative effects of schizophrenia. A group of drugs referred to as atypical neuroleptics (notably clozapine and risperidone) have become the focus of interest in recent years. They differ in their side-effect profile from the typical neuroleptics and may be effective when symptoms are resistant to typical neuroleptics.

Any therapeutic benefit of pharmacological or non pharmacological treatment is of course best demonstrated in a randomized controlled trial (RCT). The studies reported in this chapter have generally employed such methods – open studies only really having much clinical value in identifying potential adverse effects before a drug becomes widely used. This chapter can therefore be regarded as evidence based, like the following chapter on social and psychological treatments, but the sheer volume of the literature on drug therapy in schizophrenia precludes mention of each and every trial.

Typical neuroleptics

Efficacy

The most dramatic effect of the original neuroleptic drugs was their ability to treat the positive symptoms of acute schizophrenic episodes. Though their efficacy in this situation is well established (NIMH, 1964), about 30% of patients show only limited improvement in trials of acute treatment

(Davis, 1976), and about 7% of cases do not appear to show any response at all (Tuma & May, 1979; MacMillan et al., 1986).

In addition to their role in the treatment of the positive symptoms of acute episodes of schizophrenia, numerous randomized controlled trials of maintenance neuroleptics have shown their efficacy in reducing schizophrenic relapse (Leff & Wing, 1971; Hirsch et al., 1973; Davis, 1975). However, susceptibility to relapse is not entirely abolished. A two year follow-up study of patients treated with neuroleptics compared to controls treated with placebo showed relapse rates of 48% compared with 80% in the respective groups (Hogarty et al., 1974).

Though the distressing positive symptoms of acute episodes are often the most conspicuous manifestation of schizophrenia, the greatest disability is caused by the more insidiously developing defect state characterized by negative symptoms of apathy, loss of will, inability to respond emotionally or to relate to others. Negative symptoms are difficult to rate and may be confounded by other factors such as depression and drug side-effects (Owens, 1996), making research in this area problematic. Unlike positive symptoms, negative symptoms have proved resistant to pharmacological treatments (Pogue-Geile & Zubin, 1988).

Adverse effects

Neuroleptics affect a wide range of neurotransmitter and systemic organ systems. Adverse effects are therefore common, and indeed experienced in some degree by almost all patients. Side-effects may be simply classified as general, cardiovascular, endocrine and neurological.

General

Allergic and toxic reactions may occur with antipsychotics as with any other drug. Such reactions include skin rashes, photosensitivity and liver problems, which are usually benign.

Most neuroleptics are associated with dryness of the mouth, blurring of vision and urinary problems. These are principally anticholinergic effects, although anti-adrenergic actions may also be involved. Such mixed effects are probably the basis of the widespread sexual difficulties (usually anorgasmia in females and erectile impotence and ejaculatory dysfunction in males) that occur.

The term neuroleptic malignant syndrome is used to describe the sudden development of hyperpyrexia, rigidity, confusion and autonomic instability in patients on neuroleptics. Serum creatinine phosphokinase (CPK) levels are often markedly elevated. It is a rare but serious condition, the outcome of which may be death or permanent neurological damage. The nature of this syndrome is uncertain. Similar states (including the fatal outcome) have certainly occurred in psychotic patients for over a century, i.e. well before antipsychotic drugs were introduced (Mann et al., 1986). Known medical factors could account for hyperpyrexia and other features in more than half of the cases (Levinson & Simpson, 1986). Thus, although it is probable that neuroleptics are a major causative factor in some cases of this syndrome, other causes must not be overlooked. Neuroleptic malignant syndrome can be successfully treated without permanent sequelae (Levinson & Simpson, 1986).

Cardiovascular

Most neuroleptics increase heart rate, although this does not usually produce symptoms. The significant hypotension which may occur, especially with low potency phenothiazines with marked anticholinergic effects (e.g. thioridazine) can cause distressing dizziness and unsteadiness, particularly in older patients. Sudden death occurring in patients on neuroleptics is a cause of concern. Such deaths are generally thought to result from ventricular arrhythmias (Committee on Safety of Medicines, 1990).

Reports generally involve young, fit patients being treated with relatively high doses of neuroleptics for prominent positive symptoms. It is not possible to say what part autonomic activity as a direct consequence of profound mental state disturbances may play in such situations, and to what extent these deaths may be appropriately attributed to direct drug effects. These deaths are rare, but their occurrence underlines the need to adjust drug doses carefully, avoid very high doses and sudden changes, and monitor the cardiovascular state in severely psychotic patients who may be receiving high doses of neuroleptics.

Endocrine

All typical antipsychotic agents produce a marked rise in serum prolactin as a result of tubero-infundibular dopaminergic blockade. This is usually clinically insignificant, but may be associated with galactorrhoea and may contribute to the amenorrhoea which is a frequent occurrence. High prolactin levels can contribute to false positive pregnancy tests. Patients on neuroleptics frequently complain of weight gain. The causes are ill understood, but probably involve endocrine change including fluid retention and interference with hypothalamic serotonin (5-HT) systems regulating appetite.

Neurological effects

The extrapyramidal side-effects of neuroleptics are well established (Baldessarini et al., 1980). They may be classified as early (occurring within hours or days of introduction of drugs), intermediate (occurring within days or weeks to months) and late (occurring within months or years of introduction of drugs).

The early effects are acute dystonias – involuntary movements which are sustained for a variable period at the point of maximum contraction (Owens, 1990). Any muscle group can be involved, the neck and tongue being most often affected. These symptoms are extremely distressing but can be rapidly relieved by the slow intravenous injection of an anticholinergic agent such as procyclidine.

The principal intermediate neurological side-effect is Parkinsonism, of which the core features are bradykinesia, rigidity and tremor. Minor clinically insignificant degrees of this, such as reduced arm swing, can be elicited in many patients on antipsychotic agents. Treatment with anti-Parkinsonian drugs is best avoided unless clinically significant symptoms appear.

The principal late extrapyramidal effect is tardive dyskinesia – a syndrome of chronic, spontaneous, involuntary movements of a complex nature which may occur in any muscle group but which most commonly affect oro-facial, neck and upper limb muscles. The prevalence is probably around 20% (Jeste & Wyatt, 1981; Kane & Smith, 1982), but is higher if mild disorder is included. This condition is not easy to treat and may be irreversible. The pathophysiology is not fully understood but it is conventionally considered that it involves supersensitivity of dopamine receptors resulting from dopaminergic blockade.

Other problems

In addition to the clear-cut physical effects described above, many patients on neuroleptics complain of tiredness and there is evidence that, at least to some extent, their impaired performance on some psychological tests may be related to medication rather than to severity of illness (Hoff et al., 1990). A follow-up investigation of the patients who entered the Northwick Park First Episodes of Schizophrenia Study (Johnstone et al., 1990) showed significant associations between relapse and poor outcome, and between relapse and placebo medication in those patients with a shorter pre-treatment duration of illness. Nevertheless, those on the placebo medication had a significantly better outcome with regard to the work that they were able to do. This finding suggests the disquieting conclusion that the benefits of neuroleptics reducing relapse may exert a price in occupational terms.

The tiredness of which patients complain on neuroleptics may reduce their activity generally and it is usually advisable to choose a less sedative regime for patients who are in remission and wish to work or resume their domestic responsibilities. There is no consistent evidence to suggest that one mode of administration is better than another as far as social functioning is concerned and any apparent differences between different typical neuroleptics or different regimes are probably dosage effects. It is important to try to minimize all types of side-effects in order to maximize patients chances of achieving good social function. Sedative effects should be kept to a minimum. Untreated drug-induced Parkinsonism may have an adverse effect on the non-verbal aspects of social communication. While some patients do not seem to be greatly distressed by abnormalities of movement this is no reason not to attempt to treat a problem which other patients admit to finding distressing and embarrassing.

Atypical neuroleptics

As discussed in Chapter 4, the association of antipsychotic effects with extrapyramidal effects of the neuroleptic drugs led to the notion that action on the extrapyramidal system was a necessary effect of a drug that had antipsychotic properties. Both effects were thought to be mediated by blockade of the dopamine D_2 receptor. In the 1970s and early 1980s the psychopharmacology of acute schizophrenia was dominated by this idea. However, some effective antipsychotic drugs, such as thioridazine, sulpiride and clozapine, did not cause major extrapyramidal effects. As time progressed, it also became increasingly clear that dopamine D_2 receptor blockade was not necessarily associated with improvement in clinical features (Johnstone et al., 1978; 1983). Neuroleptic drugs that are not specifically targeted at dopamine D_2 receptors are referred to as atypical neuroleptics.

Commonly accepted defining characteristics of atypicality consist of criteria to be met in pre-clinical and clinical testing (Lieberman, 1993):

A. Pre-clinical criteria
1. efficacy in standard antipsychotic screening paradigms (e.g. antagonism of dopamine agonist induced stereotypes, conditioned avoidance response)

2. no induction of catalepsy
3. no up-regulation of dopamine D_2 receptors
4. no development of tolerance to increased dopamine turnover or depolarization block of A9 dopamine neurones with chronic treatment

B. *Clinical criteria*
1. antipsychotic efficacy
2. no or markedly reduced induction of acute extrapyramidal side-effects and tardive dyskinesia
3. no elevation of prolactin

These criteria have not always been rigorously applied in the reporting of new compounds, leading to some claims of atypicality when it is not warranted (Lieberman, 1993).

Atypical antipsychotic compounds in clinical usage include clozapine, risperidone, olanzapine and sertindole with zotepine, quetiapine and ziprasidone awaiting registration.

Clozapine

Clozapine is a dibenzodiazepine first synthesized in 1960. It was introduced as an antipsychotic agent in the 1970s and it was shown to be effective in schizophrenic patients, particularly the more severely ill (Fischer-Cornelson & Ferner, 1976). The administration of this drug was however found to be associated with agranulocytosis in a small percentage of cases (Idènpèèn-Heikkilè et al., 1977), and it was withdrawn from use in Great Britain, the United States and much of continental Europe. The resurgence of interest in its use followed the study by Kane et al. (1988) showing that clozapine had significantly greater benefits than a standard neuroleptic regime in treatment resistant cases.

Pharmacology

Clozapine has effects on a number of neurotransmitter systems. It is not known whether clozapine's antipsychotic properties are due to its effect on a single neurotransmitter receptor type or a particular combination of receptors of different types. Clozapine is less potent than most other antipsychotic compounds in blocking dopamine D_2 receptors (Peroutka & Snyder, 1980; Lieberman, 1993). It has greater affinity for dopamine D_1 and D_4 receptor subtypes. In addition it is more potent than typical neuroleptics in blocking muscarinic acetylcholine receptors as well as histamine, 5-HT and noradrenergic receptors (Lieberman, 1993). Hypotheses regarding clozapine's mechanism of antipsychotic action include:

1. the blockade of a combination of dopamine D_2 and 5-HT$_2$ receptors
2. the blockade of dopamine D_1 and/or D_4 receptors

Efficacy

Early acute treatment studies of clozapine were of an open-label design and were often uncontrolled. These studies gave generally favourable results, including a relative lack of extrapyramidal side-effects (Safferman et al., 1991). Subsequent double blind studies showed that clozapine was comparable to other antipsychotic agents in patients with acute schizophrenia (Van Praag et al., 1976; Shopsin et al., 1979).

Following initial reports of agranulocytosis associated with clozapine, clinical use was generally restricted (Idènpèèn-Heikkilè et al., 1975; 1977). However, the drug continued to be used in Europe where experience suggested that deaths associated with clozapine-induced agranulocytosis could be prevented by weekly blood count monitoring (Safferman et al., 1991). The results of the early studies had indicated that clozapine may be of value in patients with schizophrenia who were refractory to other antipsychotic agents. In a double blind controlled trial involving 268 patients who had failed to respond to typical antipsychotics clozapine was compared to chlorpromazine over a six week period of treatment (Kane et al., 1988). Thirty per cent of the clozapine-treated patients were judged to respond, compared to only four per cent in those receiving chlorpromazine.

After two years of follow-up of 96 patients designated as either treatment refractory (85%) or neuroleptic intolerant (15%), 62 were still on clozapine (Lindström, 1988). Forty-three per cent were significantly improved and 38% moderately improved. In a study following 216 patients for 12 years therapeutic benefit was reported in 30–50% (Povlsen et al., 1985).

Though only a limited number of studies have specifically addressed the efficacy of clozapine in relieving negative schizophrenic symptoms, the results show that clozapine is more efficacious than haloperidol in this regard (Opler et al., 1994). Reduction of negative symptoms probably takes longer to achieve than reduction of positive symptoms and may only be fully appreciated with long-term follow-up studies.

Clozapine has a low propensity to cause tardive dyskinesia and some studies have shown a beneficial effect on pre-existing tardive dyskinesia (Caine et al., 1979; Small et al., 1987; Lieberman et al., 1989b) though studies have been small and uncontrolled.

Clinical indications

Clozapine should be reserved for severely ill schizophrenic patients who have failed to respond adequately to treatment with appropriate courses of standard antipsychotic drugs. The lack of response may be because of insufficient effectiveness or the inability to achieve an effective dose due to intolerable adverse effects of the typical antipsychotic drugs. At present there are no well validated criteria for defining 'refractory' illness although operational criteria (Kane et al., 1988) and a system of levels of responsivity/resistance have been used (May et al., 1988).

Advantages

Clozapine has been shown to have greater efficacy than typical antipsychotics in the treatment of severely ill, neuroleptic-refractory schizophrenic patients. Clozapine's low propensity to cause extrapyramidal side-effects makes it more tolerable in this regard than typical antipsychotics, a factor likely to improve compliance. Clozapine may be an effective treatment for tardive dyskinesia in some patients. The absence of sustained hyperprolactinaemia with secondary effects of oligomenorrhoea or amenorrhoea may enhance compliance.

Adverse effects

Agranulocytosis is the most serious adverse effect of clozapine. Sixteen cases of agranulocytosis (out of an estimated 2500–3200 patients) were reported in Finland in the first six months of 1975 (Idènpèèn-Heikkilè et al., 1975, 1977; Amsler et al., 1977). This led to the withdrawl of clozapine from the market in some countries and its restriction in others to use in treatment-refractory patients in whom regular white blood cell (WBC) monitoring was performed. The greatest risk of clozapine-induced agranulocytosis appears to be between four and 18 weeks of starting treatment (Krupp & Barnes, 1992) with a rate of agranulocytosis in patients treated for one year of 2%. A more recent study of 11 555 patients treated with clozapine determined a 0.8% cumulative incidence of agranulocytosis after one year of treatment (Alvir et al., 1993). Mortality rate is significantly reduced if there is regular WBC monitoring and if clozapine is immediately withdrawn when agranulocytosis occurs. Any fever or sign of infection is an indication for a WBC count, especially within the first 18 weeks of treatment. Drugs that have a high likelihood of causing agranulocytosis or leukopenia, such as co-trimoxazole or carbamazepine, should not be administered with clozapine.

Clozapine causes EEG changes, predisposing to seizures in a dose related manner with a 5% incidence of seizures with doses over 600 mg per day (Safferman et al., 1991).

Sedation is a common side-effect with a reported incidence of 39% (Safferman et al., 1991). It is most prominent early in treatment but tolerance develops over the first few days or weeks (Lindström, 1988; Lieberman et al., 1989a). Other potentially troublesome side-effects include hypersalivation, dizziness, hypotension, tachycardia and weight gain.

Most side-effects can be minimized by a gradual dose titration and by using the lowest effective dose. The requirement for weekly venepuncture to check the WBC count may deter some patients from its use.

Risperidone

Risperidone is an antipsychotic compound first tested clinically in the late 1980s. It has a limited propensity to cause extrapyramidal side-effects.

Pharmacology

Risperidone is a benzisoxazole derivative that combines potent 5-HT_2 antagonism with dopamine D_2 antagonism. The development of a compound with this profile of pharmacological activity was based on the observation that the addition of a 5-HT_2 antagonist to the regimen of schizophrenic patients treated with haloperidol improved the negative symptoms, ameliorated depression and anxiety and reduced movement disorder (Livingston, 1994). Risperidone also has affinity for $\alpha1$ and $\alpha2$ noradrenergic receptors and is anti-histaminic. Although these actions are associated with side-effects, they are not thought to be relevant to the antipsychotic actions of the compound.

Evidence of efficacy

Several double blind studies have demonstrated the antipsychotic efficacy of risperidone (Chouinard & Arnott, 1993; Marder & Meibach, 1994). Some studies have also reported an improvement in negative symptoms (Marder & Meibach, 1994). There is as yet insufficient evidence to indicate whether risperidone is effective in treatment refractory or poorly responsive cases, though early studies are encouraging (Remington, 1993).

Clinical usage and advantages

At present the indications for the use of risperidone are prominent negative symptoms or interolerable movement disorder (Livingstone, 1994). Its therapeutic efficacy and limited extrapyramidal side-effect profile suggest that it may be used as a first line treatment for schizophrenia in the future, but its high cost precludes this at present.

Limitations

Risperidone produces postural hypotension due to its $\alpha 1$ adrenergic blocking effect, but the effect is mild. Treatment should be initiated gradually to avoid postural hypotension. An important side-effect is weight gain. As with other dopamine D_2 blocking drugs, risperidone causes a dose related rise in prolactin which may result in amenorrhoea, galactorrhoea, gynaecomastia and decreased libido (Livingston, 1994).

New atypical neuroleptics

Sertindole

Sertindole has a selectivity for the limbic system with effects on a number of neurotransmitter systems. It has greatest potency at dopamine D_2 receptors and 5-HT2a receptors (Lieberman, 1993). Clinical trials have shown antipsychotic efficacy superior to placebo, similar efficacy to haloperidol and a low risk of extrapyramidal symptoms (Fleischhacker & Hummer, 1997). It is associated with QTc (corrected QT interval) prolongation in the ECG and bodyweight gain.

Olanzapine

Olanzapine resembles clozapine in chemical structure and preclinical pharmacological activity. It has a broad receptor affinity profile with particular affinity for dopamine D_1, D_2, D_4, 5-HT_{2a}, 5-HT_{2c}, 5-HT_3, $\alpha 1$ adrenergic, histamine and five muscularinic cholinergic receptors (Tamminga & Lahti, 1996). It is more potent as an antagonist at 5-HT_2 than dopamine D_2 receptors (Beasley et al., 1996). In clinical trials it showed superior antipsychotic efficacy to haloperidol (10 mg per day). Negative symptoms also responded better to olanzapine than haloperidol. Extrapyramidal symptoms rates were comparable to placebo. Adverse effects include bodyweight gain and transient liver enzyme increases. Olanzapine does not appear to affect the white blood cell count (Fleischhacker & Hummer, 1997).

Zotepine

Zotepine has been available in Japan since the early 1980s and is currently being registered in various European countries. As with other atypical antipsychotics it blocks a wide range of receptors including those for serotonin, dopamine, histamine and noradrenaline. Clinical trials have demonstrated its antipsychotic efficacy as well as lower rates of extrapyramidal symptoms compared to haloperidol. Sedation, seizures and transient liver enzyme increases are reported, but there do not appear to be serious effects on white blood cell counts (Fleischhacker & Hummer, 1997).

Quetiapine

Quetiapine shows greater relative affinity for 5-HT$_{2a}$ than for dopamine D$_2$ receptors, with no appreciable affinity for muscarinic receptors. Clinical trials indicate a comparable efficacy to conventional antipsychotics in treatment of positive symptoms and a low propensity for extrapyramidal symptoms. Its effects against negative symptoms appear to be less consistent. Adverse effects include transient elevation of liver enzymes, a reduction in free thyroxine T4 levels and transient neutropenia (Fleischhacker & Hummer, 1997).

Ziprasidone

Ziprasidone is in earlier development stages than the previously mentioned atypical antipsychotics. It has high affinity for both dopamine D$_2$ receptors and a range of 5-HT receptors. Its unique neurochemical characteristic is its ability to block the noradrenergic and serotonergic reuptake sites. The clinical potential of this action is not known. Phase II studies have shown antipsychotic efficacy (Tamminga & Lahti, 1996).

Dose regimes and compliance

The dose regimes appropriate for acute episodes depend in part upon the presence or absence of behavioural disturbance. In all cases the need is to provide a drug regime which the patient can tolerate without distress, which controls non-specific symptoms such as anxiety and sleeplessness and which is flexible enough to take account of the fact that acute psychotic states fluctuate a good deal. In this situation depot medication does not really have the flexibility required. Where the patient is behaviourally disturbed or where there is a possibility of behavioural disturbance, a low potency drug which is relatively sedative is a wise choice – chlorpromazine or thioridazine in a dose of 300–600 mg/day, increasing to 800 mg if required is appropriate. Equivalent doses of sulpiride are equally suitable. Dosage adjustment every 1–2 days, taking account of amount of distress, level of sedation and the presence of side-effects is likely to be required. It will be about 14 days before antipsychotic effects become apparent in the average case (Johnstone et al., 1978), and improvements before this are likely to be non-specific or due to sedation. It is wise to have an initial regime of perhaps chlorpromazine, 75 mg twice a day and 200 mg at night, with additional dosages of 50 mg to be given up to four times per day at the nurse's discretion. The requirement for this will provide a guide to changes in the baseline regime.

In patients where behavioural disturbance is not an issue, the sedative effects of low potency neuroleptics are not helpful, and such patients will be better pleased with a high potency drug such as trifluoperazine or haloperidol. While all typical neuroleptics share the property of D_2 receptor blockade, their additional actions relating to anticholinergic effects, alpha-adrenergic blockade and sedation vary a great deal and the profile of side-effects suffered by individual patients can be a useful guide to choice of neuroleptic. If patients develop dystonic symptoms or marked Parkinsonian features in an acute episode, anticholinergic drugs should be prescribed, but they should not be given routinely. While benzodiazepines do not have antipsychotic effects, they can be very valuable in relieving anxiety and can aid sedative neuroleptics in providing adequate sleep. On an intravenous basis they provide rapid control of acute behavioural disturbance.

It is important to appreciate the time that will be required to stabilize an acute psychotic episode. Patients are generally improving after two to three weeks and become stabilized within four to six weeks, but there are often fluctuations on the road to recovery and it is important not to reduce the regime required to control the symptoms too quickly. Once a patient has achieved stability on their acute treatment regime and the florid symptoms are under control, it is appropriate to begin to consider change to a maintenance regime. Once improved, the patient will have less tolerance of relatively high neuroleptic doses and the sedation which was a benefit when the illness was acute and distressing will cause problems for a patient who is trying to regain the capacity to concentrate and organize day-to-day activities. The aim will be to achieve a simple plan with the minimum necessary number of drugs and a once or twice daily regime if possible. It is worth thinking about changing to depot, injectable neuroleptics at this stage, and certainly if compliance is known to be a problem this is advisable. It is probably wise to maintain neuroleptics for longer than 6–12 months and unless the illness has been very difficult to treat, a planned withdrawal of neuroleptics at a time when few life events would be anticipated and when a minor relapse would be less troublesome than it might be at some other times, is appropriate. In patients who have had previous episodes, evidence concerning the value of maintenance medication should be discussed with them.

There is evidence (Hoge et al., 1990) that poor compliance in patients with schizophrenia is often associated with a lack of understanding of the nature of the illness and of the purpose of maintenance medication, and that improved understanding is associated with better compliance. One of the difficulties of advocating prophylactic maintenance antipsychotic medication for patients with schizophrenia is that while the benefits of this for groups of patients are undoubted (Davis, 1975), there are some patients who will remain well without such treatment (Crow et al., 1986). Unfortunately it is difficult to identify these individuals. It was considered that patients who recovered from a functional psychotic illness (principally schizophrenic in nature) on placebo medication (Johnstone et al., 1988) might well be those who would not require antipsychotics on a maintenance basis. Follow-up over two years did not support this hypothesis (Johnstone et al., 1991) and it was concluded that recovery from an acute episode of psychosis did not identify a group of patients who could be predicted to do well without maintenance antipsychotics.

At the present time the atypical neuroleptics tend to be reserved for patients who are refractory to treatment with typical neuroleptics or who are unable to tolerate their side-effects. The potential hazard of agranulocytosis with clozapine makes it unlikely that it would have a role other than for patients with symptoms refractory to typical neuroleptics. If newer atypical neuroleptics prove to be without serious adverse effects, equally or more efficacious, and if their side-effect profile makes them more acceptable to patients, then they may gain a place in treatment of non-refractory schizophrenia.

Adjunctive medication

Antipsychotic agents are the cornerstone of psychopharmacological management of schizophrenia and their continued use unquestionably reduces the risk of psychotic relapse. However, in many patients substantial functional impairment and subjective distress persist even though florid psychosis is controlled. The addition of other medications designed to relieve some aspects of symptoms associated with schizophrenia or its treatment is often required.

Anti-Parkinsonian agents

The addition of anticholinergic medication during acute episodes will reduce the frequency of dystonic reactions and Parkinsonian symptoms. Avoidance of serious symptoms of this kind will aid future compliance and the value of this adjunctive medication is generally recognized (Lavin & Rifkin, 1991). The value of additional anticholinergics to extended maintenance antipsychotic programmes is less well established (Siris, 1993). The memory problems associated with anticholinergic use in some patients (Fayen et al., 1988) can add to the functional impairments that they have.

There is evidence that anticholinergics may have an adverse effect on positive schizophrenic symptoms (Johnstone et al., 1983; Tandon et al., 1992), though they may also reduce negative symptoms (Tandon et al., 1992). Many antipsychotic and antidepressant drugs have pronounced anticholineric properties and combinations of these drugs together with an anticholinergic drug may lead to anticholinergic toxicity. There is a danger that this may be interpreted as a worsening of psychotic symptoms leading to the use of increasing doses of the neuroleptic. The combination of anticholinergics with drugs such as clozapine which is a potent anticholinergic, may have the potential to precipitate the neuroleptic malignant syndrome (Nemecek et al., 1993).

Dopamine agonists such as L-dopa and bromocriptine may induce psychotic symptoms and are not used as anti-Parkinsonian agents in patients with schizophrenia. However, current theories that propose a cortical dopamine deficiency in schizophrenia have led to pilot studies of these agents in combination with antipsychotics. Though the studies are small, there is evidence of reduction of positive symptoms (Wolf et al., 1992; Owens et al., 1994) and improvement in cognitive function (de Beaurepaire et al., 1993).

Benzodiazepines

The use of benzodiazepines for sedation will allow very high doses of antipsychotics to be avoided. In addition, benzodiazepines may be useful in the management of antipsychotic-induced akathisia (Fleischhacker et al., 1990). These benefits have to be set against the known problems of long-term benzodiazepine use and doses should be kept to the minimum necessary and sustained use avoided if possible.

Propranolol

Propranolol is sometimes advocated as an adjunct to conventional neuro-leptic agents to enhance antipsychotic effects in schizophrenics who are not responding well (Lader, 1988), but the value of this treatment is controversial (Siris, 1993). Propranolol has been shown to be valuable in the management of akathisia (Adler et al., 1986).

Antidepressants

The occurrence of depressive symptoms in schizophrenic patients when they are not actively psychotic has been increasingly reported (McGlashan & Carpenter, 1976; Hirsch et al., 1989; Siris et al., 1994). The value of adjunctive antidepressants has been clearly demonstrated (Siris et al., 1987) and a recent trial has shown that maintenance imipramine treatment is of benefit in patients who have shown a good initial response to tricyclics (Siris et al., 1994).

Mood-stabilizers

Some investigations have shown a benefit in terms of control of psychotic symptoms for the addition of lithium to maintenance regimes (Small et al., 1975; Delva & Letemendia, 1982), although not all studies have shown positive results (Johnstone et al., 1991). Carbamazepine has not been shown to be of value as a maintenance treatment for schizophrenia (Carpenter et al., 1991) but in the acute situation its addition to neuroleptic regimes has sometimes been shown to be helpful (Christisen et al., 1991), especially in disturbed, excited patients (Klein et al., 1984).

Conclusion

Despite the limitations in understanding and the problems associated with antipsychotic drugs, pharmacological treatments have had a major impact on the management of patients with schizophrenia. Alleviation of symptoms by pharmacological means has paved the way for the discharge of patients who were previously managed by long-term custodial care and catalysed the movement towards community care. Understanding of the pharmacological mechanism of the neuroleptics has provided a basis for hypotheses about brain dysfunction in schizophrenia. The new antipsychotics hold the promise of expanding the range of options for the treatment of schizophrenia as well as raising new hypotheses about its pharmacological basis.

References

Adler, L., Angrist, B., Peselow, E., Corwin, J., Maslansky, R. & Rotrosen, J. (1986). A controlled assessment of propranolol in the treatment of neuroleptic induced akathisia. *British Journal of Psychiatry*, **149**, 42–5.

Alvir, J. J., Lieberman, J. A., Safferman, A. Z., Schwimmer, J. L. & Schaaf, J. A. (1993). Clozapine induced agranulocytosis. Incidence and risk factors in the United States. *New England Journal of Medicine*, **329**, 162–7.

Amsler, H., Leerenhovi, L., Barth, E., Harjula, K. & Vuopio, P. (1977). Agranulocytosis in patients treated with clozapine: a study of the Finnish epidemic. *Acta Psychiatrica Scandinavica*, **56**, 241–8.

Baldessarini, R. J., Cole, J. O., Davis, J. M., et al. (1980). Tardive Dyskinesia: A task force report. *American Psychiatric Press*, Washington, DC.

Beasley, C. M., Tollefson, G., Tran, P., Satterlee, W., Sanger, T. & Hamilton, S. (1996). Olanzapine versus placebo and haloperidol. Acute phase results of the North American double-blind olanzapine trial. *Neuropsychopharmacology*, **14**, 111–23.

Caine, E. D., Polinsky, R. J., Kartzinel, R. & Ebert, M. H. (1979). The trial use of clozapine for abnormal involuntary movement disorders. *American Journal of Psychiatry*, **136**, 317–20.

Carpenter, W. T., Kurz, R., Kirkpatrick, B., et al. (1991). Carbamazepine maintenance treatment in outpatient schizophrenics. *Archives of General Psychiatry*, **48**, 69–72.

Chouinard, G. & Arnott, W. (1993). Clinical review of risperidone. *Canadian Journal of Psychiatry*, **38 (suppl. 3)**, S89–S95.

Christisen, G. W., Kirch, D. G. & Wyatt, R. J. (1991). When symptoms persist: choosing among alternative somatic treatments for schizophrenia. *Schizophrenia Bulletin*, **17**, 217–40.

Committee on the Safety of Medicines (1990). Cardiotoxic affects of pimozide. *Current Problems in Pharmacovigilance*, **29**, Medicines Control Agency.

Crow, T. J., Macmillan, J. F., Johnson, A. L. & Johnstone, E. C. (1986). The Northwick Park study of first episodes of schizophrenia. II. A randomised controlled trial of prophylactic neuroleptic treatment. *British Journal of Psychiatry*, **148**, 120–7.

Davis, J. M. (1975). Overview: maintenance therapy in psychiatry I. Schizophrenia. *American Journal of Psychiatry*, **132**, 1237–45.

Davis, J. M. (1976). Recent developments in the drug treatment of schizophrenia. *American Journal of Psychiatry*, **133**, 208–14.

de Beaurepaire, C., de Beaurepaire, R., Cleau, M. & Bornstein, P. (1993). Bromocriptine improves digit symbol substitution test scores in neuroleptic-treated chronic schizophrenic patients. *European Psychiatry*, **8**, 89–93.

Delva, J. J. & Letemendia, F. J. J. (1982). Lithium treatment in schizophrenia and schizoaffective psychosis. *British Journal of Psychiatry*, **141**, 387–400.

Fayen, M., Goldman, M. B. & Moulthrop, M. A. (1988). Differential memory function with dopaminergic and cholinergic treatment of drug-induced extrapyramidal effects. *American Journal of Psychiatry*, **145**, 483–6.

Fischer-Cornelsson, K. A. & Ferner, U. J. (1976). An example of European multicenter trials. Multispecial analysis of clozapine. *Psychopharmacology Bulletin*, **12**, 34–9.

Fleischhacker, W. W. & Hummer, M. (1997). Drug treatments of schizophrenia in the 1990s. *Drugs*, **53**, 915–29.

Fleischhacker, W. W., Roth, S. D. & Kane, J. M. (1990). The pharmacologic treatment of neuroleptic induced akathisia. *Journal of Clinical Psychopharmacology*, **10**, 12–5.

Hirsch, S. R., Gaind, R., Rohde, P. D., Stevens, B. C. & Wing, J. K. (1973). Outpatient maintenance of chronic schizophrenic patients with long acting fluphenazine: double blind placebo trial. *British Medical Journal*, **1**, 633–7.

Hirsch, S. R., Jolley, A. G., Barnes, T. R. E., et al. (1989). Dysphoric and depressive symptoms in chronic schizophrenia. *Schizophrenia Research*, **2**, 259–64.

Hoff, A. L., Shukla, S., Aronson, T., et al. (1990). Failure to differentiate bipolar disorder from schizophrenia on measures of neuropsychological function. *Schizophrenia Research*, **3**, 253–360.

Hogarty, G. E., Goldberg, S. C., Schooler, S. & Ulrich, R. F. (1974). Collaborative Study Group. Drugs and sociotherapy in the aftercare of schizophrenic patients. II. Two year relapse rates. *Archives of General Psychiatry*, **31**, 603–8.

Hoge, S. K., Appelbaum, P. S., Lawlor, T., et al. (1990). A prospective multicentre study of patients' refusal of antipsychotic medication. *Archives of General Psychiatry*, **47**, 949–56.

Idènpèèn-Heikkilè, J., Alhava, E., Olkinvora, M. & Palva, I. P. (1975). Clozapine and agranulocytosis. *Lancet*, **ii**, 611.

Idènpèèn-Heikkilè, J., Alhava, E. & Olkinvora, M. (1977). Agranulocytosis during treatment with clozapine. *European Journal of Clinical Pharmacology*, **11**, 193–8.

Jeste, D. V. & Wyatt, R. J. (1981). Changing epidemiology of tardive dyskinesia: an overview. *American Journal of Psychiatry*, **138**, 297–309.

Johnstone, E. C., Crow, T. J., Frith, C. D., Carney, M. W. P. & Price, J. S. (1978). Mechanism of the antipsychotic effect in the treatment of acute schizophrenia. *Lancet*, **i**, 848–51.

Johnstone, E. C., Crow, T. J., Ferrier, I. N., et al. (1983). Adverse effects of anticholinergic medication on positive schizophrenic symptoms. *Psychological Medicine*, **13**, 513–27.

Johnstone, E. C., Crow, T. J., Frith, C. D. & Owens, D. G. C. (1988). The Northwick Park 'functional' psychosis study: diagnosis and treatment response. *Lancet*, **ii**, 119–26.

Johnstone, E. C., Macmillan, J. F., Frith, C. D., Benn, D. K. & Crow, T. J. (1990). Further investigation of the predictors of outcome following first schizophrenic episodes. *British Journal of Psychiatry*, **157**, 182–9.

Johnstone, E. C., Crow, T. J., Owens, D. G. C. & Frith, C. D. (1991). The Northwick Park 'functional' psychosis study. Phase 2: Maintenance treatment. *Journal of Psychopharmacology*, **5**, 388–95.

Kane, J., Honigfeld, G., Singer, J. & Meltzer, H. (1988). Clozapine for the treatment-resistant schizophrenic: a double blind comparison versus chlorpromazine/benztropine. *Archives of General Psychiatry*, **45**, 789–96.

Kane, J. M. & Smith, J. M. (1982). Tardive dyskinesia: prevalence and risk factors 1959–1979. *Archives of General Psychiatry*, **39**, 473–81.

Klein, E., Bental, E., Lerer, B. & Belmaker, R. H. (1984). Carbamazepine and haloperidol v. placebo and haloperidol in excited psychoses: a controlled study. *Archives of General Psychiatry*, **41**, 165–70.

Krupp, P. & Barnes, P. (1992). Clozapine-associated agranulocytosis: risk and aetiology. *British Journal of Psychiatry*, **160 (suppl. 17)**, 38–40.

Lader, M. (1988). Beta-adrenoceptor antagonists in neuropsychiatry: an update. *Journal of Clinical Psychiatry*, **49**, 213–23.

Lavin, M. R. & Rifkin, A. (1991). Prophylactic antiparkinsonian drug use. I. Initial prophylaxis and prevention of extrapyramidal side effects. *Journal of Clinical Pharmacology*, **31**, 763–8.

Leff, J. P. & Wing, L. K. (1971). Trial of maintenance therapy in schizophrenia. *British Medical Journal*, **3**, 599–604.

Levinson, D. F. & Simpson, G. M. (1986). Neuroleptic induced extrapyramidal symptoms with fever. *Archives of General Psychiatry*, **43**, 839–48.

Lieberman, J. A. (1993). Understanding the mechanism of action of atypical antipsychotic drugs. A review of compounds in use and development. *British Journal of Psychiatry*, **163 (suppl. 22)**, 7–18.

Lieberman, J., Kane, J. & Johns, C. (1989a). Clozapine: guidelines for clinical management. *Journal of Clinical Psychiatry*, **50**, 329–38.

Lieberman, J. A., Saltz, B. L., Johns, C. A., Pollack, S. & Kane, J. (1989b). Clozapine effects on tardive dyskinesia. *Psychopharmacology Bulletin*, **25**, 57–62.

Lindström, L. H. (1988). The effect of long term treatment of clozapine in schizophrenia: a retrospective study of 96 patients treated with clozapine for up to 13 years. *Acta Psychiatrica Scandinavica*, **77**, 524–9.

Livingstone, M. G. (1994). Risperidone. *Lancet*, **343**, 457–60.

MacMillan, J. F., Crow, T. J., Johnson, A. L. & Johnstone, E. C. (1986). The Northwick Park study of first episodes of schizophrenia. II. Short-term outcome in trial entrants and trial eligible patients. *British Journal of Psychiatry*, **148**, 128–33.

Mann, S. C., Caroff, S. N., Bleier, H. R., Welz, W. K. R., Kling, M. A. & Hayashida, M. (1986). Lethal catatonia. *American Journal of Psychiatry*, **143**, 1374–81.

Marder, S. R. & Meibach, R. C. (1994). Risperidone in the treatment of schizophrenia. *American Journal of Psychiatry*, **151**, 825–35.

May, P. R. A., Dencker, S. J., Hubbard, J. W., Midha, K. K. & Lieberman, R. P. (1988). A systematic approach to treatment resistance in schizophrenic disorders. In *Treatment Resistance in Scizophrenia*, ed. S. J. Denker, & F. Kulharek, pp. 22–3. Vieweg. Braunschweig, Weisbaden.

McGlashan, T. H. & Carpenter, W. T. (1976). Post psychotic depression in schizophrenia. *Archives of General Psychiatry*, **33**, 231–9.

National Institute of Mental Health (1964). Pharmacology Service Center Collaborative Study Group. Phenothiazine treatment of acute schizophrenia. *Archives of General Psychiatry*, **10**, 246–61.

Nemecek, D., Rastogi Cruz, D. & Csernansky, J. G. (1993). Atropinism may precipitate neuroleptic malignant syndrome during treatment with clozapine. *American Journal of Psychiatry*, **150**, 1561.

Opler, L. A., Albert, D. & Ramirez, P. M. (1994). Psychopharmacologic treatment of negative schizophrenic symptoms. *Comprehensive Psychiatry*, **35**, 16–28.

Owens, D. G. C. (1990). Dystonia – a potential psychiatric pitfall. *British Journal of Psychiatry*, **156**, 620–34.

Owens, D. G. C. (1996). Adverse effects of antipsychotic agents. Do newer agents offer advantages? *Drugs*, **51**, 895–930.

Owens, D. G. C., Harrison Read, P. E. & Johnstone, E. C. (1994). L-dopa helps positive but not negative features of neuroleptic-insensitive chronic schizophrenia. *Journal of Psychopharmacology*, **8**, 204–12.

Peroutka, S. J. & Snyder, S. H. (1980). Relationship of neuroleptic drug effects at brain dopamine serotonin–adrenergic and histamine receptors to clinical potency. *American Journal of Psychiatry*, **137**, 1518–22.

Pogue-Geile, M. F. & Zubin, J. (1988). Negative symptomatology and schizophrenia. A conceptual and empirical review. *International Journal of Mental Health*, **16**, 3–45.

Povlsen, U. J., Noring, U., Fog, R. & Gerlach, J. (1985). Tolerability and therapeutic effect of clozapine: a retrospective investigation of 216 patients treated with clozapine for up to twelve years. *Acta Psychiatrica Scandinavica*, **71**, 176–85.

Remington, G. J. (1993). Clinical considerations in the use of risperidone. *Canadian Journal of Psychiatry*, **38 (suppl. 3)**, S96–S100.

Safferman, A., Lieberman, J. A., Kane, J. M., Szymanski, S. & Kinon, B. (1991). Update on the clinical efficacy and side effects of clozapine. *Schizophrenia Bulletin*, **17**, 247–61.

Shopsin, B., Klein, H., Aaronsom, M. & Collora, M. (1979). Clozapine, chlorpromazine and placebo in newly hospitalized acutely schizophrenic patients: A controlled double-blind comparison. *Archives of General Psychiatry*, **36**, 657–64.

Siris, S. G. (1993). Adjunctive medication in the maintenance treatment of schizophrenia and its conceptual implications. *British Journal of Psychiatry*, **163 (Suppl. 22)**, 66–78.

Siris, S. G., Morgan, V., Fagerstrom, R., Rifkin, A. & Cooper, T. B. (1987). Adjunctive imipramine in the treatment of post-psychotic depression: a controlled trial. *Archives of General Psychiatry*, **44**, 533–9.

Siris, S. G., Bermanzohn, P. C., Mason, S. E. & Shuwall, M. A. (1994). Maintenance imipramine therapy for secondary depression in schizophrenia. *Archives of General Psychiatry*, **51**, 109–15.

Small, J. G., Kellams, J. J., Milstein, V. & Moore, J. (1975). A placebo controlled study of lithium combined with neuroleptics in chronic schizophrenic patients. *American Journal of Psychiatry*, **132**, 1315–17.

Small, J. G., Milstein, V., Marhenke, J. D., Hall, D. D. & Kellams, J. J. (1987). Treatment outcome with clozapine in tardive dyskinesia, neuroleptic sensitivity and treatment-resistant psychosis. *Journal of Clinical Psychiatry*, **48**, 263–7.

Tamminga, C. A. & Lahti, A. C. (1996). The new generation of antipsychotic drugs. *International Clinical Psychopharmacology*, **11 (suppl. 12)**, 73–6.

Tandon, R., DeQuardo, J. R., Goodson, J., Mann, N. A. & Greden, J. F. (1992). Effect of anticholinergics on positive and negative symptoms in schizophrenia. *Psychopharmacology Bulletin*, **28**, 297–302.

Tuma, A. H. & May, P. R. A. (1979). And if that doesn't work what next? A study of treatment failures in schizophrenia. *Journal of Nervous & Mental Disease*, **167**, 566–71.

Van Praag, H. M., Korf, J. & Dols, L. C. W. (1976). Clozapine versus perphenazine: the value of the biochemical mode of action of neuroleptics in predicting their therapeutic activity. *British Journal of Psychiatry*, **129**, 547–55.

Wolf, M., Diener, J., Lajeunesse, C. & Shriqui, C. L. (1992). Low-dose bromocriptine in neuroleptic-resistant schizophrenia: a pilot study. *Biological Psychiatry*, **31**, 1166–8.

11

Social and psychological treatments

Introduction

Non-pharmacological treatments for schizophrenia (and other severe psychiatric disorders) are potentially important interventions for several reasons. Antipsychotic medication is only effective for positive symptoms in most patients, is of limited benefit for a substantial minority of sufferers, has practically no effect on negative symptoms, and has a limited impact on relapse rates. Perhaps more importantly, many patients prefer talking treatments to taking drugs, and most – regardless of response to neuroleptics – will require additional help to re-integrate socially.

Of course, any treatment requires convincing evidence of its effectiveness, clinical efficacy and preferably cost-effectiveness, before it can be routinely advocated for general use. The history of psychiatry, and medicine, provides many examples of apparently promising treatments, initially proclaimed to be dramatically effective, that have subsequently failed more rigorous testing. The use of haemodialysis in schizophrenia is one recent example (Carpenter et al., 1983), but there are also numerous psychosocial interventions with similar histories. Fortunately, clinical research in this area has moved on from using the case series as a means of justifying the use of scarce resources to using more acceptable methods, i.e. randomized controlled treatment trials (RCTs). It is now possible, therefore, to evaluate the evidence base for a number of social and psychological treatments for schizophrenia in an analogous way to determining whether a particular drug therapy is worthwhile or not.

In reviewing treatment studies, it is all too easy for those with strong opinions to describe studies that support their views and ignore those that don't. Systematic review methods, with specified criteria for study selection, are obviously preferable. This review is therefore based on studies identified in a particular way, as described below, and only includes RCTs and meta-analyses of RCTs. Non-randomized controlled trials are subject to biases that increase effect sizes (Altman, 1991) and are therefore only included when no RCTs are available. The literature reviewed in this chapter is confined to English language articles, and was identified through MEDLINE and the Cochrane database. Studies are described in chronological order of the development of each approach in the management of schizophrenia, as follows: psychotherapy, milieu treatments, cognitive-behavioural interventions and various approaches to care in the community.

Psychodynamic psychotherapy

Although Freud thought that psychoanalysis was not suitable for the treatment of schizophrenia, several enthusiasts used it as the mainstay of management in the first half of this century and many therapists still use it – albeit in combination with medication. This practice was not seriously challenged until a five year follow-up study of 228 randomized patients showed that those treated with psychotherapy alone (or 'milieu therapy') stayed longer in hospital than those treated with medication or electroconvulsive therapy (ECT), (May et al., 1981). The MEDLINE search identified only one other relevant RCT (Gunderson et al., 1984), but also found a systematic review describing an additional two studies published in books and psychotherapy journals (Mueser & Berenbaum, 1990). However, patients in these studies were not randomized to particular treatments. The May studies have been criticized for using inexperienced therapists, but the Gunderson study suffered from a very high drop-out rate of 42%. Otherwise, the latter was a well conducted examination of a 'reality-adaptive supportive' (RAS) treatment focusing on practical problems and an exploratory insight orientated (EIO) therapy; although the interpretation of results was somewhat biased. Gunderson found that EIO therapy was clearly inferior to RAS treatment in terms of re-hospitalization, vocational and social adjustment – but claimed the treatments were similarly effective because 'ego functioning' was superior in the EIO group (despite no statistical differences between treatments on measures of this). Furthermore, greater time in EIO was actually associated with poorer social adjustment, suggesting that it may even have been deleterious.

Psychodynamic psychotherapy cannot therefore be recommended for schizophrenia. It is an expensive, time consuming treatment for which, at best, there is no good evidence for efficacy and which, at worst, may be harmful. This may have been obvious to most readers but needs to be stressed for at least two reasons. Firstly, when Gunderson et al. (1984) were recruiting potential collaborators for their study, many refused to participate because they felt it would be unethical to withhold psychotherapy randomly from patients. Secondly, a recent survey of patients found that most preferred brief RAS type treatment (Coursey et al., 1995). Psychotherapists interested in schizophrenia would therefore be best advised to adopt this approach or consider implementing other more effective treatments, such as 'family therapy'.

Family interventions

The term 'family therapy' reveals more about the origins of this treatment than its effects. It is derived from observations that key relatives' hostility and criticism ('expressed emotion' or EE) towards patients is a potent determinant of relapse rate in schizophrenia (Brown et al., 1972). The treatment, now more accurately called 'an intervention', has from the beginning included basic education about the illness and its treatment, as well as more psychotherapeutically inclined attempts to improve family interactions, and has sometimes incorporated other techniques such as problem solving and crisis management. Not surprisingly, therefore, although there is now very good evidence for the efficacy and acceptability of such techniques, we still do not know what are the essential components of an effective family intervention.

In the first trial, Goldstein et al. (1978) randomized 104 acutely psychotic patients, most but not all in their first episode, to one of four therapies; either with/without crisis-oriented cognitive therapy and with either high or low dose depot fluphenazine. Stratification by pre-morbid adjustment and complicated data analysis makes interpretation of the results difficult, but six month relapse rates were greatest (48%) in the low dose no therapy group and lowest (0%) in the high dose family therapy treated subjects. Family therapy in particular appeared to reduce social withdrawal generally, but any initial benefits in poorly functioning males were lost after six months. Falloon et al. (1982) compared relapse rates after family therapy or outpatient support in 36 medicated outpatients. The therapy included illness education and 'behavioural methods of problem solving' in a bid to reduce patients and family stress, and led to reduced relapse rates (6% versus 44%), shorter hospitalization and lower levels of symptomatology that were sustained two years later (Falloon et al., 1987).

In a series of reports on high EE families randomized to education and relatives' groups or family sessions, Leff and co-workers reported that relapse rates were reduced for over two years in those who remained on medication and whose families were seen (Leff et al., 1982; 1985; 1989; 1990). The authors found some evidence that the family therapy worked by reducing EE and face to face contact, but the studies can be criticized for having poorer functioning patients in the original control group (1982), excluding two patients who committed suicide in the experimental group (1985), having no normal treatment control group (1989) and using results from more than one study (1990). Nonetheless, another British group has also found some support for the idea that such behavioural intervention for families may reduce relapse rates for up to two years, at least in high EE families, by reducing criticism and over involvement (Tarrier et al., 1988, 1989), whereas simply 'counselling' parents did not have statistically significant effects (Vaughan et al., 1992).

Three further trials have developed these findings. Hogarty and colleagues (1986) examined family psychoeducation and social skills training in 103 randomized patients with schizophrenia or schizo-affective psychosis from high-EE households. Relapse rates over one year were reduced by about 20% by both treatments, with an apparent additive effect. The authors concluded that some of the benefit was attributable to a reduction of EE, but that medication was essential for patients in persistently high EE households and that the family therapy effect was to delay rather than prevent relapse. A two-year follow-up study, however, showed that the social skills training effect attenuated after one year (Hogarty et al., 1991). Glick et al. (1993) reported that family education improved symptom ratings in patients for six months, especially for females, but that the benefit was reduced at 18 months. McFarlane and co-workers (1995a,b) took the novel approach of comparing single family and multiple family treatment settings. Medication compliance was equally high in both groups, but the multiple family groups reduced relapses to 16% (versus 27%) at two years (1995a) and 50% (versus 78%) at four years (1995b). However, a multiple family group without education had a similarly low four year relapse rate (57%), suggesting that at least the bulk of the benefit may have been attributable to simple family support.

Other studies have reported similar effects from family intervention in different countries – such as China (Xiong et al., 1994; Zhang et al., 1994) – and that the benefits may be attributable to additive medication and family intervention effects (Zhang et al.,1994) or to an increased sense of control in treated families (Solomon et al., 1996). However, some groups have also reported that family treatment may actually be disadvantageous for certain patients – by symptoms exacerbation in 'less acculturated' patients (Telles et al., 1995) or by causing more frequent relapses in low EE families (Linszen et al., 1996).

A recent meta-analysis of these studies, in the Cochrane database, found that family interventions convincingly reduce relapse rates by about 50% for up to two years, that medication compliance is similarly improved and that time in employment may also increase (Mari & Streiner, 1996). This applies regardless of whether patients are treated in their first (Goldstein et al., 1978; Zhang et al., 1994; Linszen et al., 1996) or subsequent episode, and whether educational groups are given to relatives only (Hogarty et al., 1986; Tarrier et al., 1988) or to patients as well. Mari & Streiner (1996) have calculated that about six families need to be treated to prevent one relapse, but thought that relatives may find this a more acceptable success rate than doctors. Three studies which have built economic analysis into trials have found overall cost savings of 20–50% (Falloon et al., 1982; Tarrier et al.,1988; Xiong et al., 1994; reviewed by Gabbard et al., 1997) and treatment drop-out rates are usually only about 10%.

In summary, therefore, family interventions are effective but may act by generally improving family interactions, specifically reducing criticism, encouraging appropriate expectations, enhancing family support, making families feel more involved with clinical decision making, and/or improving compliance with antipsychotic medication. This uncertainty, together perhaps with resource constraints and some clinicians' lack of enthusiasm for talking treatments, may account for the far from universal provision of such a service. It remains possible that a brief discussion of the illness and its management between the professional(s) involved, the patient and their family – ideally with further contact when necessary – is as effective (and perhaps less detrimental to some) as formal 'family therapy'. Future studies will need to examine these specific questions and determine the relative value of family interventions in care plans that may include other forms of psychosocial treatment.

Milieu therapies

This now rather outmoded term is nonetheless a convenient starting point for a brief description of psychosocial approaches to treatment within institutions in the past (such as 'social therapy' and the token economy) and their latter day developments into more specific treatments (such as social skills training and illness self-management) which are generally used in outpatient settings and have much in common with cognitive–

behavioural therapies. Discussion of these treatments is hindered by problems of nomenclature (e.g. in America social therapy is known as milieu therapy), the fact that few studies seem to compare similar interventions, and that there are very few RCTs. They generally appear to have been developed as a result of concerns that institutions could harm as well as benefit individuals and are associated with the active rehabilitation and 'open doors' policies of the 1950s. Therapeutic communities (where psychodynamically inclined social analysis was the main therapeutic tool) were idealistically and enthusiastically developed, for all psychiatric patients, during the permissive 1960s but the few remaining examples now essentially only treat those with personality disorders. Such enthusiasm had no need for evidence and there is accordingly very little of any kind.

Social therapy (where facilitating socialization is the main mode and aim of treatment) has a better record of evaluation. Hogarty et al. (1974a,b) examined the effects of what they called 'major role therapy' (MRT – consisting of social casework and vocational rehabilitation) on relapse rates and community adjustment after discharge from hospital. MRT enhanced adjustment in those who complied with medication, but did not reduce relapses and even worsened adjustment in those on placebo. The comparison of a 'milieu therapy' (which simply consisted of non-specific care in hospital), psychotherapy and/or drugs, and ECT by May et al. (1976, 1981) found that milieu treatment prolonged length of stay in hospital without improving subsequent outcome over 3–5 years. An early study from Hogarty's group (1979) found that social therapy and medication had additive effects in reducing relapse rates over two years. A more recent comparison (see details below) of social milieu treatment and social skills training favoured the latter, particularly in reducing negative symptoms (Dobson et al., 1995). Overall, therefore, there is little consensus as to the potential value of non-specific milieu or social treatments for schizophrenia.

A similar conclusion appears valid for token economy (TE) programmes. No RCTs were identified on MEDLINE, although one trial used a balanced order design to compare TE and daily supportive sessions in 22 patients with schizophrenia. Both were effective but TE was more time consuming than simple support (Marks et al., 1968). Milby (1975) reviewed the literature from controlled studies on inpatients with schizophrenia. TE did seem to improve some psychotic behaviours, personal care and work within hospitals but possible interactions with medication were rarely considered and adequate community follow-up data was lacking. A rare contemporary study, from China, evaluated TE, life skills training and encouragement as compared to simple participation in the same activities in 52 randomized chronic schizophrenics who had been in hospital for at least one year (Li & Wang, 1994). The experimental intervention did reduce negative symptoms at three months but similar limitations as with previous studies apply and TE may not have been an effective component. However, Bell and colleagues (1996) have recently produced some evidence that paid work, and increases in the number of hours worked, improved positive symptoms and reduced re-hospitalization rates over six months. Of course, it remains to be seen whether such a successful programme can be replicated and whether such apparent benefits would carry over into competitive employment.

Social skills training, on the other hand, has been well evaluated and appears to confer definite benefits on recipients. Two RCTs of 'group therapy' in schizophrenia, which put an emphasis on 'tasks of daily living' (Claghorn et al., 1974) and 'communication' (Malm, 1982), effectively enhanced insight and socialization. Spencer et al. (1983) have reported that 16 hours of treatment resulted in improved conversational skills in chronic schizophrenia which were maintained at two months follow-up, whereas an equivalent length of time in drama or group discusion did not. Hogarty et al. (1986, 1991) found an additive effect of social skills and family therapy over one year, albeit less marked at two years. As briefly mentioned above, Dobson et al. (1995) randomized 33 patients to social skills or milieu and found that social skills reduced negative symptoms at three months, albeit with some decline by six months follow-up. Most convincingly, a meta-analysis of 27 studies found that social skills training improves social skills as well as assertiveness, speeds discharge and possibly reduces relapse rates; with some evidence for both generalization and maintenance of skills (Benton & Schroeder, 1990). It would appear that the greatest remaining challenge for advocates of social skills in training is to identify the essential elements of therapy for brief interventions that can be routinely used in clinical practice.

In a randomized controlled evaluation of what they called illness self-management, Eckman and colleagues (1992) incorporated many elements of these social treatments into an intensive twice-weekly group programme over six months. This included video modelling, behavioural rehearsal, role playing, resource management and problem solving activities that were delivered with focused instructions, prompting and coaching by an active group leader. Generalization was facilitated by exercises and homework and then by weekly social skills training for a further six months. Compared to a similarly intense supportive psychotherapy group, the package resulted in improved medication and self management despite little definite change in symptom levels. The authors argue that such an approach can be used to overcome the cognitive deficits of schizophrenia, but concede that they selected relatively high functioning patients and analyzed the results without including the 25–43% of treatment drop-outs. Similarly, Linszen et al. (1996) have reported that an 'individual orientated psychosocial intervention', which included problem solving for identified stressors, was as effective in reducing relapses alone as in combination with a family intervention. These treatment approaches are good examples of how social treatments have merged into evolving cognitive behavioural strategies for treating schizophrenia.

Cognitive and behavioural treatments

Two specifically behavioural treatments have been evaluated by RCT in schizophrenia. In an examination of methods to increase independent behaviours, Goldstein et al. (1973) allocated 250 inpatients to modelling and/or instruction or neither. Instruction alone was as effective as the combination with modelling in the laboratory setting, but this was not tested in a more everyday situation. Pharr & Coursey (1989) examined the efficacy of muscle relaxation training via electromyographic (EMG) bio-feedback from the frontalis and forearm extensor muscles, as compared to progressive relaxation and no treatment, in 30 chronically hospitalized patients. Over six sessions, the patients receiving EMG training had signifi-cantly lower EMG recordings than both groups, and significantly im-proved on nurses' ratings of social competence and social interest. This observation, however, does not appear to have been taken any further.

The application of cognitive behavioural therapy (CBT) for schizo-phrenia is a comparatively new development, with only a handful of RCTs being found by the search strategies. Tarrier et al. (1993) randomly assigned 27 patients with residual positive symptoms after medication to coping strategy enhancement or problem solving, while a further 22 patients were assigned to a waiting list control condition. Both treatments reduced positive symptoms, with a suggestion that coping strategy enhancement was superior to problem solving, but there was no evidence for generaliz-ation to negative symptoms or social functioning. Hodel & Brenner (1994), however, found no definite benefits of several cognitive therapy techniques in 21 patients with schizophrenia in a mirror design study. Finally, Kemp et al. (1996) have suggested that CBT can be adapted to improve compli-ance with medication. Forty seven patients were randomized to four to six sessions of CBT or non-specific counselling and monitored for six months. CBT led to improved attitudes to and compliance with medication, greater insight into illness, and overall social functioning – all of which persisted over the follow-up period.

Another recent application of CBT principles is into cognitive remediation or neuropsychological rehabilitation programmes. Benedict et al. (1994) compared 16 patients who received 15 hours of computerized vigilance task training and 17 who received no treatment; although the training improved task performance, symptom levels were unchanged. In an interesting comparison of the effects of two card-sorting tasks on hallucination intensity, Gallagher et al. (1995) found that vocalizing the card colour led to greater improvements than simple card-sorting – suggesting that some aspect of producing a verbal response was more important than simple distraction. Similarly, another study has found that performance on the Wisconsin Card Sort Test could be improved by training on it (Vollema et al., 1995), although patients randomized to monetary reinforcement actually did less well and generalizability was not examined. Lastly, Corrigan et al. (1995) have compared the effects of a one hour session of vigilance, with or without memory training, on social cue recognition in 40 randomized patients and reported that combined training had greater benefits which were maintained 48 hours later.

Thus, cognitive techniques appear to have potential benefits on symptom levels, compliance and neuropsychological deficits and clearly merit and require more rigorous testing. For example, the relative importance of greater therapist attention, behavioural strategies that bypass deficits in memory and attention, and possible actual improvements in cognition need to be evaluated.

Community care

The final broad category of management approaches to schizophrenia is as much about the setting of treatment as what is actually provided. The psychiatric profession's interest in alternatives to hospitalization can be traced back to concerns about how to avoid institutionalization and implement social treatments. However, this has been given an added political and social imperative in the past five to ten years as a result of a small number of dramatic failures of community care, giving rise to more intensive approaches such as assertive community treatment and case management.

Several RCTs provide convincing evidence that there are many suitable alternatives to chronic hospitalization for acute psychiatric illness, although comparatively few studies have studied schizophrenia specifically (Hargreaves et al., 1977; Hoult & Reynolds, 1984; Burns & Raftery, 1991; Wiersma et al., 1991). Nonetheless, psychosis can generally be successfully treated: in open wards (Jin, 1994); with short inpatient stays (Glick et al., 1975; Hargreaves et al., 1977); day care (Glick et al., 1986; Wiersma et al., 1991, 1995); in the patient's home (Fenton et al., 1979, 1984; Hoult & Reynolds, 1984; Burns & Raftery, 1991; Muijen et al., 1992; Audini et al., 1994); and even in foster (Linn et al., 1977; Haveman & Maaskant, 1990) or residential homes (Dickey et al., 1986; Mosher et al., 1995). These studies have found that the outcome of such care is generally as good as hospital treatment and perhaps better for subsequent social adjustment, with only one exception (Linn et al., 1985), that overall costs may be cut and that patients and their relatives prefer these approaches (Fenton et al., 1979, 1984; Burns & Raftery, 1991; Wiersma et al., 1991). However, a substantial number of patients are simply too ill to be treated in these ways.

The more intensive approaches to community care (developed for frequent users of inpatient services and/or those at risk to themselves and others) suffer from a confusing array of similar terms and definitions. In general, assertive community treatment (ACT) refers to management by a multidisciplinary team of mental health professionals, with a high patient: staff ratio, who work with particular patients individually when their particular skills are called for – with an emphasis on 'assertive' means of compliance, facilitating independent living skills and avoiding hospital admissions if possible. Confusingly, this has in the past often been called 'intensive case management', whereas 'standard case management' or just 'case management' is used to describe a completely different approach. The principles of case management (CM) – and the care programme approach (CPA) – are that a designated 'keyworker' assesses needs, writes a care plan and regularly reviews progress in meeting those needs through the care obtained from a number of outside agencies. Unfortunately, CM and CPA for all patients with long-term psychiatric disorders have been imposed on mental health services by government directives in England (although such management remains flexibly applied in other parts of the UK) despite little evaluation, while ACT has been generally found beneficial in several studies but remains essentially unused.

In a comparison of ACT and CM in the USA, in a group of 105 mentally ill homeless patients leaving jail, it was found that re-incarceration was common in both groups, but the researchers noted that CM could easily deteriorate into simple monitoring rather than rehabilitation (Solomon et al., 1994). Essock & Kontos (1995) reported that ACT halved admissions and increased numbers with a permanent residence as compared to CM. Three further trials of intensive case management or community care (i.e. ACT) and standard care have all reported reduced inpatient service use, while also reducing overall care costs (Rosenheck et al., 1995; Quinlivan et al., 1995), as well as reducing the burden on relatives and increasing the patients' social networks (Aberg-Wistedt et al., 1995). The latter Swedish report was the only one to exclusively study patients with schizophrenia, but the equivalent performance of CM and a family management programme that actually increased symptoms in another study of schizophrenics (Telles et al., 1995) is in keeping with the other studies and suggests that their results can be generalized to schizophrenia. Further evidence for the ineffectiveness and possibly harmful effects of CM comes from a single British study of CPA implementation. Four hundred patients on a special needs register were randomized to close supervision by a nominated keyworker or to standard care. The CPA reduced loss from follow-up, but resulted in more admissions (Tyrer et al., 1995).

Final confirmation of the negative impression one gets of CM from these studies comes from a meta-analysis in the Cochrane database. Marshall et al. (1997), reviewing nine high quality studies, found that CM does lead to some increase in regular contact with patients, but that it also doubles the rates of admission to hospital and does not provide any definite improvements in symptom levels or social functioning. Clinicians are perhaps therefore best advised to apply standard CM to only the most vulnerable of their patients, to seek new approaches to CM or to try to secure adequate funding for implementing ACT (for which the original studies look generally positive and a meta-analysis is in preparation).

Conclusions

In summary, there appears to be good evidence that family interventions and social skills training offer definite benefits to patients with schizophrenia and their families, although the means of achieving these effects in routine clinical practice requires elucidation. It may be that suitably trained nurses, relatives and even recovered patients could provide such services more enthusiastically and less expensively than doctors. Various cognitive strategies and assertive community treatment look to have promising possibilities, but require further RCT testing; while psychotherapy, non-specific social treatments and case management appear to be of little value and may even worsen various aspects of the illness.

It is concerning that the development of various psychosocial management approaches has followed fashionable notions in psychology and sociology rather than objective evidence for their effectiveness. This has resulted in a substantial wastage of professional resources and patients' time. Fortunately, as this review demonstrates, latter day developments are generally being well evaluated – apart from the notable exception of some political directives – with the gold standard of medical experimentation, the randomized controlled trial.

References

Aberg-Wistedt, A., Cressell, T., Lidberg, Y., Liljenberg, B. & Osby, U. (1995). Two-year outcome of team-based intensive case management for patients with schizophrenia. *Psychiatric Services*, **46**, 1263–6.

Altman, D. G. (1991). Randomisation – essential for reducing bias. *British Medical Journal*, **302**, 1481–2.

Audini, B., Marks, I. M., Lawrence, R. E., Connolly, J. & Watts, V. (1994). Home-based versus out-patient/in-patient care for people with serious mental illness. Phase II of a controlled study. *British Journal of Psychiatry*, **165**, 204–10.

Bell, M. D., Lysaker, P. H. & Milstein, R. M. (1996). Clinical benefits of paid work activity in schizophrenia. *Schizophrenia Bulletin*, **22**, 51–67.

Benedict, R. H., Harris, A. E., Markow, T., McCormick, J. A., Nuechterlein, K. H. & Asarnow, R. F. (1994). Effects of attention training on information processing in schizophrenia. *Schizophrenia Bulletin*, **20**, 537–46.

Benton, M. K. & Schroeder, H. E. (1990). Social skills training with schizophrenics: a meta-analytic evaluation. *Journal of Consulting and Clinical Psychology*, **58**, 741–7.

Brown, G. W., Birley, J. L. T. & Wing, J. K. (1972). Influence of family life on the course of schizophrenic disorders. *British Journal of Psychiatry*, **121**, 241–58.

Burns, T. & Raftery, J. (1991). Cost of schizophrenia in a randomized trial of home-based treatment. *Schizophrenia Bulletin*, **17**, 407–10.

Carpenter, W. T. Jr., Sadler, J. H., Light, P. D., et al. (1983). The therapeutic efficacy of haemodialysis in schizophrenia. *New England Journal of Medicine*, **308**, 669–75.

Claghorn, J. L., Johnstone, E. E., Cook, T. H. & Itschner, L. (1974). Group therapy and maintenance treatment of schizophrenics. *Archives of General Psychiatry*, **31**, 361–5.

Corrigan, P. W., Hirschbeck, J. N. & Wolfe, M. (1995). Memory and vigilance training to improve social perception in schizophrenia. *Schizophrenia Research*, **17**, 257–65.

Coursey, R. D., Keller, A. B. & Farrell, E. W. (1995). Individual psychotherapy and persons with serious mental illness: the clients' perspective. *Schizophrenia Bulletin*, **21**, 283–301.

Dickey, B., Cannon, N. L., McGuire, T. G. & Gudeman, J. E. (1986). The Quarterway House: a two-year cost study of an experimental residential program. *Hospital & Community Psychiatry*, **37**, 1136–43.

Dobson, D. J., McDougall, G., Bucheikin, J. & Aldous, J. (1995). Effects of social skills training and social milieu treatment on symptoms of schizophrenia. *Psychiatric Services*, **46**, 376–80.

Eckman, T. A., Wirshing, W. C., Marder, S. R., et al. (1992). Technique for training schizophrenic patients in illness self-management: a controlled trial. *American Journal of Psychiatry*, **149**, 1549–55.

Essock, S. M. & Kontos, N. (1995). Implementing assertive community treatment teams. *Psychiatric Services*, **46**, 679–83.

Falloon, I. R., Boyd, J. L., McGill, C. W., Razani, J., Moss, H. B. & Gilderman, A. M. (1982). Family management in the prevention of exacerbations of schizophrenia: a controlled study. *New England Journal of Medicine*, **306**, 1437–40.

Falloon, I. R., McGill, C. W., Boyd, J. L. & Pederson, J. (1987). Family management in the prevention of morbidity of schizophrenia: social outcome of a two-year longitudinal study. *Psychological Medicine*, **17**, 59–66.

Fenton, F. R., Tessier, L. & Struening, E. L. (1979). A comparative trial of home and hospital psychiatric care: one-year follow-up. *Archives of General Psychiatry*, **36**, 1073–9.

Fenton, F. R., Tessier, L., Struening, E. L., et al. (1984). A two-year follow-up of a comparative trial of the cost-effectiveness of home and hospital psychiatric treatment. *Canadian Journal of Psychiatry*, **29**, 205–11.

Gabbard, G. O., Lazar, S. G., Hornberger, J. & Spiegel, D. (1997). The economic impact of psychotherapy: a review. *American Journal of Psychiatry*, **154**, 147–55.

Gallagher, A. G., Dinan, T. G. & Baker, L. V. (1995). The effects of varying information content and speaking aloud on auditory hallucinations. *British Journal of Medical Psychology*, **68**, 143–55.

Glick, I. D., Hargreaves, W. A., Raskin, M. & Kutner, S. J. (1975). Short versus long hospitalization: a prospective controlled study: III. Results for schizophrenic inpatients. *American Journal of Psychiatry*, **132**, 385–90.

Glick, I. D., Fleming, L., DeChillo, N., et al. (1986). A controlled study of transitional day care for non-chronically-ill patients. *American Journal of Psychiatry*, **143**, 1551–6.

Glick, I. D., Clarkin, J. F., Haas, G. L. & Spencer, J. H. Jr. (1993). Clinical significance of inpatient family intervention: conclusions from a clinical trial. *Hospital & Community Psychiatry*, **44**, 869–73.

Goldstein, A. P., Martens, J., Hubben, J., et al. (1973). The use of modeling to increase independent behavior. *Behaviour Research & Therapy*, **11**, 31–42.

Goldstein, M. J., Rodnick, E. H., Evans, J. R., May, P. R. & Steinberg, M. R. (1978). Drug and family therapy in the aftercare of acute schizophrenics. *Archives of General Psychiatry*, **35**, 1169–77.

Gunderson, J. G., Frank, A. F., Katz, H. M., Vannicelli, M. L., Frosch, J. P. & Knapp, P. H. (1984). Effects of psychotherapy in schizophrenia: II. Comparative outcome of two forms of treatment. *Archives of General Psychiatry*, **10**, 564–98.

Hargreaves, W. A., Glick, I. D., Drues, J., Showstack, J. A. & Feigenbaum, E. (1977). Short vs long hospitalisation: a prospective controlled study. VI Two-year follow-up results for schizophrenics. *Archives of General Psychiatry*, **34**, 305–11.

Haveman, M. J. & Maaskant, M. A. (1990). Psychiatric foster care for adult patients: results of a study in the Netherlands. *International Journal of Social Psychiatry*, **36**, 58–67.

Hodel, B. & Brenner, H. D. (1994). Cognitive therapy with schizophrenic patients: conceptual basis, present state, future directions. *Acta Psychiatrica Scandinavica*, **S384**, 108–15.

Hogarty, G. E., Goldberg, S. C., Schooler, N. R. & Ulrich, R. F. (1974a). Drug and sociotherapy in the aftercare of schizophrenic patients. II. Two-year relapse rates. *Archives of General Psychiatry*, **31**, 603–8.

Hogarty, G. E., Goldberg, S. C. & Schooler, N. R. (1974b). Drug and sociotherapy in the aftercare of schizophrenic patients. III. Adjustment of nonrelapsed patients. *Archives of General Psychiatry*, **31**, 609–18.

Hogarty, G. E., Schooler, N. R., Ulrich, R., Mussare, F., Ferro, P. & Herron, E. (1979). Fluphenazine and social therapy in the aftercare of schizophrenic patients. Relapse analyses of a two-year controlled study of fluphenazine decanoate and fluphenazine hydrochloride. *Archives of General Psychiatry*, **36**, 1283–94.

Hogarty, G. E., Anderson, C. M., Reiss, D. J., et al. (1986). Family psychoeducation, social skills training, and maintenance chemotherapy in the aftercare treatment of schizophrenia. I. One-year effects of a controlled study on relapse and expressed emotion. *Archives of General Psychiatry*, **43**, 633–42.

Hogarty, G. E., Anderson, C. M., Reiss, D. J., et al. (1991). Family psychoeducation, social skills training, and maintenance chemotherapy in the aftercare treatment of schizophrenia. II. Two-year effects of a controlled study on relapse and adjustment. *Archives of General Psychiatry*, **48**, 340–7.

Hoult, J. & Reynolds, I. (1984). Schizophrenia: A comparative trial of community orientated and hospital orientated psychiatric care. *Acta Psychiatrica Scandinavica*, **69**, 359–72.

Jin, Z. (1994). Effect of an open-door policy combined with a structured activity programme on the residential symptoms of schizophrenic in-patients. A six-month randomised controlled trial in Yanbian, Jilin. *British Journal of Psychiatry*, **24**, supplement, 52–7.

Kemp, R., Hayward, P., Applewhaite, G., Everitt, B. & David, A. (1996). Compliance therapy in psychotic patients: randomized controlled trial. *British Medical Journal*, **312**, 345–9.

Leff, J., Kuipers, L., Berkowitz, R., Eberlein-Vries, R. & Sturgeon, D. (1982). A controlled trial of social intervention in the families of schizophrenic patients. *British Journal of Psychiatry*, **141**, 121–34.

Leff, J., Kuipers, L., Berkowitz, R. & Sturgeon, D. (1985). A controlled trial of social intervention in the families of schizophrenic patients: two-year follow-up. *British Journal of Psychiatry*, **146**, 594–600.

Leff, J., Berkowitz, R., Shavit, N., Strachan, A., Glass, I. & Vaughn, C. (1989). A trial of family therapy v. a relatives group for schizophrenia. *British Journal of Psychiatry*, **154**, 58–66.

Leff, J., Berkowitz, R., Shavit, N., Strachan, A., Glass, I. & Vaughn, C. (1990). A trial of family therapy versus a relatives' group for schizophrenia. Two-year follow-up. *British Journal of Psychiatry*, **157**, 571–7.

Li, F. & Wang, M. (1994). A behavioural training programme for chronic schizophrenic patients. A three-month randomised controlled trial in Beijing. *British Journal of Psychiatry*, **524**, 32–7.

Linn, M. W., Caffey, E. M., Klett, C. J. & Hogarty, G. (1977). Hospital versus community/foster care for psychiatric patients. *Archives of General Psychiatry*, **34**, 78–83.

Linn, M. W., Gurel, L., Williford, W. O., et al. (1985). Nursing home care as an alternative to psychiatric hospitalization. A Veterans Administration cooperative study. *Archives of General Psychiatry*, **42**, 544–51.

Linszen, D., Dingemans, P., Van der Does, J. W., et al. (1996). Treatment, expressed emotion and relapse in recent onset schizophrenic disorders. *Psychological Medicine*, **26**, 333–42.

McFarlane, W. R., Lukens, E., Link, B., et al. (1995a). Multiple-family groups and psychoeducation in the treatment of schizophrenia. *Archives of General Psychiatry*, **52**, 679–87.

McFarlane, W. R., Link, B., Dushay, R., Marchal, J. & Crilly, J. (1995b). Psychoeducational multiple family groups: four-year relapse outcome in schizophrenia. *Family Process*, **34**, 127–44.

Malm, U. (1982). The influence of group therapy on schizophrenia. *Acta Psychiatrica Scandinavia*, (S) **297**, 1–65.

Mari, J. J. & Streiner, D. (1996). Family intervention for those with schizophrenia. In Schizophrenia Module of *The Cochrane Database of Systematic Reviews* [updated 02 December 1996]. ed. C. Adams, J. De Jesus Mari & P. White. Available in *The Cochrane Library* [database on disk and CDROM]. The Cochrane Collaboration; Issue 2. Oxford: Update Software; 1996. (See also: *Psychological Medicine*, (1994) **24**, 565–78 and *Evidence-based Medicine*, (1996. **1**, 121).

Marks, J., Sonoda, B. & Schalock, R. (1968). Reinforcement versus relationship therapy for schizophrenics. *Journal of Abnormal Psychology*, **73**, 397–402.

Marshall, M., Gray, A., Lockwood, A. & Green, R. (1997). Case management for people with severe mental disorders. In *Schizophrenia Module of The Cochrane Database of Systematic Reviews* [updated 02 December 1996], ed. C. Adams, J. De Jesus Mari & P. White. Available in *The Cochrane Library* [database on disk and CDROM]. The Cochrane Collaboration; Issue 1. Oxford: Update Software; 1997. Updated quarterly. (See also *Evidence-Based Medicine*, (1995) **1**, 30).

May, P. R., Tuma, A. H., Yale, C., Potepan, P. & Dixon, W. J. (1976). Schizophrenia – a follow-up study of results of treatment. *Archives of General Psychiatry*, **33**, 481–6.

May, P. R., Tuma, A. H., Dixon, W. J., Yale, C., Thiele, D. A. & Kraude, W. H. (1981). Schizophrenia. A follow-up study of the results of five forms of treatment. *Archives of General Psychiatry*, **38**, 776–84.

Milby, J. B. (1975). A review of token economy treatment programs for psychiatric inpatients. *Hospital & Community Psychiatry*, **26**, 651–8.

Mosher, L. R., Vallone, R. & Menn, A. (1995). The treatment of acute psychosis without neuroleptics: six-week psychopathology outcome data from The Soteria Project. *International Journal of Social Psychiatry*, **41**, 157–73.

Mueser, K. T. & Berenbaum, H. (1990). Psychodynamic treatment of schizophrenia: is there a future? *Psychological Medicine*, **20**, 253–62.

Muijen, M., Marks, I. M., Connolly, J., Audini, B. & McNamee, G. (1992). The daily living programme. Preliminary comparison of community versus hospital-based treatment for the seriously mentally ill facing emergency admission. *British Journal of Psychiatry*, **160**, 379–84.

Pharr, O. M. & Coursey, R. D. (1989). The use and utility of EMG biofeedback with chronic schizophrenic patients. *Biofeedback & Self Regulation*, **14**, 229–45.

Quinlivan, R., Hough, R., Crowell, A., Beach, C., Hofstetter, R. & Kenworthy, K.

(1995). Service utilization and costs of care for severely mentally ill clients in an intensive case management program. *Psychiatric Services*, **46**, 365–71.

Rosenheck, R., Neale, M., Leaf, P., Milstein, R. & Frisman, L. (1995). Multisite experimental cost study of intensive psychiatric community care. *Schizophrenia Bulletin*, **21**, 129–40.

Solomon, P., Draine, J. & Meyerson, A. (1994). Jail recidivism and receipt of community mental health service. *Hospital & Community Psychiatry*, **45**, 793–7.

Solomon, P., Draine, J., Mannion, E. & Meisel, M. (1996). Impact of brief family psychoeducation on self-efficacy. *Schizophrenia Bulletin*, **22**, 41–50.

Spencer, P. G., Gillespie, C. R. & Ekisa, E. G. (1983). A controlled comparison of the effects of social skills training and remedial drama on the conversational skills of chronic schizophrenic inpatients. *British Journal of Psychiatry*, **143**, 165–72.

Tarrier, N., Barrowclough, C., Vaughn, C., et al. (1988). The community management of schizophrenia. A controlled trial of a behavioural intervention with families to reduce relapse. *British Journal of Psychiatry*, **153**, 532–42.

Tarrier, N., Barrowclough, C., Vaughn, C., et al. (1989). Community management of schizophrenia. A two-year follow-up of a behavioural intervention with families. *British Journal of Psychiatry*, **154**, 625–8.

Tarrier, N., Beckett, R., Harwood, S., Baker, A., Yusupoff, L. & Ugarteburu, I. (1993). A trial of two cognitive-behavioural methods of treating drug-resistant residual psychotic symptoms in schizophrenic patients: I. Outcome. *British Journal of Psychiatry*, **162**, 524–32.

Telles, C., Karno, M., Mintz, J., et al. (1995). Immigrant families coping with schizophrenia. Behavioral family intervention v. case management with a low-income Spanish-speaking population. *British Journal of Psychiatry*, **167**, 473–9.

Tyrer, P., Morgan, J., Van Horn, E., et al. (1995). A randomised controlled study of close monitoring of vulnerable psychiatric patients. *Lancet*, **345**, 756–9.

Vaughan, K., Doyle, M., McConaghy, N., Blaszczynski, A., Fox, A. & Tarrier, N. (1992). The Sydney intervention trial: a controlled trial of relatives' counselling to reduce schizophrenic relapse. *Social Psychiatry & Psychiatric Epidemiology*, **27**, 16–21.

Vollema, M. G., Geurtsen, G. J. & van Voorst, A. J. (1995). Durable improvements in Wisconsin Card Sorting Test performance in schizophrenic patients. *Schizophrenia Research*, **16**, 209–15.

Wiersma, D., Kluiter, H., Nienhuis, F. J., Ruphan, M. & Giel, R. (1991). Costs and benefits of day treatment with community care for schizophrenic patients. *Schizophrenia Bulletin*, **17**, 411–19.

Wiersma, D., Kluiter, H., Nienhuis, F. J., Ruphan, M. & Giel, R. (1995). Costs and benefits of hospital and day treatment with community care of affective and schizophrenic disorders. *British Journal of Psychiatry*, **S**, **27**, 52–9.

Xiong, W., Phillips, M. R., Hu, X., et al. (1994). Family-based intervention for schizophrenic patients in China. A randomised controlled trial. *British Journal of Psychiatry*, **165**, 239–47.

Zhang, M., Wang, M., Li, J. & Phillips, M. R. (1994). Randomised-control trial of family intervention for 78 first-episode male schizophrenic patients. An 18 month study in Suzhou, Jiangsu. *British Journal of Psychiatry*, **S24**, 96–102.

12

Service provision: the economic perspective

Introduction

In all Western countries in recent years, regardless of the way in which health care is financed, the percentage of the gross domestic product allocated to health care expenditure has been increasing (Moscarelli, 1994; OECD, 1993). The rate of growth in real health care expenditure per person, however, has been steadily falling (Schieber & Poullier, 1989) and as governments have struggled to meet the ever increasing and competing demands for health care from within limited resources, there has been a growing awareness of the need both to control health care costs and to ensure that the resources which are available are used efficiently and cost-effectively.

In Britain, mental disorders are the largest contributor to the health care costs (Department of Health, 1991) and approximately 1.6% of the resources that are allocated to mental health are used to provide services for those who suffer from schizophrenia (Davies & Drummond, 1994). Irrespective, therefore, of whether services are hospital or community based considerable resources are currently being deployed in providing care for patients with schizophrenia and the magnitude of both the direct and the indirect costs associated with this condition are such that it is probably the most costly of all the mental illnesses which psychiatrists treat (Andreasen, 1991).

The substantial expenditure which is required in order to provide for patients with schizophrenia reflects both the epidemiology of the illness and the lack of efficacious treatments (Wasylenki, 1994); the majority of patients become unwell in early adult life, will remain significantly disabled as a result of both the positive and negative symptoms of the illness and will therefore require access to a range of services in the longer term.

Although the costs incurred in providing such services are indeed 'staggering' (Wasylenki, 1994), the direct treatment costs are only one of the factors which contribute to the heavy economic burden associated with the

238

illness. The indirect costs which result from lost productivity for the patient, their carers and society have consistently been shown to outweigh the service costs (Fein, 1958; Andrews et al., 1985; Davies & Drummond, 1990; Wyatt et al., 1995). The opportunity costs (the loss of gains which could have been expected had funds been available for investment elsewhere) and the intangible costs (the social and psychological costs experienced by patients and family members) are also considerable (Moscarelli & Capri, 1991; Andreasen, 1991).

In attempting to evaluate the costs associated with this illness, it is thus important to recognize that it is not only monetary considerations and the direct costs of treatment which are important. The effects which the illness and its treatment have had on the quality of life of both the patient and their family and the wider economic implications for society in providing care for those who have this condition must also be taken into account. Economic evaluations which fail to assess such costs may wrongly attribute changes in the magnitude of costs to a particular intervention, when in fact the burden of costs has merely been shifted from one sector to another (Weisbrod, 1983). Such limited evaluations may thus arrive at conclusions which are misleading (O'Donnell, 1991).

In the UK the National Health Service has undergone recent reforms (House of Commons, 1990) which have focussed attention upon economic issues. The role of purchaser has been separated from that of provider and an 'internal market' created. This has promoted an increased awareness of the importance and the value of economic evaluations in both service planning and the delivery of services. Those charged with responsibility for purchasing services must be able to prioritize competing therapies and to target resources at those individuals who will be expected to get the greatest incremental benefit per unit of additional costs. Thus, while purchasers do require data on the total economic burden associated with the illness, in itself such data is of limited value (Mooney et al., 1992). Additional information is needed on the effectiveness of health care programmes, their impact on health status and the cost-effectiveness of alternative services, especially at the margin. Those providing services also require accurate cost data on the resource implications of the care they are delivering, if they are to be able to provide services in an efficient and cost-effective manner (Hallam et al., 1994).

These issues are causing concern on a world wide scale to those attempting to deliver mental health services. In the UK, since the reforms it is clear that there is a need for those on both sides of the purchaser/provider split to have access to detailed information on the costs and the outcomes of care. It is also necessary for mechanisms to be developed which will enable the costs and the benefits of alternative means of providing health and social care services to be determined systematically and explicitly.

Although the need for such information has clearly been recognized there is scant evidence that an evaluative culture is developing (Freemantle et al., 1993). While there has been a steady growth in the number of economic analyses which have been conducted in recent years (Hurley, 1990) there have been relatively few cost-effectiveness studies on service provision. Those that have been conducted have focused on selected groups of patients, often for relatively short periods of time, and few have comprehensively assessed both direct and indirect costs.

In part, the lack of robust cost data which is currently available reflects the problems that are encountered in studying such a complex and chronic illness where as yet there is no possibility of a cure. Patients' symptoms vary considerably and it is therefore difficult to obtain a truly representative sample of individuals and to place research findings in a local context. Few indicators of outcome have been developed as it has proved problematic to identify, measure and value outcomes which are so varied and multidimensional in nature (Knapp et al., 1992). Researchers have therefore rarely employed a full range of outcome measures (Avison & Speechley, 1987) and have tended to focus on indicators of outcome which reflect service measures. The number of admissions or patients' lengths of stay are measures which while they may be easy to determine do not adequately reflect the effects of the illness upon both the patient's life and that of his/her relatives. The development of better measures of outcome and in particular measures which include an assessment of quality of life (Rosser & Kind, 1978; Heinrichs et al., 1984; Nord 1992; Wilkinson et al., 1992) would be a welcome advance in service evaluation.

At present, we still lack a clear understanding of the costs involved in caring for patients with schizophrenia, of the way in which costs relate to outcome and perhaps most importantly, given the current economic climate, of the potential benefits which may be gained by an increase in service expenditure or a change in the configuration of a service. Without such information it will not be possible to rank alternative interventions and to attempt to rationalize resources effectively. At both local and national levels therefore, there is a pressing need for more accurate and detailed cost and activity data, for a comprehensive database of evaluative studies to be established which can inform purchasing and resource allocation decisions and can guide providers so that they may operate more efficiently and effectively within a contracting environment.

Methods of economic evaluation

The aim of economic evaluations in service provision is to make the costs and the benefits related to choices more transparent and thus to enable informed decisions to be made on resource allocation (Capri, 1994).

If this aim is to be realized then the measures employed to determine costs should be broad and extended in time (Beecham et al., 1991). The evaluations of different methods of treatment must be based on an appraisal of all the services involved in patient care, of the actual outcomes in patients rather than on just the price of a particular treatment (Moscarelli et al., 1991).

There are four basic rules, therefore, in evaluating service provision (Knapp & Beecham, 1990). Firstly, the costing has to be comprehensive. It should include an assessment of the direct costs, which must now include an allowance for the capital costs of the buildings and the costs of the service infrastructure as well as the recurrent costs of the particular treatments (Andrews, 1991; Secretary of State, 1989). In addition to the direct costs, an assessment must also be made of the opportunity costs had resources been used elsewhere, the costs associated with lost productivity and of particular importance given the ongoing development of community care policies, the intangible costs of pain, suffering and lost opportunities borne by both patients and their relatives.

As well as identifying and measuring costs, the sources of variation in costs will need to be examined. It is important to ensure that, in evaluating alternative approaches to care, like is being compared with like, and that all costs are assessed in relation both to the needs of individual patients and to the outcomes associated with the care received. This applies particularly to a condition as heterogeneous as schizophrenia where average costings have been shown to be of limited value (Lang et al., 1997). In our study of service provision in an urban Scottish district, costs of care over a six month period were equivalent to the annual income of a person earning the proposed legal minimum wage; individual care costs ranged from less than 50% to more than 300% of this sum (Lang et al., 1997). Clearly, therefore, when evaluating the costs associated with the illness it is essential to disaggregate the data, to look within the data set for sources of variation and to relate and inter-relate the cost data to measures of need and outcomes in order to identify and to explain differences between patients (Beecham et al., 1991).

Prevalence and incidence based costing

In determining costs there are two approaches which can be taken. The easiest approach and the one which is most readily applied to a chronic condition such as schizophrenia is that of prevalence based costing; a cohort of individuals is identified and costs are determined over a defined period of time. Both the direct costs and the productivity losses are assigned to the years in which they occur and it is therefore possible to identify the major contributors to current expenditure.

A more informative approach is that of incidence based costing. Although often difficult to undertake, this method is to be preferred when evaluating a chronic condition such as schizophrenia where a life course perspective is essential for developing policies for financing care. Using an incidence based approach to costing, all present and future direct and indirect costs are assigned to the year in which the costs began. Future expenditures and lost productivity must thus be translated into current values using the technique of discounting. By means of incidence based costing it is possible to make predictions about the likely long-term impact of interventions (Capri, 1994) and this approach is therefore the most appropriate one to choose for the purposes of making decisions about which treatment to implement.

Study design

Cost of illness studies

The earliest attempt to assess the costs of schizophrenia took the form of descriptive, cost of illness studies (Fein, 1958). Such studies aim to determine the overall economic burden to society by identifying, valuing and then totalling the direct, indirect and intangible costs for a given treatment approach. Data are collected on a cohort of individuals and the results then extrapolated to a population of cases. Costing can be either incidence or prevalence based, but in assessing costs, no attempt is made to match costs to outcomes or to compare alternative uses of resources. Cost of illness studies are therefore of limited value when decisions are required on the allocation of resources between competing interventions.

Despite their limitations, cost of illness studies have provided valuable information on the expenditure which is being incurred in caring for patients with schizophrenia. Such studies have highlighted the wide variation which exists in individual care costs (Andrews et al., 1985; Davies & Drummond, 1994; Hallam et al., 1994; Knapp et al., 1990; Lang et al., 1997).

Clearly, therefore, average costs should be treated with caution and more detailed figures, especially lifetime estimates of costs, according to the severity of the disease, are required if future decisions on service planning and resource allocation are to be better informed.

If such information is to be obtained, more sophisticated methods of analysis must be employed whereby the sources of variation within costing totals can be determined, costs can be related to outcome and we can identify the particular characteristics of the subgroup of patients who are consuming the majority of the expenditure (Davies & Drummond, 1994; Lang et al., 1997), and for whom treatments which have the potential to reduce dependence and disability are most likely to have the largest impact on costs.

Cost–benefit and cost-effectiveness studies

Cost–benefit analysis and cost-effectiveness studies which incorporate the descriptive element of cost of illness methodology into an analytical frame-work are two methods of evaluation which can provide such detailed information.

In a cost–benefit study the aim is to compare all costs and outcomes across different interventions and to express them in monetary terms. In practice, this is difficult to do and attempts to value health consequences in this way have tended to fall into one of two categories. Individual or societal preference can be determined in terms of willingness to pay to obtain a benefit, to avoid a state of disability or conversely, willingness not to fund a treatment and thus to accept a loss or reduction in service. Alternatively an assessment can be made of human capital, that is a valuation of an individual's worth to society based on their present and future earnings. It is not always possible, however, to relate worth to productivity and this approach does tend to overestimate productivity losses as these are usually valued against average earnings. In response to such criticism a technique known as the friction cost method has been devised (Koopmanschap & Van Ineveld, 1992) whereby production losses are confined to the period needed to replace a sick worker, depending on the unemployment rate, the industrial and organizational structure of the economy and the labour market.

In valuing outcomes in a cost–benefit analysis it is also important to recognize that decisions on spending imply an expression of time prefer-ence and must therefore be subjected to discounting. It must also be borne in mind that while techniques of evaluation based on individuals' reports of willingness to pay for a treatment or to accept a loss of benefit may accurately reflect individual preferences, the application of such values to the wider public may be inappropriate.

Cost-effectiveness studies assess the most efficient way of achieving an objective and thus allow alternative forms of care to be evaluated. Recently this approach to evaluation has been further refined with the development of cost utility studies whereby the measures employed to determine outcome combine an assessment of both quantity and quality of life. Such measures therefore reflect individuals' preferences for health status and their judgements of the relative values of the outcome of interventions. At present cost utility analysis is the most sophisticated method of economic evaluation available to inform decisions on resource allocation.

Factors relating to cost

Untimately the most effective way of reducing the costs of schizophrenia would be to prevent it from occurring (McGuire, 1991). Currently, however, primary prevention is not possible. Given that we cannot reduce the incidence of the illness, reduction of expenditure and enhanced cost-effectiveness of services must depend upon the development of improved treatment and service provision in order to reduce relapse rates and minimise symptoms and levels of disability.

At present there are three aspects of patient care which have an impact on costs: relapse rates, current approaches to patient management and the use of antipsychotic medication.

Relapse prevention

In schizophrenia the occurrence of relapse depends upon two main factors:
– lack of treatment efficacy and patients' non-compliance with antipsychotic medication.

There is now a general consensus that 5–25% of patients are clinically unresponsive to standard antipsychotic therapy (Brenner et al., 1990), and monthly relapse rates of 3.5% per month for patients on maintenance neuroleptics have been reported (Weiden & Olfson, 1995). As many as 50% of patients may fail to comply with antipsychotic medication (Bebbington, 1995), non-compliance rates in community settings have been found to be of the order of 7.6% per month (Weiden & Olfson, 1995) and relapse rates of 11% per month have been reported in studies of patients who have discontinued medication (Weiden & Olfson, 1995).

Given such figures, it is perhaps not surprising that it has been estimated that about one half of the costs of schizophrenia could be saved through relapse prevention (Kissling, 1993) and the reduction in the use of inpatient care which could thus be achieved. Non-compliance is one of the main factors which contribute to the rehospitalization of frequently hospitalized patients (Green, 1988) and lack of treatment efficacy can account for as much as 60% of rehospitalization costs (Weiden & Olfson, 1995).

Both lack of efficacy and non-compliance therefore act synergistically on relapse and thus on patients' need for both hospital and community services. Considerable cost savings could thus be realized if it were possible to improve treatment efficacy and to combine advances in pharmacological approaches to patient management with educational programmes for patients and their families. These have been shown to be of benefit in improving compliance with maintenance medication (Penn & Mueser, 1996; Anderson & Adams, 1996; McFarlane et al., 1995; Kemp et al., 1996).

Current service provision

Although it is now generally accepted that the disadvantages of institutional care outweigh the advantages (Shepherd et al., 1996), patients are continuing to make significant use of inpatient services; 37% of schizophrenic patients in a recent study of service provision in Scotland had been treated in hospital on at least one occasion in the previous six months and 14% had spent the entire six months in hospital. (Lang et al., 1997).

Given such figures and the high costs associated with the provision of inpatient care, it is perhaps not surprising that inpatient care still accounts for the majority of the total costs incurred in managing the illness (Kiesler, 1982; Lang et al., 1997). As attempts have been made to increase community based services, therefore, there has been considerable research interest in evaluating both the costs and the benefits associated with approaches to patient management which are not hospital based and a growing awareness that the present distribution of expenditure often disguises the considerable contributions which other agencies are making to patient care (Kavanagh et al., 1995, Hallam et al., 1994).

The early studies which were conducted did conclude that community care was less expensive but they failed to take account of the costs and benefits to patients and their families (Cassell et al., 1972; Murphy & Datel, 1976; Sharfstein & Natziger, 1976). While the results of more recent work have clearly demonstrated that providing care outwith of hospital can be cost-effective (Goldberg, 1991; Hafner & an der Heiden, 1989; Knapp &

Beecham, 1990; Knapp et al., 1990; Dauwalder & Compi, 1995; William & Dickson, 1995), the cost savings are only of the magnitude of 4–25% (Marks et al., 1994) and although patients do not appear to have a poorer outcome when they are cared for in the community, any improvements in outcome are 'incremental rather than dramatic' (Burns & Santos, 1995).

The studies of alternatives to hospital treatment have in the main been conducted in one of two ways. The naturalistic approach has been to compare cohorts of patients in receipt of different programmes of care with regards to their social and clinical outcomes and then to relate these outcomes to the costs incurred. The alternative approach which has been adopted has been to randomly assign patients to different treatment programmes and then to compare the outcomes and costs associated with each (Goldberg, 1994). While from a scientific perspective such randomized controlled trials may be considered to be the 'gold standard', the results of these trials must be treated with caution as in practice when they are conducted in a psychiatric setting it is difficult for raters to be blind, and all the studies of this nature which have been undertaken have excluded many patients. It is therefore often difficult to determine to what extent, if any, the results of such trials can be generalized.

Three alternatives to traditional hospital care have been extensively evaluated; day care, often preceded by a short admission (Creed et al., 1991; Wiersma et al., 1991); home based care (Burns & Raftery, 1991; Burns et al., 1993; Knapp et al., 1994); and assertive community treatment (Weisbrod et al., 1980; Fenton et al., 1982; Hoult et al., 1984; Knapp et al., 1990; Marks et al., 1994).

While all three approaches to patient management have been shown to be cost-effective in comparison to the care that is hospital based, in some studies patient outcomes have not been significantly different when patients have been cared for in the community (Fenton et al., 1982; Burns et al., 1993; Knapp et al., 1990). In others the direct costs have been greater in the community programmes (Weisbrod et al., 1980) but these higher unit costs have been associated with higher levels of observed need, with greater achievements in reducing such need (Knapp & Beecham, 1990) and thus with an improvement in outcome. Innovations in service delivery, therefore, while they may initially generate greater treatment costs, can be better for society in the longer term (Goldberg, 1991).

Current policies mean that an increase in the number of patients with severe levels of disability who are cared for in the community and in hospital is to be anticipated and thus the average treatment costs in both settings will rise. In planning services, therefore, it cannot be assumed that today's money will buy the same services for tomorrow's clientele (Knapp, 1990). It is important that those patients whose care costs are greatest and who are responsible for the majority of the overall expenditure on service provision are identified in order that resources may be targeted efficiently and effectively.

More than just information on patient populations will be required. Limited understanding of community treatment programmes must also be addressed. Currently, although such treatments are known to be effective, there is little understanding of the basic assumptions which underlie the elements of the programmes (Knudson, 1996). We do not know which approaches should be targeted at which subgroups of patients, and for what period of time any one intervention should be provided.

Antipsychotic drugs

New pharmacological approaches to patient management, if they can treat patients symptoms more effectively and can minimize the side-effects associated with conventional neuroleptic drugs, may improve patients' compliance with medication, enable them to engage more readily with community services, and thus reduce relapse rates.

The atypical antipsychotic agents have been shown to be effective in a proportion of patients who respond poorly or not at all to traditional drugs (Kane et al., 1988; Meltzer et al., 1989) and are less likely to induce extrapyramidal side effects which commonly result in non-compliance (Van Putten, 1974). These preparations, however, while they may be a useful addition to patient care, are expensive in comparison with standard neuroleptics and it is therefore essential that their use is subject to rigorous economic evaluation.

Although medication accounts for only 5% of the direct costs of treating patients with schizophrenia (Davies & Drummond, 1994) and is therefore relatively inexpensive in comparison to the high costs of hospital care, the overall spend in the UK Health Service on medication is considerable (Office of Health Economics, 1992). It is therefore important that there is adequate data available, on both the costs of new products and the benefits which they may afford in patient care, to inform prescribing practice.

Of the atypical agents, clozapine has been the most widely studied and the research findings clearly illustrate the complex nature of the issues to be considered when evaluating such new products.

When it was launched in 1989 clozapine was 8–15 times more expensive than conventional neuroleptics due to the costs which were involved in patient monitoring. Understandably, the economic implications which it was envisaged would arise were the drug to be introduced into routine clinical practice caused considerable alarm (Griffith, 1990; Salzman, 1990). Since then, however, it has been possible to reduce the monitoring costs and studies have shown that the administration of clozapine can afford a better outcome for some patients in terms of psychopathology (Meltzer, 1992; Brier et al., 1994), social and cognitive functioning (Jonsson & Walinder, 1995; Hagger et al., 1993), and quality of life (Meltzer et al., 1990; Meltzer et al., 1993; Davies & Drummond, 1993) and that patients treated with this drug are less likely to develop tardive dyskinesia (Lieberman et al., 1991). There is also some evidence to suggest that clozapine may be associated with reduced suicide rates (Meltzer & Okayli, 1995) and data provided by the manufacturers indicate that the majority of patients once established on maintenance treatment comply in the longer term (Sandoz, 1996).

While it may be argued that the package of management associated with the hospital administration of clozapine, which involves regular assessments of the patient and blood monitoring, enhances the benefits afforded by the drug itself the use of clozapine has been associated with the return to the community of patients previously resident in hospital (Lindström, 1988).

Although this drug is still more expensive than conventional neuroleptics, the savings which it produces in hospital costs (Revicki et al., 1990; Meltzer et al., 1993; Reid et al., 1994) have been shown in some circumstances to at least balance the costs of community care and of clozapine itself (Davies & Drummond, 1993: Matheson, 1994). In determining cost-effectiveness, however, discharge rates and dose regimen are crucial; it has been estimated that if the discharge rate falls below 16% or the average dose is more than 300 mg per day, then the drug will no longer be cost-effective. (Davies & Drummond, 1993). Furthermore, it now appears that it may be some time before the full benefits of the treatment are realized (Jonsson & Walinder, 1995). Initially, therefore, there may be some patients who need additional outpatient support or continue to require inpatient treatment and in the short-term, at least, the use of clozapine may increase the average care costs and thus not appear to be cost-effective (Lang et al., 1997).

Administrators who are concerned with immediate cost, may thus require some persuasion to look beyond the immediate financial implications which will result from the use of the drug and may need considerable encouragement to 'reset their drug cost thermostat' in order that sufficient additional funds can be made available or existing budgets restructured to finance the use of such new products (Reid, 1994).

Conclusions

In schizophrenia, analyses of costs and management patterns are particularly important given the considerable degree of suffering associated with the illness and the heavy and enduring economic burden experienced by patients, their families and society (Moscarelli & Capri, 1991).

Despite the growing awareness of the contribution which such analyses can make to decision making they are not, as yet, undertaken as a matter of routine and the economic data which are available do not reflect the diversity of treatment approaches or the differences which exists between patients.

In evaluating service provision, therefore, there are still many challenges to be overcome; practical approaches to health needs assessment must be developed. Mechanisms are required by which performance monitoring and standard setting, which are as yet poorly developed (Frank & Huskamp, 1996), can be improved and robust indicators of outcome need to be devised. Only then will it be possible to ensure that we are investing in those interventions which yield the maximum health gain per unit of expenditure and that we are therefore deploying the resources that are available to their best effect.

Given the present level of demand for health care and the finite resources that are available in all countries it is inevitable that at all levels of decision making choices will have to be made. While UK government policies currently place much emphasis on the active involvement of local people in decision making (NHS Executive, 1992), concern has been expressed that those with the least power and ability to press their case will be disadvantaged. No clear guidance has been given as to how it may be possible to resolve the conflicts which will arise between what the public want and what can be afforded and between the lay and professional perceptions of what constitutes the optimum allocation of resources.

The British press recently highlighted a case where a 10 year old girl (Child B) suffering from lymphoblastic leukaemia had treatment withheld. Both the parents and the public were evidently outraged by this medical decision. Such differences in opinion on the use of resources often arise as a result of public's misperception that when clinicians decide to withhold a treatment that they are doing so not on clinical grounds but on the basis of the cost. This may in part reflect the way in which such high profile cases are reported in the media and in the case of 'Child B', while the national newspapers varied greatly in the way in which they covered the story (Entwistle et al., 1996), headlines such as 'Condemned by bank balance' (*The Sun*, 11th March 1995), 'A price too high to pay' (*Daily Mirror*, 11th March 1995) undoubtedly fuelled public concern that it was on financial grounds that the child was being denied the care that she 'needed'.

Thus while increased public involvement in debates on health care may be desirable, it would seem that ways of informing the public, other than through the media, will need to be found if the public are to be provided with an appropriate understanding of the complexity of the issues involved when decisions are to be made on treatment and resource allocation.

Even were such informed debate to be possible, human nature being what it is, it would still be likely that there would be cases such as that of 'Child B' where in the face of objective evidence to the contrary, the public would demand that treatment be given. Economic evaluations, no matter how sophisticated, cannot fully capture the devastating human dimensions of an illness and in seeking to develop an optimal service it is important to recognize that economic efficency is only one of the objectives which should be pursued, and that consideration must also be given to issues of equity and humanity (Jefferson et al., 1996).

Such comprehensive evaluations, however, will not bring about improvements in care unless the findings of such analyses are translated into clinical practice. This may be difficult to achieve. Advances in knowledge have always been slow to be incorporated into clinical practice, the majority of interventions which have been developed have not been scientifically proven (Black, 1984; Cochrane, 1972; Eddy & Billings, 1988) and it has long been recognized that individual clinicians differ considerably in the way in which they treat patients with similar or identical conditions.

If the best use of scarce resources is to be made then such variations in clinical practice require measurement and challenge. Ideally this should be achieved by there being a strong collaboration between clinicians and economists. To date, however, although economists have been convinced of the value of involving all those concerned with patient care in service evaluation (Williams, 1980; Mooney, 1986), clinicians have been very reluctant to acknowledge the need for their work to be economically appraised and have tended to view any attempts to do so with much suspicion, fearing that such exercises represent an attempt on the part of managers and planners to cut existing budgets.

If there is to be any prospect of developing an evaluative culture then clinicians will have to rethink their views and reappraise their attitudes to clinical freedom. Economic evaluations involving clinicians are likely to be beneficial. If clinicians are not proactive, then they may find themselves in a situation where purchasers will use their power to lever changes in clinical practice by insisting on evaluations and refusing to fund inefficient practices (Maynard, 1993). The age of the economist has now dawned and may well last for some time.

References

Anderson, J. & Adams, C. (1996). Family intervention in schizophrenia. *British Medical Journal*, **313**, 232–6.

Andreasen, N. C. (1991). Assessment issues and the cost of schizophrenia. *Schizophrenia Bulletin*, **17**, 475–81.

Andrews, G. (1991). The cost of schizophrenia revisited. *Schizophrenia Bulletin*, **17**, 389–94.

Andrews, G., Hall, W., Goldstein, G., Lapsley, H., Barlets, R. & Silove, D. (1985). The economic costs of schizophrenia. *Archives of General Psychiatry*, **42**, 537–43.

Avison, W. R. & Speechley, K. N. (1987). The discharged psychiatric patient: a review of social, social-psychological and psychiatric correlates of outcome. *British Journal of Psychiatry*, **144**, 10–18.

Bebbington, P. E. (1995). The content and context of compliance. *International Clinical Psychopharmacology*, **9 (5)**, 41–50.

Beecham, J., Knapp, M. & Fenyo, A. (1991). Costs, needs and outcomes. *Schizophrenia Bulletin*, **17**, 427–39.

Black, A. D. (1984). *An Anthology of False Antithesis* (*Rock Carling Fellowship*). London: Nuffield Provincial Hospitals Trust.

Brenner, H. D., Dencker, S. J., Goldstein, M. J., et al. (1990). Delivering treatment refractoriness in schizophrenia. *Schizophrenia Bulletin*, **16**, 557–62.

Brier, A., Buchanan, R. W., Kirkpatrick, B., et al. (1994). Effects of clozapine on positive and negative symptoms in outpatients with schizophrenia. *American Journal of Psychiatry*, **151**, 20–6.

Burns, T. & Raftery, J. (1991). Cost of schizophrenia in a randomised trial of home-based treatment. *Schizophrenia Bulletin*, **17**, 407–10.

Burns, B. J. & Santos, A. B. (1995). Assertive community treatment: an update of randomized trials. *Psychiatric Services*, **46**, 669–75.

Burns, T., Raftery, J., Beadsmore, A., McGuigan, S. & Dickson, M. (1993). A controlled trial of home based psychiatric services. II Treatment patterns and costs. *British Journal of Psychiatry*, **163**, 55–61.

Capri, S. (1994). Methods for evaluation of the direct and indirect costs of long-term schizophrenia. *Acta Psychiatrica Scandinavica*, **89 (382)**, 80–3.

Cassell, W. A., Smith, C. M., Grunberg, F., Boan, J. A. & Thomas, R. F. (1972). Comparing costs of hospital and community care. *Hospital and Community Psychiatry*, **23**, 197–200.

Cochrane, A. L. (1972). *Effectiveness and Efficiency: Random Reflections on Health Services*. London: Nuffield Provincial Hospitals Trust.

Creed, F., Black, D., Anthony, P., et al. (1991). Randomised controlled trial of day and inpatient psychiatric treatment. *British Journal of Psychiatry*, **158**, 183–9.

Dauwalder, J. P. & Cimpi, L. (1995). Cost-effectiveness over 10 years. A study of community-based social psychiatric care in the 1980s. *Social Psychiatry and Psychiatric Epidemiology*, **38 (4)**, 171–84.

Davies, L. M. & Drummond, M. F. (1990). The economic burden of schizophrenia. *Psychiatric Bulletin*, **14**, 522–5.

Davies, L. M. & Drummond, M. F. (1993). Assessment of costs and benefits of drug therapy for treatment-resistant schizophrenia in the United Kingdom. *British Journal of Psychiatry*, **162**, 38–42.

Davies, L. M. & Drummond, M. F. (1994). Economics and schizophrenia: the real cost. *British Journal of Psychiatry*, **165 (25)**, 18–21.

Department of Health. (1991). *The Health of the Nation*, **Cm 1523**, London: HMSO.

Eddy, D. M. & Billings, J. (1988). The quality of medical evidence. *Health Affairs*, **7 (1)**, 19–32.

Entwistle, W. A., Watt, S. I., Bradbury, R. & Pehl, L. J. (1996). Media coverage of the child B case. *British Medical Journal*, **312**, 1587–91.

Fein, R. (1958). *The Economics of Mental Illness*. New York: Basic Books.

Fenton, F. R., Tessier, L., Contandriopoulos, A. P., et al. (1982). A comparative trial of home and hospital psychiatric treatment: financial costs. *Canadian Journal of Psychiatry*, **27**, 177–87.

Frank, R. G. & Huskamp, H. A. (1996). Shaping national policy: delegation and decentralisation of mental health care. *Current Opinion*, **9**, 171–4.

Freemantle, N., Watt, I. & Mason, J. M. (1993). Developments in the purchasing process in the NHS: towards an explicit politics of rationing. *Public Administration*, **71 (4)**, 535–48.

Goldberg, D. (1991). Cost-effectiveness studies in the treatment of schizophrenia: a review. *Social Psychiatry and Psychiatric Epidemiology*, **26**, 139–42.

Goldberg, D. (1994). Cost-effectiveness in the treatment of patients with schizophrenia. *Acta Psychiatrica Scandinavica*, **89 (382)**, 89–92.

Green, J. H. (1988). Frequent rehospitalisation and non-compliance with treatment. *Hospital and Community Psychiatry*, **39**, 963–6.

Griffith, E. E. H. (1990). Clozapine: problems for the public sector (letter). *Hospital and Community Pscychiatry*, **41**, 337.

Hafner, G. & an der Heiden, W. (1989). Effectiveness and cost of community care for schizophrenia patients. *Hospital and Community Psychiatry*, **40**, 59–63.

Hagger, C., Buckley, P., Kenny, J. T., et al. (1993). Improvement in cognitive functions and psychiatric symptoms in treatment-refractory schizophrenic patients receiving Clozapine. *Biological Psychiatry*, **34**, 702–12.

Hallam, A., Beecham, J., Knapp, M. & Fenyo, A. (1994). The costs of accommodation and care – community provision for former long-stay psychiatric hospital patients. *European Archives of Psychiatry and Clinical Neurosciences*, **243**, 304–10.

Heinrichs, D. W., Hanlon, T. E. & Carpenter, W. T. (1984). The quality of life scale; an instrument for rating the schizophrenic deficit syndrome. *Schizophrenia Bulletin*, **10**, 388–98.

Hoult, J., Rosen, A. & Reynolds, I. (1984). Community orientated treatment compared to psychiatric hospital orientated treatment. *Social Science and Medicine*, **18**, 1015–20.

House of Commons. (1990). *The National Health Service and Community Care Act*. London: HMSO.

Hurley, S. (1990). A review of cost-effectiveness analysis. *Medical Journal of Australia*, **153**, 20–3.

Jefferson, T., Demicheli, V. & Mugford, M. (1996). Elementary Economic Evaluation in Health Care. *British Medical Journal*, Publishing Group, BMA House, Tavistock Square: London.

Jonsson, D. & Walinder, J. (1995). Cost-effectiveness of clozapine treatment in therapy-refractory schizophrenia. *Acta Psychiatrica Scandinavica*, **92**, 199–201.

Kane, J., Honigfield, G., Singer, J., et al. (1988). Clozapine for the treatment-resistant schizophrenic *Archives of General Psychiatry*, **45**, 789–96.

Kavanagh, S., Opit, L., Knapp, M. & Beecham, J. (1995). Schizophrenia: shifting the balance of care. *Social Psychiatry and Psychiatric Epidemiology*, **30**, 206–12.

Kiesler, C. A. (1982). Mental hospitals and alternative care: non institution-alisation as a potential public policy for mental patients. *American Psychologist*, **37**, 349–60.

Kemp, R., Hayward, P., Appelwhaite, G., et al. (1996). Compliance therapy in psychotic patients: random controlled trial. *British Medical Journal*, **312**, 345–9.

Kissling, W. (1993). The importance of relapse prevention. *9th World Congress of Psychiatry Abstracts*. *World Congress of Psychiatry*, 208.

Knapp, M. (1990). The direct costs of community care of chronically mentally ill people. In *Comprehensive Mental Health Care*, ed. J. H. Henderson. London: Gaskell.

Knapp, M. & Beecham, J. (1990). Costing mental health services. *Psychological Medicine*, **20**, 893–908.

Knapp, M., Beecham, J., Anderson, J., et al. (1990). The TAPS Project: Predicting the community costs of closing down mental hospitals. *British Journal of Psychiatry*, **157**, 661–70.

Knapp, M., Cambridge, P., Thomson, C., Beecham, J., Allen, C. & Darton, R. (1992). *Care in the Community: Challenge and Demonstration*. Aldershot: Ashgate.

Knapp, M., Beecham, J., Kontsogeorgopolou, V., et al. (1994). *A Controlled Study of Home Versus Hospital Based Care for People with Serious Mental Illness: Service Use and Costs. PSSRU Discussion paper OP969/2*. Canterbury: PSSRU.

Koopmanschap, M. A. & Van Ineveld, B. M. (1992). Towards a new approach for estimating indirect costs of disease. *Social Science and Medicine*, **34**, 1005–10.

Knudsen, H. C. (1996). Rehabilitation and care of mentally ill patients. *Current Opinion*, **9**, 167–70.

Lang, F. H., Forbes, J. F., Murray, G. D. & Johnstone, E. C. (1997). Service provision for patients with schizophrenia. I. A clinical and economic perspective. *British Journal of Psychiatry*, **171**, 159–63.

Lieberman, J. A., Saltz, B. L., Johns, C. A., et al. (1991). The effects of Clozapine on tardive dyskinesia. *British Journal of Psychiatry*, **158**, 503–10.

Lindström, L. (1988). The effect of long term treatment with Clozapine in schizophrenia: a retrospective study in 96 patients treated with Clozapine for up to 13 years. *Acta Psychiatrica Scandinavica*, **77**, 524–9.

Marks, I. M., Connolly, J., Muijen, M., Audini, B., McNamee, G. & Lawrence, R. E. (1994). Home-based versus hospital care for people with serious mental illness. *British Journal of Psychiatry*, **165**, 179–94.

Matheson, L. A. (1994). Value for money – care for patients with schizophrenia. *British Journal of Medical Economics*, **71**, 25–34.

Maynard, A. (1993). Never mind the quality, count the numbers. *Health Service Journal*, **103 (5343)**, 21.

McFarlane, W. R., Link, B., Dushay, R., Marshal, J. & Crilly, J. (1995). Psychoeducational multiple family groups: four year relapse outcome in schizophrenia. *Family Process*, **34 (2)**, 127–44.

McGuire, T. G. (1991). Measuring the economic costs of schizophrenia. *Schizophrenia Bulletin*, **17**, 375–88.

Meltzer, H. Y. (1992). Dimensions of outcome with Clozapine. *British Journal of Psychiatry*, **160 (17)**, 46–53.

Meltzer, H. Y. & Okayli, G. (1995). Reduction of suicidality during clozapine treatment of neuroleptic resistant schizophrenia: impact on risk–benefit assessment. *American Journal of Psychiatry*, **182**, 183–90.

Meltzer, H. Y., Bastani, B., Young Koon, K., Ramirez, L. F., Burnett, S. & Sharpe, J. (1989). A prospective study of clozapine in treatment resistant schizophrenic patients. 1. Preliminary Report. *Psychopharmacology*, **99**, 68–72.

Meltzer, H. Y., Burnett, S., Bastani, B., et al. (1990). Effect of six months of clozapine treatment on the quality of life of chronic schizophrenic patients. *Hospital and Community Psychiatry*, **41**, 892–7.

Meltzer, H. Y., Cola, P., Way, L., et al. (1993). Cost-effectiveness of Clozapine in neuroleptic-resistant schizophrenia. *American Journal of Psychiatry*, **150**, 1630–8.

Mooney, G. H. (1986). *Economics, Medicine and Health Care*. Brighton: Wheatsheaf Books.

Mooney, G. H., Hall, H., Donaldson, C. & Gerard, K. (1992). Re-weighing heat. *Journal of Health Economics*, **11(2)**, 105–215.

Moscarelli, M. (1994). Health and economic evaluation in schizophrenia: implications for health policies. *Acta Psychiatrica Scandinavica*, **89 (382)**, 84–8.

Moscarelli, M. & Capri, S. (1991). The cost of schizophrenia: editor's introduction. *Schizophrenia Bulletin*, **17**, 367–73.

Moscarelli, M., Capri, S. & Neri, L. (1991). Cost evaluation of chronic schizophrenic patients during the first 3 years after the first contact. *Schizophrenia Bulletin*, **17**, 421–6.

Murphy, J. G. & Datel, W. E. (1976). A cost-benefit analysis of community versus institutional living. *Hospital and Community Psychiatry*, **27**, 165–70.

NHS Management Executive. (1992). *Local Voices: The Views of Local People in Purchasing for Health*, January 1992.

Nord, E. (1992). Methods for quality adjustment of life years. *Social Science and Medicine*, **34**, 559–69.

O'Donnell, O. (1991). Cost-effectiveness of community care for the chronic mentally ill. In *Evaluation of Comprehensive Care for the Chronic Mentally Ill*, ed. H. Freeman & J. Henderson. London: Gaskell.

Office of Health Economics. (1992). *Compendium of Health Statistics*. London: Office of Health Economics.

Organisation for Economic Co-operation and Development. (1993). *OECD Health Data*. Paris: OECD.

Penn, D. & Mueser, K. (1996). Research update on the psychosocial treatment of schizophrenia. *American Journal of Psychiatry*, **153**, 607–17.

Reid, W. H. (1994). The treatment of psychosis: resetting the drug cost 'thermostat'. *Journal of Clinical Psychiatry*, **55 (B)**, 166–8.

Reid, W. H., Mason, M. & Toprac, M. (1994). Saving in hospital bed stays related to treatment with clozapine. *Hospital and Community Psychiatry*, **45**, 261–4.

Revicki, D. A., Luce, B. R., Washler, J. M., et al. (1990). Cost-effectiveness of clozapine for treatment-resistant schizophrenic patients. *Hospital and Community Psychiatry*, **41**, 850–4.

Rosser, R. & Kind, P. (1978). A scale of valuation of states of illness: is there a social consensus? *International Journal of Epidemiology*, **7 (4)**, 347–58.

Salzman, C. (1990). Notes from a state mental health director's meeting on Clozapine. *Hospital and Community Psychiatry*, **41**, 838–9, 842.

Sandoz Pharmaceuticals. (1996). Data on File (1) Sandoz Pharmaceuticals (UK) Ltd, December 1996.

Schieber, G. J. & Poullier, J. P. (1989). International health-care expenditure trends. *Health Affairs*, **8 (3)**, 169–77.

Secretary of State for Health, Wales, Northern Ireland and Scotland. (1989). *Working for Patients*. London: HMSO.

Sharfstein, S. S. & Natziger, J. C. (1976). Community care: costs and benefits for a chronic patient. *Hospital and Community Psychiatry*, **27**, 171–3.

Shepherd, G., Muijen, M., Dean, R. & Cooney, M. (1996). Residential care in hospital and in the community – quality of care and quality of life. *British Journal of Psychiatry*, **168**, 448–56.

Van Putten, T. (1974). Phenothiazine – induced compensation. *Archives of General Psychiatry*, **30**, 102–5.

Wasylenki, D. A. (1994). The cost of schizophrenia. *Canadian Journal of Psychiatry*, **39 (2)**, 65–9.

Weiden, P. J. & Olfson, M. (1995). Cost of relapse in schizophrenia. *Schizophrenia Bulletin*, **21**, 419–29.

Weisbrod, B. A. (1983). A guide to benefit cost analysis as seen through a controlled experiment in treating the mentally ill. *Journal of Health Politics, Policy and Law*, **7 (4)**, 809–45.

Weisbrod, B. A., Test, M. & Stein, L. (1980). An alternative to mental hospital treatment: II economic benefit cost analysis. *Archives of General Psychiatry*, **37**, 400–5.

Wiersma, D., Kluiter, H., Nierihuis, F., et al. (1991). Costs and benefits of day treatment with community care for schizophrenic patients. *Schizophrenia Bulletin*, **17**, 411–19.

Wilkinson, G., Williams, B., Krekonan, H., McLees, S. & Falloon, I. (1992). QUALY'S in mental health: a case study. *Psychological Medicine*, **22**, 725–31.

William, R. & Dickson, R. A. (1995). Economics of schizophrenia (review) *Canadian Journal of Psychiatry*, **40 (2)**, 60–7.

Williams, A. H. (1980). Health economics: the end of clinical freedom? *British Medical Journal*, **297**, 1183–6.

Wyatt, R. J., Hunter, I., Leary, M. C. & Taylor, E. (1995). An economic evaluation of schizophrenia, *Social Psychiatry and Psychiatric Epidemiology*, **30**, 196–205.

13

Legal and ethical issues

The definition and diagnosis of psychiatric disorders, as well as their treatment, have long been the subject of philosophical debate and continue to give rise to ethical concerns. Legal considerations play an increasing role in influencing the delivery of psychiatric services. The importance of these issues is intensified by current concerns about the management of individuals with active major mental illness, who may be perceived as socially undesirable, difficult or dangerous, but who are no longer closely supervised. They are living outside of the confines of large, seemingly entirely safe and suitably distant state run mental hospitals (for these are no longer available) and now reside in the almost mythical, widely discussed but still undefined 'community'. Historically, attitudes about the origins of mental illness and towards the care of those suffering from such disorders has swung dramatically from custodial warehousing to wholesale asylum, to the 'open door' liberalization of hospitals and now to care in the community. Along the way there have been periods of great enlightenment, but also times when the mentally ill have tended to be criminalized and in some parts of the world they are still. They have been isolated from society as a whole and deprived of basic rights and considerations. During its evolution modern psychiatry has had to face challenges from many quarters in order to maintain standards of care for some of the most damaged and deprived individuals alive. Even nowadays there is a tendency, reflected in the media, to reject those affected by mental illness, particularly when they are most disturbed. This applies not only to the general population but also at times, to professional groups and even those concerned with mental health care themselves (Lewis & Appleby, 1988).

This chapter explores just some aspects of the current legal and ethical issues raised by the diagnosis and treatment of patients with mental disorders, in particular schizophrenia, and especially in relation to compulsory care, civil liberties and the right to treatment.

The mentally ill are, in general, set apart from the majority of those with other forms of ailment by virtue of the very nature of the disorder from which they suffer in that in many instances it can impair insight and affect judgement. This is nowhere more the case than in relation to major psychotic disorders where these disabilities may lead to the necessity for confinement and treatment against the patient's expressed wishes. This has been one of the reasons for the emergence of a specific, and in some places extensive, legal framework governing compulsory measures of care in such circumstances which also offer the protection of important rights to both service users and providers. Historically the perception of the mentally ill has been dependent upon the predominant religious culture and tradition, as well as upon the work of social reformers, and standards of treatment have evolved accordingly. For a long time, little consideration was given to the rights of the sufferer as an individual citizen. Thus there was no perceived need for legal, or any other forms of safeguard (Gostin, 1977) for those considered not only to be 'lunatics' but also dangerous. Now civil compulsory commitment standards throughout much of the world are enshrined in statutory law. These take a wide variety of different forms (Curran & Harding, 1978). The majority of those have been formulated or revised in the most recent past and are founded on the premise that each individual has the right to voluntary, non-coercive treatment for psychiatric disorder with due consent. In addition, however, many provide for compulsory measures given certain prescribed limits, including confinement, deprivation of liberty, together with loss of some other civil rights and responsibilities and even the imposition of physical treatments if judged to be necessary, all ultimately against the will of the individual.

The assumption that mental disorder is linked in some of its forms to an inability to recognize one's own need for care and treatment has been, and continues to be, challenged. The status of mental illness itself, so called 'sanity' and 'insanity', has been questioned and examined in detail, particularly in this context, throughout the second half of the twentieth century. The very nature of psychiatric practice and diagnosis has been extensively considered and some people (often called anti-psychiatrists) still hold the view that psychiatrists and psychiatry exist solely as a result of the apparent need to maintain the social and moral status quo. Those holding such views consider that psychiatric practice sanctions the medicalization of normal personal and interpersonal phenomena and in particular identifies and marginalizes those who exhibit aberrant behaviour which is in fact simply the product of every day human diversity (Szasz, 1974; Reich, 1976). Psychiatric 'diagnosis' has been variously described as a means of alleviating guilt, avoiding responsibility, obtaining reassurance, imposing punishment, dehumanizing or excluding (Reich, 1981). Nevertheless, one of the basic beliefs of anti-psychiatry, namely that without physical evidence of disease none exists, except in the mind of the physician in the form of this 'diagnosis', has increasingly been shown to be incorrect, perhaps most convincingly of all in the case of schizophrenia with the emergence of more and more compelling evidence for the presence of specific structural and functional abnormalities associated with the symptoms, signs and course of the condition (Johnstone et al., 1976; Weinberger & Kleinman, 1986; see Chapter 5). Despite this, and specifically as a result of concerns over civil rights arising out of a range of issues, there continues to be a powerful lobby in favour of the abolition of compulsory measures for the treatment of psychiatric disorder. This is centred upon the notion that in many if not all cases, the basis on which individuals are frequently first compelled to be in hospital against their will is really the differences (identified consciously or otherwise) between the 'patient' and socially acceptable norms, and also the dislike of the psychiatrist for the individual concerned. It is implied that rather than a true illness having been identified and then found to require containment or compulsory treatment, psychiatric 'diagnosis' follows the decision to confine and control essentially as a means of justifying the action (Szasz, 1987). In reality huge efforts have been put into improving classificatory systems and the diagnostic process for mental disorders over the past 30 or more years and this has resulted in highly sophisticated systems for making very clearly defined diagnoses (World Health Organization, 1992; American Psychiatric Association, 1994).

Major mental illnesses such as schizophrenia, with all the evidence which now clearly supports their existence as in effect just another manifestation of the anatomical and physiological abnormalities associated with any other autonomous disease process, continue to ravage the lives of sufferers and carers alike and they impose huge burdens upon health and social services and, for some patients, necessitate treatment of a very particular nature in specific settings unique in the spectrum of health care facilities (Fraser, 1994). It is generally believed that both the restrictive and facilitative aspects of statutory mental health legislation need to inform practice and provide structure and guidance for professionals as well as safeguards for patients (Gostin, 1986). It is essential that the care of vulnerable, damaged and seriously ill people who, unable to look after themselves or appreciate the degree to which they are affected by their illness, should be carefully and comprehensively monitored and governed. This is perhaps best done by those who are not intimately concerned with the provision of treatment. Specialist mental health workers should, however, understand the need and rationale for such structures and their effective policing, which needs to be independent but practical. Supervisory systems ought not be so daunting as to be limiting, over prescriptive or adversarial but should seek to protect the rights of all those concerned and in particular address the needs of individual patients, particularly those deprived of the right to choose for themselves, either by others or by the severity of their illness.

In recent times it seems that the balance has swung away again from the civil libertarian view that each individual had the right, to some extent at least, to determine his or her own fate, mentally ill or not. It might be argued that a more restrictive view has gradually emerged and seems increasingly to predominate. This is evidenced by the introduction of more and more legislation placing certain limits and sanctions upon patients including those restored to life outside of hospital and by the high expectations of mental health professionals and the heavy and sometimes impractical responsibilities placed upon them (Mental Health (Patients in the Community) Act 1995). This apparent change has arisen out of the situation existing in the UK and the United States, where the vast asylums of the earlier part of this century have gradually dwindled in size and population with advances in treatment, standards of care, social change and expectations. Only recently has there been the realization that for some mentally ill people the concept of asylum, even in the form that it had taken previously, might be in some way positive. It might be important, comforting, even helpful and possibly necessary if not altruistically desirable, or suitable to satisfy the most sensitive of social consciences. Some authorities now question the ability of drastically reduced hospital based services to care adequately for the most seriously mentally unwell (Coid, 1996; Mechanic, 1994; Okin, 1995) and this has been reflected in very recent times in the way the political climate has changed to embrace the idea of a 'spectrum' of care implying a range of services, rather than a single, somewhat rigid and impracticable ideal intended to provide for a whole range of different circumstances at different points in time (Eastman, 1995). In the United States a great deal of concern has centred upon the issue of overall policy in mental health care programmes, particularly in the light of state responsibility for services and the differences which may exist as a result (Rochefort, 1996).

Schizophrenia is an illness which does indeed impair insight at times and is associated with disturbed and occasionally dangerous behaviour (Johnstone et al., 1991; Humphreys et al., 1992), but which can usually be effectively treated given time and the right circumstances. Compulsory measures must sometimes form a part of that spectrum of care. In the same way that facilities for care and treatment of the mentally unwell vary across the world so too are there quite considerable differences of emphasis in the law relating to the care of the mentally disordered in different countries and jurisdictions, even where the underlying principles, definitions and standards are essentially similar. These differences reflect a combination of historical factors, societies' attitudes to the mentally ill and practical matters such as the availability of services. As examples of such differences, the Mental Health Act 1983 which applies to England and Wales, defines the term 'mental disorder' very broadly for the purposes of compulsory admission for assessment only but requires the presence of one of four more clearly specified categories, mental illness, mental impairment, severe mental impairment or psychopathic disorder, to be identified for the purposes of an order which then allows actual treatment to be imposed (Mental Health Act 1983). The use of short term urgent measures for compulsory admission is discouraged under this same Act and seldom used. In contrast the situation which applies to Scotland is that the equivalent provision, emergency detention for up to 72 hours, has become the main means by which formal admission is pursued. Furthermore, mental disorder is defined even less precisely in the Scottish legislation and is all that is required to enable treatment to be enforced once a further period of detention is deemed necessary after the initial three days (Mental Health (Scotland) Act 1984). In the United Kingdom as a whole, in addition to the presence of some form of mental disorder, there is a requirement before an individual may be detained that they should require care in the interests of their own health or safety or for the protection of other people. There is not, however, as there is in many parts of the United States, a formal requirement to consider potential dangerousness. This may be an immensely important issue for patients suffering from schizophrenia (Humphreys et al., 1992; Johnstone et al., 1991). The only place in which an explicit consideration of the threat which the dangerously mentally ill person might pose in a more general sense in the United Kingdom is found within the provision for the care of those involved in criminal proceedings and even then only in relation to a court's deliberations over whether special restrictions should be placed on the individual's future movements and eventual discharge from hospital.

In some parts of the world compulsory admission is still the norm for the majority, if not all, of psychiatric hospital patients. In others all compulsory admissions must be sanctioned by an independent psychiatrist and elsewhere agreed by a magistrate or a judge.

Leaving aside civil detention the fact is that the mentally disordered sometimes commit offences (see Chapter 9) and this may be particularly so for those with schizophrenia. This not only has practical implications in terms of the need for specialist resources, but poses major ethical questions. Should the individual be charged in the first place, given the presence of a mental illness, or even appear in court at all? If he (or she) does appear is he/she fit to be there and can he/she understand the legal procedure and what might be expected of him/her? Can we assess how their illness influenced his/her actions at the time of commission of the offence and how it affected his/her responsibility for his/her behaviour? Should he/she be punished in the same way as someone in similar circumstances who is mentally well? Practice varies even within the same jurisdiction and courts may proceed very differently dependent upon a whole range of matters, legal precedent, public interest or simple expediency and the need to deal with a particular case quickly. Even where a mentally disordered offender appears before a court in very similar circumstances but at different times in a different political climate or a separate legal framework the outcome may not be the same at all. In some states or countries psychiatrists are content to address psychiatric issues alone and resist the temptation to speculate on matters such as guilt, criminal responsibility or the expression of remorse, but in others they are happy to be drawn into speculation about areas such as this. As a result, courts become confused and lawyers come to expect guidance, or press for opinions in areas where the psychiatric witness has no expertise or experience beyond that of the person in the street. Pronouncements that he/she makes in these circumstance may have a profound effect, not only on the judge and jury, but also on the life of the person in the dock.

There is a danger of blurring the boundaries between the need for care and treatment on the one hand, and on the other, a requirement for some form of retribution to be exacted through the criminal justice system where the person concerned has come before a court and been convicted of a serious offence. The two do not sit comfortably together (Bean, 1986) and while there is, quite rightly, a reluctance to sentence the mentally ill to prison (Verdun-Jones, 1989), the alternatives may be even more restrictive (Ashworth & Gostin, 1985). Maximum security psychiatric hospitals, which for many might be the only available alternative, are not without their own problems (Report of the Committee of Enquiry into Complaints about Ashworth Hospital; Bluglass, 1992; Hamilton, 1985). The great majority of those detained in such hospitals are suffering primarily from schizophrenic illness (Maden et al. 1995; Thompson et al., 1997). Many of them may be incarcerated for years 'without limit of time'. They subsequently carry the stigma not only of mental illness as well as offending behaviour but also of commitment to a high security facility. The process of rehabilitation and reintegration into society, already severely compromised by an illness of particularly malignant course with violent or antisocial behaviour, is thus further compounded.

The idea of self-determination and control over one's own life in the case of patients with serious psychotic disorders is compromised not only by legal provision and control but sometimes by medical paternalism. The idea that the doctor knows best not only goes with the use of compulsory powers, but actually underlies the whole concept of involuntary treatment. Arguably this is reflected most clearly in the apparent ignorance on the part of doctors in general, but more particularly psychiatrists themselves, of the law and how it affects their practice. There is increasing evidence from all over the world that psychiatrists' knowledge of statutory provision for care, detention and treatment of mentally disordered patients is lacking (Peske & Wintrob, 1974), and that this may not simply be due to lack of training or failure in understanding, but is equally likely to be the result of complacency (Affleck et al., 1978). This is borne out by the fact that the deficiencies identified are irrespective of seniority or experience and seemingly present however straightforward and simple the law itself might be. In the first systematic studies of psychiatrists' knowledge of mental health legislation undertaken in the United Kingdom there was clear evidence that those in training as well as senior practitioners were limited in terms of their detailed knowledge (Humphreys, 1994). This extended not only to the more complex parts of the relevant legislation, but included an inability to describe accurately basic definitions, simple terminology and provision for urgent compulsory admission and emergency, potentially life-saving treatment (Humphreys, 1998). Of equal concern in relation to this work was the fact that so few of these doctors, who were regularly using the legislation, and admit patients compulsorily to hospital, and enforce treatment, were not only willing to admit that they had never read the relevant Act, but seemed unashamed of this.

There is evidence from elsewhere that in making decisions about compulsory hospitalization, doctors act very much on the basis of 'needs' rather than 'rights' (Schwartz et al., 1984). In doing so, more often than not they reach the correct conclusions and pursue the right course of action (Soothill et al., 1990), frequently remaining within the bounds of the law (Lidz et al., 1989). In many ways though psychiatrists are in the unique position of having to operate within clear statutory confines in a particular area of their practice and whatever else they do must be able to justify their actions not simply in clinical terms, but in those imposed by the law as well. The responsibility, but also the power, afforded to the practitioner is difficult to over-emphasize.

One of the problems arising out of the reduction in psychiatric hospital facilities is the fact that even though in the judgement of the clinician a patient suffering from a serious mental illness may be unable to care for her/himself adequately and require treatment in hospital, no place is available for him/her. This is an increasingly common scenario in parts of the United Kingdom and is further complicated when the patient is unwilling to agree to informal admission to hospital and compulsory measures have to be considered. It is difficult to justify detaining someone against their will if there is nowhere for them to go. However up to date and potentially effective mental health legislation might be, its value is limited by lack of facilities for care. In addition the issue of whether a patient is, or is not, competent to make the decision to agree to informal admission to hospital, particularly if deluded, seriously depressed or intellectually handicapped, has recently become an issue of great concern to psychiatrists in the United States. This has centred on the fact that it might be wrongly assumed since patients suffering from a psychotic illness or other serious form of disorder do not actively oppose voluntary hospitalization, that they are in agreement with it. A further question is whether or not they have the legal capacity to give consent to informal admission. Paradoxically, assuming a fairly stringent test of competency was applied in each case, it is possible that this might lead to a dramatic increase in the number of patients formally detained. This problem persists although various approaches have been explored in an attempt to alleviate the obvious difficulties, including the possibility of reducing the degree of mental capacity required for agreement to informal inpatient care. This runs the risk, however, of being seen as simply a matter of convenience and a way not only of undermining the rights of those mentally ill people who warrant hospital care, but also of reinforcing the paternalism and power of the detaining doctors and undermining the gravity and importance of the whole process. One only has to observe for a short period the care of moderately disturbed patients who initially seem agreeable to being in hospital who then, for whatever reason, become equivocal or change their mind about remaining there, to understand that it may very well be much easier in those circumstances to make the individual subject to formal detention than to attempt to continue to build a trusting relationship and maintain their informal legal status. The reasons for imposing one's own will upon a mentally ill individual in these and many other situations are highly complex and the decisions which relate to whether or not an individual should be detained against their will are sometimes arbitrary and unrelated to strict legal, or even clinical considerations. On occasions heavy reliance must be placed upon professional standards and integrity, as well as independent scrutiny.

There are many ethical and legal issues which impinge upon the care of those with mental disorder, especially those with a psychotic illness, the most common of these being schizophrenia. It is evident that there must be adequate legal provision and protection for patients and professionals alike, but that these are of little value without adequate training and balanced and responsible attitudes to the care of patients who are, or may be, incapable of caring for themselves.

References

Affleck, G. G., Peske, M. A. & Wintrob, R. M. (1978). Psychiatrists' familiarity with legal statutes governing emergency involuntary hospitalisation. *American Journal of Psychiatry*, **135**, 205–9.

American Psychiatric Association. (1994). *Diagnostic and Statistical Manual of Mental Disorders*, 4th edn. Washington, DC: American Psychiatric Association.

Ashworth, A. & Gostin, L. (1985). Mentally disordered offenders and the sentencing process. In *Secure Provision*, ed. L. Gostin, pp. 211–35. London: Tavistock Publications.

Bean, P. (1986). *Mental Disorder and Legal Control*. Cambridge: Cambridge University Press.

Bluglass, R. (1992). The special hospitals. *British Medical Journal*, **305**, 323–4.

Coid, J. W. (1996). Dangerous patients with mental illness: increased risks warrant new policies, adequate resources, and appropriate legislations. *British Medical Journal*, **312**, 965–9.

Curran, W. J. & Harding, T. W. (1978). *The Law and Mental Health: Harmonising Objectives*. Geneva: World Health Organization.

Eastman, N. (1995). Anti-therapeutic community mental health law. *British Medical Journal*, **310**, 1081–2.

Fraser, K. (1994). Resource requirements in forensic psychiatry. *Journal of Forensic Psychiatry*, **5**, 478–82.

Gostin, L. (1977). *A Human Condition*. London: MIND.

Gostin, L. (1986). *Mental Health Services – Law and Practice*. London: Shaw & Sons Ltd.

Hamilton, J. R. (1985). The special hospitals. In *Secure Provision*, ed. L. Gostin, pp. 84–125. London: Tavistock Publications.

Humphreys, M. S. (1994). Junior psychiatrists and emergency compulsory detention in Scotland. *International Journal of Law and Psychiatry*, **17**, 421–9.

Humphreys, M. S. (1998). Consultant psychiatrists' knowledge of mental health legislation in Scotland. *Medicines, Science and the Law*, (in press).

Humphreys, M. S., Johnstone, E. C., Macmillan, J. F. & Taylor, P. J. (1992). Dangerous behaviour preceding first admissions for schizophrenia. *British Journal of Psychiatry*, **161**, 501–5.

Johnstone, E. C., Crowe, T. J., Frith, C. D., Husband, J. & Kreel, L. (1976). Cerebral ventricular size and cognitive impairment in chronic schizophrenia. *Lancet*, **II**, 924–6.

Johnstone, E. C., Leary, J., Frith, C. D. & Owens, D. G. C. (1991). Disabilities and circumstances of schizophrenic patients – a follow up study. VII: Police Contact. *British Journal of Psychiatry*, **159 (Suppl. 13)**, 37–9.

Lewis, G. & Appleby, L. (1988). Personality disorder: the patients psychiatrists dislike. *British Journal of Psychiatry*, **153**, 44–9.

Lidz, C. W., Molvy, F. P., Applebaum, P. S. & Cleveland, S. (1989). Commitment: the consistency of clinicians and the use of legal standards. *American Journal of Psychiatry*, **146**, 176–81.

Maden, T., Curle, C., Meux, C., Burrows, S. & Gunn, J. (1995). *Treatment and Security Needs of Special Hospital Patients*. London: Whurr Publishers.

Mechanic, D. (1994). Integrating mental health into a general health care system. *Hospital and Community Psychiatry*, **45**, 893–7.

Mental Health Act (1983). London: HMSO.

Mental Health (Scotland) Act (1984). London: HMSO.

Mental Health (Patients in the Community) Act. (1995). London: HMSO.

Okin, R. L. (1995). Parity is not enough. *Hospital and Community Psychiatry*, **46**, 211.

Peske, M. A. & Wintrob, R. M. (1974). Emergency commitment – a transcultural study. *American Journal of Psychiatry*, **131**, 36–40.

Reich, W. (1976). Brainwashing, psychiatry and the law. *Psychiatry*, **39**, 400–3.

Reich, W. (1981). *Psychiatric Diagnosis as an Ethical Problem in Psychiatric Ethics*, ed. S. Block & P. Chodoff. Oxford: Oxford University Press.

Report of the Committee of Enquiry into Complaints about Ashworth Hospital, (1992). Vol. I + II. London: HMSO.

Rochefort, D. A. (1996). Mental health reform and inclusion of the mentally ill: dilemmas of US policy-making. *International Journal of Law and Psychiatry*, **19**, 223–37.

Schwartz, H. I., Applebaum, P. S. & Kaplan, R. D. (1984). Clinical judgements in the decision to commit. Psychiatric discretion and the law. *Archives of General Psychiatry*, **41**, 811–15.

Soothill, K., Kupituksa, P. & Macmillan, J. F. (1990). Compulsory hospital admissions: dangerous decisions? *Medicine, Science and the Law*, **30**, 17–25.

Szasz, T. S. (1974). *The Myth of Mental Illness: Foundations of a Theory of Personal Conduct*. New York: Harper & Rowe.

Szasz, T. S. (1987). *Insanity*. New York: John Wiley & Sons.

Thompson, L. D. G., Bogue, J., Humphreys, M. S., Owens, D. G. C. & Johnstone, E. C. (1997). The State Hospital survey: a description of patients in conditions of special security in Scotland. *Journal of Forensic Psychiatry*, **81**, 263–84.

Verdun-Jones, S. N. (1989). Sentencing the partly mad and the partly bad; the case of the hospital order in England and Wales. *International Journal of Law and Psychiatry*, **12**, 1–27.

Weinberger, D. R. & Kleinman, J. E. (1986). Observations on the brain in schizophrenia in psychiatry update. *The American Psychiatric Association Annual Review*, Vol. 5, ed. A. J. Francis & R. E. Hayles, Washington, DC: American Psychiatric Press.

World Health Organization. (1992). *Diagnostic and Statistical Manual of Mental Disorders*, 4th edn. Washington, DC: American Psychiatric Association.

Index